LYLE CREELMAN

The Frontiers of Global Nursing

Lyle Creelman

The Frontiers of Global Nursing

SUSAN ARMSTRONG-REID

UNIVERSITY OF TORONTO PRESS
Toronto Buffalo London

© University of Toronto Press 2014
Toronto Buffalo London
www.utppublishing.com
Printed in Canada

ISBN 978-1-4426-4705-3

Printed on acid-free, 100% post-consumer recycled paper
with vegetable-based inks

Library and Archives Canada Cataloguing in Publication

Armstrong-Reid, Susan, 1950–, author
Lyle Creelman : the frontiers of global nursing / Susan Armstrong-Reid.

Includes bibliographical references and index.
ISBN 978-1-4426-4705-3 (bound)

1. Creelman, Lyle, 1908–2007.   2. World Health Organization – Officials
and employees – Biography.   3. United Nations Relief and Rehabilitation
Administration – Officials and employees – Biography.   4. World health.
5. Nurses – Canada – Biography.   I. Title.

RT37.C73A75 2014   610.73092   C2013-905686-6

This book has been published with the help of a grant from the Canadian
Federation for the Humanities and Social Sciences, through the Awards
to Scholarly Publications Program, using funds provided by the
Social Sciences and Humanities Research Council of Canada.

University of Toronto Press acknowledges the financial assistance
to its publishing program of the Canada Council for the Arts
and the Ontario Arts Council.

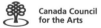
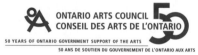

University of Toronto Press acknowledges the financial support of the
Government of Canada through the Canada Book Fund
for its publishing activities.

All photos courtesy of UBC Archives.

Contents

Contents

Illustrations follow page 44

Preface

Throughout her long and distinguished career, Canadian nursing leader Lyle Morrison Creelman commanded wide-reaching respect. Actively engaged in the key issues and events that transformed modern nursing from the Great Depression to the Cold War, and considered one of the most important international nursing leaders of the twentieth century, Creelman strove to improve provincial, national, and international nursing standards and championed a more modern approach to public health within Canada and abroad. Her career encompassed the rapid transformation of modern nursing and reflected its struggle to gain an effective voice within the global health-care system of the post-war era.

Unusually well educated, Creelman began her career in 1936 as a public health nurse in northern British Columbia just as the provincial Liberal government of T.D. Pattullo sought to wield greater state authority over public health. By 1941, she had been appointed the director of nursing of the recently formed Metropolitan Health Committee in Vancouver. An early leader in community-based public health in Canada, Creelman parlayed her executive positions on both the Registered Nurses Association of British Columbia (RNABC) and the Canadian Nurses Association (CNA) into an assignment on the international stage. In 1944 she joined the United Nations Relief and Rehabilitation Administration (UNRRA), the pioneering post-war liberal international organization, whose health mandate was considered foundational for enduring peace and prosperity. As the chief nurse of the British Zone of Occupied Germany, she orchestrated the provision of nursing services for millions of displaced persons awaiting repatriation or resettlement. After her return home in 1947, Creelman was granted a leave from the Metropolitan Health Committee to co-author with Dr J.H. Baillie a landmark study that, coinciding with the emergence of the Canadian welfare state, set new directions for public health practice in Canada for years to come and was basic to her own vision of global health. This vision, in short, was tightly tied to an understanding of individual social responsibility and political citizenship that had been recast in the wake of the Great Depression and by the mobilization of the Canadian state to win the war and fashion an enduring peace, a period in history when social-security systems were conceived as a pathway for providing preventative medicine. During this time, Creelman was preparing for the transformational role she was to play on the international scene.

In 1949 she joined the World Health Organization (WHO) as a nursing consultant in maternal and child health and subsequently served as the organization's chief nursing officer (CNO) from 1954 to 1968. An effective communicator and astute administrator, Creelman skilfully promoted the profession within the WHO and, to advance its interests worldwide, articulated nursing's unique contribution to health promotion among both medical and nonmedical professionals. A collaborative but sometimes intimidating leader, role model, mentor, and visionary, she formed strong relationships and networks with nurses around the world to share, refine, and realize her vision. Together, she and her colleagues defined new directions for international nursing and conceptualized plans of action. As CNO, Creelman pioneered a transcultural approach to international nursing that valued individual countries' diversity and need for self-sufficiency in health care. She consistently advocated tailoring programs to local context and norms rather than imposing them from above by international aid agencies. Hence, long before the WHO adopted primary health care as a global strategy in the 1978 Declaration of Alma-Ata, Creelman actively promoted it as an efficient model for improving health-care delivery on a sustainable basis, especially within developing countries.

I first met Lyle Creelman in 2004 at Hollyburn House, Vancouver, where she resided during her last years until her death in 2007. While completing *Armies of Peace: Canada and the UNRRA Years*, I had come to speak with her about her UNRRA assignment and its impact on her future career. During those few hours, as she recalled her work with UNRRA and the WHO, both great experiments with unprecedented international health tasks, I glimpsed the strong, intelligent, reserved woman already described to me by friends and colleagues. I left convinced that her intriguing story, one whose accomplishments, disappointments, and failures embraced the lives of ordinary nurses around the world, needed to be told.

Later, in undertaking Lyle Creelman's biography, I remembered one defining moment in that first visit. Creelman bent across the tea table to reach for my hand, feeling compelled to correct my statement about her adept administrative leadership, especially when compared with the difficulties that other

UNRRA chief nurses experienced elsewhere in Germany. "Oh my dear, my chief contribution was not as an administrator; I was always an educator first and foremost."[1] It became obvious that this statement was key to unlocking her story. Her career casts light on the way that new knowledge, education, and work were woven together in the reconceptualization of nursing's role in the middle decades of the twentieth century. Education became a critical professionalizing strategy for a generation of nursing leaders who aspired to achieve self-direction and self-regulation and, ultimately, to gain effective representation in health-care policy formation.

All this was clear to me at an early stage. Yet, even so, deciding how to tell Creelman's story raised critical issues of methodology. As nursing history has matured from simply adding nurses to historical accounts or celebrating the lives of "great nurses," biographies have been sidelined in a "new nonsubject-centred" historiography focused on race, gender, and class. In these circumstances, nursing biographers have been compelled to rethink the purpose of such works, as well as the audience for which they are intended.[2] But the determination of whether a subject – whether "great" or "ordinary" – is "worthy" of a biography must equally consider such a study's value as a contribution to the field.[3] The number of scholarly works covering either Canadian public health nursing or post-war nursing's contribution to global health is surprisingly small. In this context, in spite of their vital contribution, nurses "are not identified as key stakeholders at the health policy table."[4] Symptomatically, in 2012, the International Council of Nurses decried the appalling decline in nursing leadership positions within the WHO since 1968, "which if it continues will result in no posts by the end of 2016."[5] At a time when vibrant nursing leadership – at all levels of the health-care system – is vital to improving the equity and access to health care and addressing the continuing global shortage of nurses, a biography that explores the challenges of nursing leadership from the local to the global arena is well suited to contextualize and inform current policy debates and options. Creelman's expansive career offers historical perspective on nursing's contemporary values, responsibilities, and challenges as the largest group of front-line health-care caregivers, nationally and globally. As important, previously untapped sources, interviews, private papers, diaries, photographs, and archival collections allow the author to acknowledge Creelman's legacy while bringing to light the diversity of "ordinary" nurses' experiences, agency, and leadership.

Creelman waged a lifelong campaign to improve nursing services by raising the standards of nursing education and thereby equipping it to contribute to and function in a more complex society. She pursued and promoted the advantages of university-based nursing education over hospital-based training.

She viewed education not only as a route to personal intellectual growth, financial security, and professional advancement but also as an instrument for social change. But she never elevated collegiate nursing education to the status of a universal model. As her own education and administrative experience as a public health nurse broadened, Creelman gained a deeper understanding of the various socio-economic factors that underlay the delivery of community nursing services and the development of nursing education in a particular country. Seizing every opportunity to champion the unique role of public health nursing in improving health across the care continuum, she consistently used public health as the litmus test not only of a country's health-care system but also of its sense of social and civic responsibility.

Since Creelman always defined herself as an educator, a complete portrait of the forces that shaped her views, on education generally and on nursing in particular, must include the value her family placed on education, her early schooling, and the experiences and connections that she acquired while teaching before entering nursing school. But it was her years at the University of British Columbia (UBC) and Teachers College (TC), Columbia University, that laid the foundations both for her philosophy of nursing and for her continued social and professional development.

During Creelman's early nursing career, a number of factors helped to form both the woman and the nurse, including her mentors, the diverse professional activities in which she immersed herself, and the expanded professional network that emerged as a result. In fact, neither Creelman's views on nursing nor her leadership role in Canada and abroad can be fully understood without reference to the transnational networks of professional and personal relationships that eventually connected her to nurses at all levels around world. As the WHO's CNO, Creelman would act as a catalyst in the creation of new transnational networks that connected nurses beyond the established North Atlantic leadership circles and empowered them to advance nursing's interests worldwide. In turn, her own personal and philosophic nursing values were formed, enriched, tempered, and altered within these networks. Contextualizing these professional relationships, which crossed linguistic, geographic, and cultural boundaries, within the larger socio-economic landscape is crucial for understanding the complexity of the discourse in which issues of professional identity, nursing knowledge, and collective political action were debated throughout Creelman's nursing career. Creelman worked tirelessly to help nurses communicate more effectively across borders, functioning as what is now commonly referred to as a cross-cultural broker. Her role within these transnational nursing networks between 1949 and 1968 provides an important historical portal into the transformational forces that fashioned a more diversified twentieth-century nursing community. In short, power and authority within these networks was multidirectional, contested, and brokered.

"Good international history," Geertje Boschma suggests, "is historical scholarship that contributes to the exploration of diversity in local contexts, helps to unsettle parochial assumptions about nursing and healthcare, and most of all assists us in reaching a deeper understanding of what it means to be different."[6] In this vein, postcolonial critics have perceptively challenged the "binary othering"[7] that Eurocentric discourse invoked, including among nurses, to perpetuate imperialism and racism. They have documented the role of eugenics in underpinning imperialism. They have shown how the U.S. government rolled out medical interventions and sanitation campaigns to complement political and diplomatic strategies.[8] To the extent that WHO nursing has been examined, it has been seen primarily within a postcolonial frame or as an adjunct of American foreign policy.[9] Recently, however, international-relations scholars have cautioned against the assumption that "those from outside a particular state or region are 'inauthentic knowers' and actors who cannot understand or share in struggles outside of locales from which they come."[10] I agree. Analysing Creelman's struggle to articulate and implement a "social approach" to international nursing within developing countries – rather than one predicated on the biological model – uncovered the unexpected. Contrary to the prevailing postcolonial portrait, not all international nurses acted as agents of Western cultural imperialism during the post-war era.[11] Post-war nursing's vibrant but contested effort to challenge a hegemonic approach to nursing within other countries with very different cultures was a far more complex and fascinating story. Rather than being entirely top-down and donor-driven, the WHO's nursing programs were both more experimental and more highly negotiated than previously acknowledged.

Creelman's career also places in historical context some of the most enduring issues of knowledge, authority, scope of clinical practice, and professional identity that influenced nursing's evolution from 1930 until 1970. Nurse-historian Sylvia D. Rinker has noted, "The primacy of practice is the overarching concept in nursing that unites the diversity of nursing's educational programs, research agendas, knowledge paradigms, and various practice initiatives."[12] But historians have been decreasingly satisfied merely to chronicle what nurses did and have sought to examine critically "why their care took the form it did ... They tease out the threads of common interests around which nurses joined to maintain a sustainable work culture. They cast patients as equally important actors in shaping the work of nurses."[13] And, most significantly, they consider the implications of gender, class, race, and, more recently, place for nursing identity and work. Nurse-historian Pat D'Antonio has extended the scope of historical inquiry by repositioning identity as well as work at the centre of her scholarship to explore how nursing allowed men and women to "trade work that transformed nursing care … for the knowledge that changed their identity; their sense of themselves and their social place." Instead of casting nurses as victims, she focuses on the ways that nurses "renegotiated the terms of their experience and to reshape their own sense of worth, value and power." In so doing, D'Antonio has found that "the idea of place as a geographical, political, cultural and liminal space really mattered to the experiences of nurses and to the development of the profession."[14] In my own research, I also found that place proved an important historical lens through which to situate Creelman's experience as a young public health nurse within the larger provincial nursing service and to differentiate WHO nurses' vastly different experiences in sharing their knowledge across borders. As important, acknowledging the role of place permitted the inclusion of indigenous nurses' activism and agency to construct a more nuanced portrait of the power relations undergirding international nursing. Creelman's career, spanning both the national and international nursing worlds, provides important insights into the historical antecedents of many of the ambiguities, challenges, and accomplishments of modern-day nursing transnationally and globally.

That few were aware of Creelman's contribution to international nursing at the time of her death in 2007 is not surprising. Nursing's role is sanitized within the WHO's and UNRRA's celebratory official histories, and, symptomatically, it is invisible in the latest biography of the WHO's first director general.[15] These institutional histories provide a truncated version of the WHO's historical past, describing the values and activities of physicians but marginalizing the indispensable contribution of nurses. That nursing has been sidelined reflects its low status historically; because it was long viewed as an extension of feminine work, it was not greatly valued in medical circles. Even for the most successful WHO nurses, their careers were very different from those of their male colleagues. That said, however, the literature fails to consider how nurses navigated the gendered environment within the WHO's sprawling operations or whether nurses, through the different ways in which they worked and defined issues, influenced the actual implementation of WHO projects at the ground level.

Despite the increasingly multidisciplinary and global perspective underlining recent revisionist nursing scholarship,[16] significant lacunae remain in our historical understanding of the global dimensions of nursing's past in the post-war era. Perhaps this is in part because the new nursing scholarship until recently has largely excluded the work of international-relations scholars.[17] As a historian, I find that my methodology remains firmly grounded in the rich private and public archival sources illuminating Creelman's life and work. In co-authoring *Armies of Peace*, however, I began to move beyond a state-centric approach for their interpretation, thinking instead about the transnational circulation of ideas, values, process, peoples, resources, and practices. Constructing the Creelman biography as a window on the global transformation of twentieth-century nursing – part of an effort to "restore to their rightful place [nurses] who have been ignored, misunderstood or forgotten"[18] – made it necessary to incorporate recent historiographical trends that situate race, gender, ethnicity, place, and post-colonialism in a framework informed by the rich body of international-relations scholarship.

My book engages with theoretical work examining the increasing complexities of global health governance. These scholars helped me contextualize the complex roles that transnational nursing networks played in shaping Creelman's personal and professional life, as well as nursing's challenges in directing global health care within postwar liberal international organizations. Since nursing as a historical phenomenon is a tapestry of relationships constructed within specific cultural, socio-economic, and international political contexts, one model cannot explain all the phases of Creelman's career from student-nurse to international nursing leader. My point here is not to foreground theory but to preview how my biography of Creelman is framed.

Creelman's life story requires a transnational analytical framework that ceases to privilege the nation state as a historical paradigm for understanding nursing's past. A transnational framework implicitly rejects the notion, inherent in the state-centric approach, that only decisions negotiated at the highest levels establish the direction of global health policy and that these decisions are consistently reflected at the operational level. It abandons a narrow definition of politics as an exclusively public sphere or as solely governmental activities in order to challenge the view that the only subjects worthy of historical inquiry are the nation state or its representatives operating as unitary actors at the level of high politics.[19] Instead, a transnational framework admits an increasingly important array of new non-state actors – such as international institutions and non-governmental organizations (NGOs), and new forums, such as private-public partnerships, transnational agency and information networks, and knowledge-based communities – into the vibrant discourse that determined the contours of twentieth-century nursing generally and, more particularly, Creelman's international career. It profoundly alters the concept of power and authority and thus potentially permits a more nuanced portrait of nurses' agency and activism outside formal politics. This approach allows me to more seriously consider whether nurses as women exercised influence in a manner different from that of their male colleagues. This biography does not ignore the preponderance of national power or the interstate rivalry engendered in the pursuit of national security and economic aggrandizement during the Cold War. Rather, it seeks to understand how, in tandem with decolonization, globalization, and the rise of the modern administrative state, the advent of new global actors rendered nursing's position within global-health governance progressively more complex in the post-war era. Creelman's difficulties in brokering nursing's interests within this increasingly fragmented global health-care system foreshadowed the profession's continued challenges in navigating global-health governance in the twenty-first century.

The influences upon Creelman's views on nursing and her subsequent career as a nursing leader can be understood only within a transnational framework that looks beyond the nation state to consider the lively traffic of ideas, people, and resources within the worldwide nursing networks, a process that shaped the practice, knowledge, sense of agency, and, ultimately, professional identity of modern nursing. A biography of Creelman invites an approach that views nursing as a "world-wide social activity,"[20] both a creative force and a constructed social entity contextualized in time and space. Her life and work cannot be extricated from the constraints and prejudices that shape Western civil society; she had to consider how health problems intersected with power, gender, race, and social class in an era of rapid decolonization at the height of the Cold War. A study of her life permits a discriminating portrait of nursing organizations, one that depicts the clashes of ethnicity, race, gender, and professionalism that accompanied nursing's transformation in the mid-twentieth century.

The WHO offered Creelman the greatest potential to influence nursing worldwide and her most challenging leadership role. How did she, along with other nursing leaders, exercise power to advance nursing's professional agenda within the physician-dominated global and national health-care policy-making circles? Membership within the transnational network of nursing leaders remained a constant factor, both moulding Lyle Creelman's philosophy of nursing and determining the trajectory of her international career. In the post-war era, however, both the nature of the nursing networks and Creelman's role within them would change. To enhance nursing's sense of international agency and professional identity, Creelman would lead in the development of three specialized nursing networks: a policy advocacy network, an administrative intelligence network, and a grass-roots advocacy and information network. Designed to monitor policies, exchange information, and build solidarity, all were directed at addressing nursing's under-representation and lack of status within the gendered global health community, as well as the inadequate resources that these weaknesses entailed.

International nursing can never be divorced from domestic or institutional politics. The perspectives offered by Robert Keohane, a pioneer of transnational analytical frameworks since 1977 and a leading institutionalist,[21] highlight the potential constraints and determining characteristics of liberal international institutions that affected Creelman's exercise of transnational leadership during these years. Viewing institutions like the WHO "both as created by human action and as structuring that action,"[22] Keohane contends that, while interdependence breeds discord that in turn gives rise to the need for institutions, institutions themselves can be oppressive, restraining the behaviour of both member governments and non-state actors alike.[23] Institutions, such as the WHO, are important for promoting social justice and human security, but do they incorporate biases that constrain their members or other non-state actors, such as international nursing organizations, from taking an independent stance to achieve these goals? That perspective opened the door to explore how the Cold War shaped the WHO's policies in a manner that conflicted with Creelman's views on the appropriate development of WHO's nursing programs. Further, Keohane's work raises another pertinent question: what options did Creelman have to forward a different agenda for international nursing? From this perspective, the paradigm of "complex interdependence"[24] provides an analytical framework well suited "for analyzing multiple transnational issues and contacts" in organizations like the WHO where "force is not a useful instrument of policy."[25] In a global system characterized by "complex interdependence," "states use institutions to reduce the costs of making, monitoring and enforcing rules – transaction costs – provide information, and facilitate the making of credible commitments."[26] Keohane's concept of complex interdependence suggests that power can still be exercised when an actor's ability to leverage traditional sources of power (economic or military) is constrained, if more powerful actors deem the outcomes to be in their interest. Extending this concept of power, by drawing on recent scholarship on social networking, opens an intriguing perspective on nursing organizations' ability to frame nursing issues in a manner that leveraged power within the WHO's decision-making circles with the intent of influencing policy formation within their individual nations' gendered health-care systems.

Keohane's underestimation of the effect of both domestic politics and ideas on global politics[27] led me to consider the writings of other international scholars, whose emphasis on subjectivity and the role that norms, culture, and ideas have on world politics affords a more sophisticated historical lens through which to examine the complex intersection of personal motivations and liberal idealism that influenced the views of the post-war nursing leadership and the founding figures of the WHO. This work also helps situate the transnational nursing networks within a specific cultural, socio-economic, and international political context, viewing them as contingent on convention, perception, shared values, and educational and social experience.[28]

Recent global-governance literature enhances Keonane's valuable insights into the cross-cultural strategies that Creelman and her fellow nurses employed to navigate the political corridors of health care as part of a broader effort to influence nursing's future direction, whether at home or abroad. Cross-cultural brokerage, a fundamental prerequisite of any transnational network, is broadly understood as the linking of two or more previously unconnected social sites by an international actor that mediates their relations with one another and with other international actors. Several works that studied transnational networks and the role of cross-cultural brokers within them offered useful perspectives for investigating the tensions that Creelman experienced during her WHO tenure, tensions that flowed from the cleavages within nursing networks.[29] Others provided important insights into the leadership qualities within trans-national advocacy networks necessary for effective brokerage.[30] Many of these qualities – such as legitimate authority and the ability to act as an educator and to use common documents to establish a common framework and to codify commitments – proved especially apposite to Creelman's career with the WHO.

This literature prompted further investigation of how nurses used social and professional networks to identify common grievances and to organize in pursuit of international alternatives – a process termed "a globalization from below."[31] In particular, the notion that transnational advocacy networks blur, in a "boomerang pattern,"[32] the boundaries between a state's relations with its own nationals and the recourse both citizens and states have to the international sys-tem to influence state behaviour is applicable to the role of the WHO's expert committees, conferences, and technical reports. Within these, nurses used a variety of tactics still employed by agency networks to harness the WHO's authority in the interest of establishing international standards and best prac-tices and then effecting similar changes within their own nation states.[33]

Taken as a whole, international-relations scholarship reinforces a frame-work in which nursing is no longer marginalized within the narrative of global health as a minor player in a top-down and donor-driven process. Instead, Creelman's personal and professional relationships with nursing leaders, rank-and-file nurses, international organizations, and other non-state actors are seen as central to the transformation of modern nursing. Seeking a more textured understanding of international nursing's past, to paraphrase Pat D'Antonio, I took up the challenge to find "a new way to redefine and recapture the power inherent in the way [nurses like Lyle Creelman] chose to define their lives."[34] Framing Creelman's story within the broader nursing networks permits a nuanced approach to writing the biography of a major nursing leader, one that recognizes her significant achievements without ignoring the shortcomings or limitations of her leadership. Nor does it exclude the activities and agency of nursing colleagues of all nations and ranks that shaped her legacy.

Since nursing defined Creelman's personal and professional life, this biography focuses on the years that she was active in her chosen profession. The first three chapters explore the formative influences of, and her rise within, the North American nursing leadership network. Chapters 4 and 5 chronicle her emergence as a nursing leader within the North Atlantic nursing network during and after the Second World War and set the stage for understanding the philosophy of nursing that would guide her post-war international career. Chapters 6 through 11 cover the WHO years, with chapter 11 providing a retrospective of this part of her life. They examine Creelman's emergence as cross-cultural broker within a more diversified global nursing network as nursing struggled to define its role in global health in the context of the Cold War and decolonization. A brief epilogue looks at her post-nursing career and reflects on the salience of her life and work today.

Acknowledgments

Deciding to write a modern biography of one of the foremost nursing leaders of the twentieth century as a window into the larger social and political forces that redefined nursing worldwide launched a fascinating six-year journey of historical discovery. As on any such journey, the story of both the woman and the dramatic transformation of her chosen profession took many unexpected turns. Unravelling the public and private life story proved additionally challenging for the biographer of Lyle Morrison Creelman. She was both intensively private and astutely aware that nursing was political. She governed her private and public discourse accordingly.

To unpack the complete story of Lyle Creelman's contribution to the development nursing worldwide therefore required considerable detective work to uncover privately held letters, diaries, memories, and mementos that complemented the succinct official reports and memos prepared on the job that are located in the Lyle Creelman Fonds (University of British Columbia, Vancouver) and in the extensive manuscript collections housed at the World Health Organization Archives (Geneva), the United Nations Archives (New York), the Rockefeller Foundation Archives (Tarrytown), the Howard Gotlieb Archival Research Centre (Boston), and Library and Archives Canada (Ottawa). Research trips to these collections never seemed long enough. I owe a great debt to the hard-working and knowledgeable archivists for what was accomplished during these trips. But special thanks are due to Chris Hives, Leslie Fields, and Candice Bjur at the University of British Columbia Archives, Thomas Allen and Marie Villemin at the World Health Organization, and Diane Gallagher at the Howard Gotlieb Archival Research Centre.

This biography, however, would not have been possible without the generosity of the many nurses who shared their personal nursing stories, their memories of Lyle Creelman, and, as importantly, their extensive knowledge of the history of nursing and its hidden archival sources. They opened their private diaries and letters and provided introductions to colleagues across the country and overseas. It was through my encounters with Mary Abbott, Barbara Barton, Barbara Bubb, Kay Dier, Dr Beverly DuGas, Dr Helen Mussallem, Dr Dorothy Hall, Eva (Billie) Williamson, Dr Verna Huffman Splane, Dr Shirley Stinson, and Dame Sheila Quinn that I first glimpsed the power of the transatlantic nursing network in action.

I am especially grateful for the friendship and support that the Faculty of Nursing at University of British Columbia, especially, Dr Geertje Boschma and Dr Glennis Zilm gave to this project. The British Columbia History of Nursing Society, especially those members who participated in the oral history project, also deserves special recognition for its foresight and ongoing support of nursing scholarship.

My manuscript benefited from the careful reading and comments of colleagues with different perspectives. Dr Sonya Grypma, Dr Wendy Mitchinson, Dr James Snell, Dr David Murray, and Dr Richard Reid provided valuable advice and encouragement for the manuscript's overall improvement at various stages of its development. Curtis Fahey offered sage editorial advice throughout the manuscript review. All helped me immeasurably in improving the manuscript.

In preparing the manuscript for publication, I was delighted to work with Len Husband and Frances Mundy, two extremely supportive and capable editors. Every manuscript benefits immensely from working with a good copy editor; I was fortunate to work with Ian MacKenzie, an exceptionally discerning and judicious copy editor. Many thanks also to Noeline Bridge for her meticulous work on the index.

And finally, the researching and writing of this book would not have been as enjoyable without the good-humoured culinary and editorial support of my husband, Richard, the senior historian in the family.

LYLE CREELMAN

The Frontiers of Global Nursing

Chapter One

The Formative Years, 1908–1936

Lyle Creelman was born on 14 August 1908 in Upper Stewiacke, Nova Scotia, the heart of the local agrarian and lumbering community. The only child of a second marriage, she was the youngest of eleven children. Six years after his first wife, Marianna (née McDonald), died in 1901, Lyle's father, Samuel, then fifty-four, married a distant cousin, Laura Creelman of Portaupique, Nova Scotia.[1] At first it appeared that baby Lyle might share the fate of her four stepsisters – all of whom had died before her birth. Years later, the nurse who attended Laura recalled the complications surrounding Lyle's entry into the world: "She was premature and very delicate. I stayed with her mother all one night – not knowing whether the baby would live through the night."[2]

Lyle Creelman survived to emerge as Canada's foremost international nursing leader – as, from the beginning, hers would be a life journey filled with triumphs, disappointments, and tangled relationships. This chapter focuses on the formative experiences and identities that provided the scaffolding upon which the Canadian nurse would reframe her personal and professional identities as a woman of influence well beyond the nation state.

Lyle's early years, typical of rural life in the valley, centred on church and school. Both were important vehicles to socialize Canadian children into moral, productive citizens. She was raised in a loving but strict Presbyterian family. Each morning she joined the daily parade of children ranging from six to eighteen who attended the two-room white schoolhouse, built in 1866. The teacher had little tolerance for mischievous children who couldn't work independently.[3] In other respects, Lyle's early childhood diverged from that of the youngest child in a large rural family. Laura Creelman never developed a close relationship with her stepsons. The youngest son, Prescott, went to live with an aunt after his father's remarriage; Hugh, James, and Ralph sought employment in British Columbia. Given the age differences and geographical separation, Lyle was in essence raised during her early childhood as an only child in a very adult world – a factor that may have reinforced her natural reserve.

In mid-August 1920 Samuel Creelman uprooted his family and left the province his grandfather had helped settle. Many of the immediate family ties that bound the couple to the Maritimes had by then been severed. Laura Creelman's father had died in 1919; her brothers, James and Forest, had already relocated in Saskatchewan; and her sister, Mrs A.C. Thompson, was living in British Columbia. Whether Lyle's father was lured by the prospect of a better life or urged west by his sons remains unclear. Certainly, the death of his son James, who left behind a widow, Lydia, with three small children, Kay, Hazel, and Arthur, in Vancouver, influenced the family's decision to locate nearby.[4] After visiting Laura's brothers and spending the winter in North Vancouver with James's widow, the family resettled the next spring in Steveston, British Columbia, a fishing port southwest of Vancouver, known as the salmon capital of the world.

On their first stroll along Steveston's cannery row, the Creelman family would have seen little resemblance between the boisterous fishing port's vibrant and ethnically diverse population, which included the largest Japanese community in British Columbia, and their former hometown. On summer evenings, thousands of seasonal Asian, Aboriginal, and European fishers and cannery workers jammed the boardwalk, eager to enjoy the social activities offered in the numerous saloons and gambling and opium dens. Despite a string of bad fishing seasons and the disastrous fire of 1918 that closed several canneries, Steveston served as a natural hub for the expanding regional market.[5] Accordingly, Sam Creelman purchased a modest two-bedroom cottage on two acres of land directly opposite the Cottage Station on the Interurban Electric Railway just outside the town. He resumed mixed farming and Laura cultivated a large vegetable garden for the family's use and to sell in the local farmers' market. Later, as Lyle's father sought to expand his farming activities on rented land, the family faced increased competition from the Japanese farmers, who turned to market gardening on small acreages as a result of the federal government's policy after 1924 restricting the number of Japanese fishing licences. Awareness of racial discrimination became part of the Creelman family's new life in Steveston.

After a period of home schooling to bring her up to grade level, Lyle entered Lord Byng Elementary School in Steveston that May.[6] Her arrival in Steveston coincided with renewed demands from the Japanese community for integration within the local school system. But it was not until 1923, by which time Lyle had entered high school, that an agreement was reached with the Japanese community whereby Lord Byng would accept Japanese children in return for financial aid to complete the building's construction. Apparently, no Japanese students joined Lyle and her Steveston classmates at Bridgeport High School in nearby Richmond. The matriculation class of 1926, of which Lyle was one of nineteen students, was exclusively Anglo-Saxon and predominantly female.

During these years, Lyle developed a strong relationship with the family of her stepbrother James. She quickly dispelled any notion that his children should refer to her as "Auntie Lyle"; Kay, the eldest daughter, was only five years her junior. In many respects, Lyle and Kay's relationship was more akin to that of young siblings. Kay's humorous account of being Lyle's first patient provides a window on that relationship as well as Lyle's character. Once, while their mothers visited Laura's family on the prairies, the two teens decided to seek refuge from the summer night's heat by sleeping on the porch. Unfortunately, Kay became violently ill during the night, creating, in her own words, quite a mess. Knowing that "Uncle Hughie" would be dropping by early the next morning to check in on them, Lyle calmly took control of the situation. Both her young niece and the porch were quickly washed off with the nearby garden hose! For Kay, Lyle would always be a take-charge, intelligent, dependable woman, as well as a cherished companion.[7]

In 1926, having graduated from Bridgeport High School with the highest marks in the province, Lyle, now intent on a career in medicine, was awarded a one-year scholarship to the University of British Columbia (UBC).[8] By this time, she was poised to enjoy the promise of improved access to higher education and respectable paid work when family circumstances thwarted her plans. After completing the first year of a liberal-arts program at UBC in 1927, Lyle left to attend the BC Provincial Normal School, the teachers training college. In all likelihood, the death of her father from pneumonia on 16 October 1926 forced her change of course. Samuel Creelman had made a modest provision for his daughter's support and continued education – a lump-sum payment of $200 for her education and a further $200 per year until she reached twenty-four years of age. While the stipend indicated the importance placed upon education within the Creelman family, the amount was not sufficient to allow Lyle to pursue her educational dreams.

Lyle's diaries, written years afterwards, are silent about her feelings towards her father and do not even mention his death. One diary entry does reveal, however, that an illness of another unidentified family member prevented Lyle from starting her teaching career until 1929, the year following her graduation from Normal School.[9] A pattern had been set. In the future, as the only daughter, her career decisions would be balanced against concerns about her mother's well-being.

Lyle's first appointment was to the staff of the Lord Byng Public School in Steveston, where she would continue to teach until the summer of 1932.[10] Her class at Lord Byng included many Japanese children, and Hideko Hyodo, the only Japanese teacher employed by a public school board in British Columbia, had been teaching an all-Japanese grade one class since 1924.[11] While Lyle's photo albums of her teaching years indicate that she enjoyed the camaraderie of Hyodo and her male colleagues outside the classroom, not much is known of her time as a schoolteacher. Her private diary simply recorded, "Taught school in Steveston. Had my first love affair."[12]

Lyle's teaching experience, while short, shaped her attitudes towards her future career in public health nursing. She would remain a staunch advocate of using teachers as a vehicle for promoting healthy living. At the same time, educated within a racially segregated educational system, and then working within it, the ambitious young career woman increased her awareness of the barriers of race as well as gender that non-Anglo-Saxon women faced in pursuing their professional aspirations.

Creelman always made it clear to her superiors that she never considered teaching small children as her final vocation but rather a method to fund her goal of studying medicine. Yet, once again, financial considerations dictated her career path. Nursing offered a more challenging career than teaching while being less prohibitively expensive than medical training. Even though funding her tuition would have been difficult for Creelman, the university offered a busy, privileged, and socially homogenous setting. The "racialization of femininity" in Canadian nursing, of "Whiteness and White womanhood" documented elsewhere applied to UBC / Vancouver General Hospital (VGH) schools of nursing as well.[13] The first nurses of Asian origin, admitted to UBC in the diploma public health program, graduated in 1937, the year after Creelman.[14]

Lyle Creelman's choice of the public health option in the five-year UBC degree program was ideally suited to her independent temperament, keen intellect, and quest for financial autonomy. The BASc(N) degree offered the ambitious young woman the prospect of upward career mobility, leading to a teaching or administrative appointment. In the interim, as a public health nurse, Creelman would be better paid and face less economic uncertainty. During the Great Depression, many private-duty nurses were forced to combine nursing with non-nursing employment to survive, whereas public health nursing expanded to meet the changing health needs associated with urbanization, industrialization, and immigration – challenges that were severely exacerbated by social dislocation as millions of Canadians became either unemployed or underemployed. Public health nursing promised a more professionally and socially satisfying career. Public health's practice setting required enhanced critical thinking skills, more adaptability, and greater initiative in order to meet diverse and unique challenges that private-duty nurses seldom faced. There were other advantages as well for a single, independently minded young woman. The private-duty nurse was hired by and lived on a twenty-four-hour basis with the family of the patient for whom she was providing care; the public health nurse visited several patients a day and lived independently, leaving more time for a social life. As nurse-historian Cynthia Connolly has observed, "Since the class relationship between patient and nurses was usually reversed from that of the private duty nurse and the care was subsidized by a third party, public health nurses held more authority than did other nurses."[15] Just as important, public health nursing refocused nursing from its curative role to include teaching about proper hygiene, disease prevention, and healthy living. The goal was to foster citizenship within the whole community as the preferred vehicle for social reform – a particularly appealing role for the former teacher.

One of the youngest universities within the British Empire, UBC had been the first to establish a combined degree program in nursing in 1919. Dr Henry Esson Young, the provincial health officer from 1916 until his death in 1939, played a pivotal role in the founding of UBC's nursing school. Across Canada, as in other countries worldwide, public health activities quickened when large numbers of their men were found unfit for military service and when their soldiers later returned home from the First World War, bringing with them the Spanish influenza of 1918–19 that swept across the world throughout the 1920s.[16] Young seized the opportunity presented by the heightened public interest in the preventative aspects of public health and the enhanced image of nurses as first-line responders in the wake of the influenza epidemic to establish a nursing department at UBC during the 1919–20 academic year.

Despite the financial restraints of the 1930s, UBC's nursing courses, especially in public health, evolved, as enrolment increased to meet the growing demands for more and better-trained public health nurses.[17] The interwar period was a time of activism, growth, and development for community health nursing in British Columbia.[18] There, corporate and industrial sponsorship of public health nursing services found a ready ally in the provincial government. The increasing pressure exerted on all levels of government to reduce appalling and ubiquitous rates of tuberculosis and infant and maternal mortality opened new opportunities for public health nurses, as prenatal clinics, classes, and screening services offered by Metropolitan Life and the Victorian Order of Nurses and provincial nursing services expanded. The growth of community nursing was also funded by individual industries determined to provide a safe and healthy workforce to increase productivity.

The province's more scattered population forced the government to take direct action early, rather than delegating the responsibility to the municipalities, as other provinces chose to do.[19] In response, British Columbia's physicians were re-casting their medical authority as purveyors of state-directed progressive social reform. Young supported the dramatic expansion of public health nursing programs to meet the changing needs of the Provincial Nursing Services. The introduction of the idea of patient education and patient responsibility changed the role of public health nursing. To contain the social ills associated with industrialism, immigration, and urbanization, the state needed competent nurse agents to preach the gospel of prevention. In British Columbia, as elsewhere, public health nurses' new role as the state's messengers of care, cleanliness, character, and citizenship demanded a better-educated nursing profession that could function within demanding and more autonomous practice settings. Young would become Creelman's employer and mentor in her first public health role as the conveyer of and model for clean living and citizenship.

Lyle's entrance into UBC baccalaureate nursing program in 1932 coincided with several interesting developments signalling the shift in the focus of public health work from the treatment of disease to the promotion of overall health. Those changes left an indelible imprint on Creelman's lifelong approach to public health nursing. The new breed of policymakers and politicians fostered an educational environment more closely aligned with the concept of a liberal welfare state. The political climate in British Columbia was receptive to changes that marked a shift away from the reform movement adroitly orchestrated by Dr Henry Esson Young in the 1920s, the earlier approach being a blend of progressive reform, maternal feminism, and science.[20] The new social-reform impulse heralded the shift from voluntarism to the age of the social scientist as academic and policymaker in the state-directed economic and social regeneration.[21] Following the election of the Liberal government of Premier Duff Pattullo in 1933, Young remained an important but not the dominant figure driving the reorganization of health services. Premier Pattullo, regarded elsewhere in Canada as a maverick in regard to his social-welfare program,[22] recruited Dr Grégoire Amyot, Dr George Weir, Dr Harry Cassidy, Dr J.W. McIntosh, Dr George Davidson, and John Marshall to implement the Liberal Party's ambitious health program. At the provincial level, these reformers' initiatives sought to replace voluntarism with professionally educated public health officials, to centralize administrative hierarchies, and to promote community education and the inspection of target groups at risk.[23]

More immediately, these men all taught Creelman and her fellow nursing students at UBC regularly. In their final year at UBC, Creelman and her fellow public health nurses were exposed to Amyot's views in his lectures on acute communicable diseases and epidemiology. His social validation of the preventative function of modern nursing and his identification of teaching as public health nursing's cardinal social responsibility served as the architectural scaffolding around which Creelman would construct her own view of the unique role of the modern public health nurse in the care continuum. Collectively, their ideas became the twin pillars of Creelman's approach to public health at home and abroad: first, education was the key to improved community health, and second, good communication networks – which depended on the communication skills nurtured by education – were vital to the spread of the gospel of public health.[24]

As important, Amyot would dramatically influence Creelman's career trajectory. A former Rockefeller Foundation (RF) travelling fellow, he already had extensive public health field experience in Canada and the United States before his appointment as the first director of the North Vancouver Health Unit in 1930. Considering the close personal connections of British Columbia's civil servants and the substantial funding the province received from the Rockefeller Foundation, it is not surprising that Amyot and others echoed the RF's views on public health as a well-organized, rational system that would employ medical science to protect and promote a healthy, productive public.[25] The creation of the Metropolitan Health Committee of Greater Vancouver in 1936 – long regarded as Amyot's most significant legacy of bureaucratic centralization – amalgamated six health departments, five independent school-health services, and UBC's Medical Services Department. As a new UBC graduate that year, Creelman would have more than a casual interest in Amyot's plans to develop the Metropolitan Health Unit of Greater Vancouver. He would be her second employer and sponsor for a Rockefeller Foundation fellowship.

The third influential figure in public health during Creelman's time at UBC was George Weir. Appointed as provincial secretary and minister of education in Pattullo's Cabinet in 1933,[26] Weir campaigned for new directions in public health policy and had already spotlighted the need for more well-educated public health nurses as a prerequisite for the expansion of public health initiatives. Weir's views on an activist state, professionalism, and the importance of a scientific approach to socio-economic problems dovetailed with the new liberal paradigm that informed politics in British Columbia, the rest of Canada, Britain, and the United States during this era. Weir shared Young's belief that the prevention of disease was a less costly option than treating those who became charges of the state through illness, but he raised that view to a new level in his overriding concern for bureaucratic efficiency through centralization and fiscal management rather than humanitarianism. According to Megan Davies,

"Positive public health," the catchword of British Columbia public health officials in the 1930s, "fit well with the individualistic focus of both Weir's own philosophy and the broader shift in public health away from the concept of dirt to
an interest in personal hygiene." Shortly after his appointment to the provincial
Cabinet, Weir predicted that Creelman's generation of nurses would be part of a
future, "which would include more public health nursing, more psychiatry and
more preventive work." The state would provide each individual with the education and services to attain good health; individuals then had the obligation to
be healthy and productive.[27] Strands of those beliefs, stressing the individuals'
responsibility for their own well-being, would underpin Creelman's understanding of the role of public health nursing throughout her career. It was also
an early statement of the principle of "helping people to help themselves" that
would guide her international work in the years to come.

As importantly, nursing leaders had identified George Weir as the ideal progressive reformer to advance their professional agenda the next step. As Julia
Kinnear points out, Canadian nursing leaders had already fostered a spirit of
cooperation with progressive physicians, such as Henry Esson Young, during the 1920s to reform nursing education.[28] Physicians' disposition to view
nursing as an "extension of the natural female role" prompted the College of
Physicians to comment, when a nursing department at the University of British
Columbia was proposed in 1919, that "overtraining nurses is not desirable and
results in their losing their usefulness."[29] In British Columbia, as elsewhere in
North America, the ambivalence about broadening liberal education opportunities for women triggered anxiety about its destabilizing implications.[30]
Nursing leaders' efforts to promote more rigorous scientific education, and to
gain legal self-regulation and adequate financial compensation, continued to
bring them into conflict with physicians. Paternalistic attitudes, fear that nurses
would become economic competitors, and territorial disputes over the control
of new scientific knowledge would fuel physicians' negative attitude towards
granting nursing greater professional autonomy.[31] The nursing elite was determined to forge new political alignments with progressive physicians to set a
new direction for nursing education.

When Creelman entered UBC, Canadian nursing leaders, like their British
and American colleagues, were vigorously debating the state of nursing education. By 1920, university programs had been established at Dalhousie, McGill,
Toronto, Alberta, and British Columbia; most offered only postgraduate diplo-
mas to hospital-trained graduates in administration, public health, or education. Nursing leaders were anxious to consolidate these gains to garner wider
acceptance for university-based nursing education.[32] The Canadian nursing
elites had identified the apprenticeship system – wherein the training schools

functioned as the nursing department of the hospitals and the students provided cheap labour to deliver the majority of the hospitals' nursing services –
as the crux of the problem. The hospital focused on the "care of the patient
today," but modern nursing education needed to "include the care of the patient
of tomorrow."[33] As long as service was the primary mission of the hospital,
forward-looking education would be a secondary consideration in these training schools. The Canadian leadership followed their American neighbour's
campaign to curtail the power of hospitals over nursing education and to raise
nursing standards embodied in the ground-breaking Goldmark Report (1923),
sponsored by the Rockefeller Foundation.[34] These transnational trends, however, were interpreted within local contexts.[35] The Canadian nursing elites were
determined to conduct an independent assessment of the educational standards and programs that met national needs and conditions.[36]

Consequently, the Canadian Nurses Association (CNA) collaborated with
the Canadian Medical Association (CMA) to appoint George Weir, then
still a professor of education at UBC, to conduct the most extensive study
of Canadian nursing education undertaken to date. The *Survey of Nursing
Education in Canada* (1932), commonly referred to as the Weir Report, was a
blueprint for the next generation of Canadian nursing leaders, including Lyle
Creelman. It would be major reference point for her future public health studies
and writings. UBC's Mabel Gray, appointed president of the CNA in 1927, and
VGH's Kathleen Ellis, its director from 1922 to 1929, had been instrumental
in guiding the Weir Report to a successful conclusion. It vindicated nursing
leaders' concerns about the uneven quality of nursing education across the
country, finding that while hospital-nursing schools turned out a disciplined
workforce, many small hospital-schools failed to provide the sufficient breadth
or depth of clinical experiences necessary for a highly competent nurse. Weir
recommended integrating nursing education into the general education system, rather than leaving it under the control of the hospitals. The Weir Report
made many far-reaching recommendations for public health nursing, including doubling the number of public health nurses in Canada over five to ten
years, setting a minimum educational qualification of a one-year course in
public health nursing offered by an approved university nursing school following the three-year general training, and establishing cost-sharing agreements
between provincial governments and municipalities to meet the costs of public
health services. Nurse historians Zilm and Warbinek argue that although the
report "had identified some terrible conditions in nursing education, the depth
of the Depression set back most of its recommendations."[37] The report's recommendation that nursing education ultimately be offered only at the university
level would be debated for decades before it was fully implemented in Canada.

The stage would change, but nursing leaders' concerns had a familiar refrain. The belief that nurses, wherever possible, should be offered a broad liberal education within a university setting remained the cornerstone of Creelman's enduring approach to nursing education in Canada and abroad. It was not surprising, therefore, that the mature Creelman would support nursing leaders' efforts worldwide to improve traditional hospital-focused training as an interim measure.

Given the limited number of university programs in nursing available in the 1930s, the majority of nurses continued to be trained in hospital-schools. Students entering university courses were carefully selected to receive a broader liberal education, to prepare them for their future roles as administrators and educators or for work in specialized fields such as public health. In the five-year combined UBC program, the traditional hospital-training program at the Vancouver General Hospital was sandwiched between the first two years of general academic training and the final year during which the nursing students specialized in either teaching and supervision or public health nursing. Creelman chose the latter. Between the second and third year, Lyle spent a probationary period of four months at VGH. The third and fourth years were also spent at VGH. Her life at VGH was a carefully orchestrated daily routine of classes and ward work – seven days a week, ten hours a day. Class were often held in the off-duty hours or on the half-day off. The scope of UBC's nursing program – embracing social work, mental hygiene, sociology, psychology, education, and public health, and offering perspectives on teaching, administration, and even parliamentary procedure – was very progressive for the era. Creelman's fieldwork ran concurrently with her two years at VGH. During the final year of her program, her placements – half of each week and the final four weeks of the second term – was divided among the Victorian Order of Nurses, the Vancouver Rotary Clinic for Diseases of the Chest, the Provincial Mental Hospital at Essondale, the Provincial Department of Health, the Medical Department of the Vancouver School Board, the Government Venereal Disease Clinic, the provincial sanatorium, and the Department of Child Hygiene for the city of Vancouver.

Lyle Creelman benefited from her professional and personal encounters with the talented and influential nurses who taught her at both Vancouver General Hospital and University of British Columbia. Mabel Gray, Grace Fairley, and Margaret Kerr were known for their progressive views on women's ability to shape modern society constructively – views that they brought to bear on nursing education. All reflected the belief common among the North American nursing leadership that "a particular combination of character and content defined professional nursing."[38] Accordingly, the first two years of the combined

UBC program provided students with "an introduction to the general cultural subjects and a foundation in the sciences underlying the practice of nursing"[39] and "were intended to prepare the student for citizenship as well as to awaken a love of learning."[40]

A number of considerations weighed on the minds of those responsible for developing UBC's nursing program. They were mindful of the criticisms that university education did not improve the level of care given, particularly in respect to bedside nursing.[41] It was not sufficient that university nursing education, imbricated in the latest scientific discoveries, would allow UBC's future graduates to better protect patient health and to deliver superior bedside care; their feminine respectability and professional integrity were equally paramount. University-based nursing programs, Fairley believed, bore a special social responsibility that distinguished nursing from other professional groups within Canadian universities: "Is there any other school where the pupil, from the first day to her last day of training, is carrying in her hands the lives of her fellow man?"[42]

Consequently, Creelman had to satisfy both Mabel Gray at UBC and Grace Fairley at VGH that she not only met the academic requirements for admission but was "personally fit for the profession of nursing."[43] As Gray explained, the prospective student "must measure up to all standards set by the [VGH's] nursing school, with respect to such factors as physique, character, intelligence, personality and adaptability."[44] Moreover, since there was no residence on campus, women were expected to choose from a list of approved homes, and their living companions and subsequent conduct outside the hospital were carefully monitored to ensure that social propriety was maintained. Little changed after graduation. Public health nurse Creelman, as the state's role model of healthy living, would be expected to have impeccable moral credentials.

As the superintendent of nursing at VGH from 1929 until her retirement in 1943, Grace Fairley[45] pioneered many progressive changes, including the introduction of clinical experiences that reflected her belief that nursing had a role beyond the hospitals. These were "a real innovation at the time." Known for her "keen mind," "crispness of thought," and "ready wit and rare sense of humour,"[46] Fairley was a steadfast supporter of higher education for nurses.[47] She encouraged her students to see that "the patient was the focus rather than the disease or the technique ... [and] stressed that the students must not be robots and work by rote, but were expected to question and not just to follow orders."[48] As historian Julie Kinnear noted, the Canadian nursing elite advocated a professional identity that attempted to reconcile "the conflicting elements of science and reward on one hand, and caring and sacrifice on the other."[49] Fairley passionately believed that the nurse had a great responsibility to the community as a professional and as a citizen: she "was a very courageous person, and when convinced for the need for change, she was not afraid to take the difficult road."[50] Consequently, over the years, she set the standard for her students by remaining active in provincial, national, and international nursing bodies.[51] Creelman herself was content to be known as one of "Fairley's girls"; their paths would intertwine long after Lyle graduated from UBC. She, too, expected nurses to be self-motivated, socially engaged, and forward looking.

Yet the progressive views of VGH's staff did not reflect the stark reality of Creelman's clinical experience. When VGH students provided service on wards, they were exposed to a work culture of submission, precision, routine, duty, and accountability. Creelman worked long, gruelling days; she was expected to perform hospital cleaning duties in addition to her nursing work, as well as giving bed baths, making beds, and serving meals. Many of the treatments then used entailed heavy physical exertion. Here, as in other cases, Fairley did not shy away from confronting VGH's hospital board when its actions jeopardized her students' ability to acquire the skills, knowledge, and composure that she believed were required to evaluate and deliver effective patient care. During Creelman's student days at VGH, overcrowding on the general wards had become so chronic that Fairley complained that it "did not permit professional poise or the calm thinking that is essential to GOOD NURSING."[52] After working in an overcrowded hospital and living in an unattractive nurses' home, Creelman would welcomed the more expansive personal and intellectual opportunities afforded by life away from the hospital, as she entered her final year at UBC.

Although Dr Hibbert Hill acted as titular professor and head of the university's Department of Nursing and Health, the department's real head from 1925 until 1941 was Mabel F. Gray. Lacking a degree, however, she could never assume leadership. A seasoned administrator and a forceful advocate of improving student nurses' working conditions, Gray had honed her considerable political skills while guiding the Winnipeg General Hospital (WGH) School of Nursing towards greater financial independence during the First World War.[53] Having taken postgraduate courses at Simmons College in Boston and at Teachers College (TC), Columbia, she remained well connected with American nursing educators. With her "lady-like" reputation, she was the ideal prophet of the gospel of health within the nursing community. Gray's approach to education was "fearless and enlightened" but also "eminently practical and sane."[54] Like other progressive reformers, she was a strong proponent of collegiate schools of nursing, ones connected to a university leading to a degree.[55] She too campaigned against the hospital training schools' insatiable demand for patient care at the expense of the students' educational experience.

She contended that, since the nursing school was "a professional school – not a trade school or factory," its students "should have the same freedom to develop the course and carry out essential practice in the hospital wards as any other group of professional students."[56]

Placing nursing on a scientific basis, Gray believed, would help legitimize its professional status within the medical community. She condemned the idea that science courses should be watered down for nursing students: it prevented nurses "from applying scientific methods to the solution of nursing problems" and left them ill-prepared to assume the teaching of science in nursing schools.[57] Instead, she encouraged Creelman's classmates to enrol in full science courses in their pre-clinic years. Once they were armed with the language and knowledge of science, she then expected UBC graduates to act with initiative and authority. She urged Creelman and her fellow students to be "teachers of health to let the scientific knowledge you possess on the cause of illness, modes of transmission, modes of protection or immunization, influence your outlook and enable you to bring science to bear on solving the problem of how to improve the nation's physical health."[58] Positioning nursing knowledge as scientifically grounded directly challenged the lingering view that nursing was an extension of women's domestic work. As nurse historian Pat D'Antonio reminds us, American nursing educators similarly looked to science to mediate gendered relationships within the medical community.[59] Creelman's interest and ability in science classes was acknowledged when she was awarded the applied-science scholarship in her third year – an early indication of her life-long interest in empirical nursing research as a professional strategy to advance nursing's claims to knowledge and distinctive professional identify.

Expecting UBC public health nurses to become women of "vision and initiative,"[60] Mabel Gray prepared her students for this role by introducing them to the latest trends in nursing and the related social sciences. Gray regularly invited guest lecturers in "social case work" and "mental hygiene" as well as other prominent nursing educators, such as Isabel Maitland Stewart of TC. Changes were also introduced in the clinical experience offered to UBC nursing students. Gray concurred with Weir's recommendation that nurses would be prepared to evaluate and meet the communities' needs only if their hospital-based training was expanded to include clinical experience in health centres, in tuberculosis sanatoriums, and at state mental hospitals as well as through home visiting with the Victorian Order of Nurses (VON). Without this broad clinical experience, a public health nurse lacked the "viewpoint of the prevention of illness which she [Gray] believed every nurse should have."[61]

Another figure in the UBC nursing department at this time who had the most enduring influence on Creelman was Margaret E. Kerr. Appointed a public health nursing instructor in 1929[62] and later promoted to assistant professor, a position that she held until leaving in 1944 to become the editor of the *Canadian Nurse*, Kerr helped to shape the thinking and understanding of generations of nursing students.[63] An early graduate of UBC, she completed a master's degree on a RF fellowship at TC. Although Kerr and Gray were polar opposites – one casual and friendly and the other decorous and reserved – they functioned well together. Known for her vigour, keen mind, sense of humour, and powerful public-speaking skills, Kerr set her course with determined enthusiasm. It made her a formidable figure in the eyes of colleagues and students alike.

In an article written in 1930 for the *Canadian Nurse*, Kerr defended the importance of postgraduate public health training and defined its unique educational requirements. She began by challenging the common notion that a public health nurse was "educated for her life work"; the expression, she argued, "can be carried further – 'education is life.' It is the keynote to all public health work." She argued that competent public health nurses needed to have both hospital and community experience – a innovative position that bore the imprint of the Goldmark Report. The article was a stinging indictment of the apprenticeship method used in hospital schools of nursing. Their practice "to train the nurse to do precisely what she is told" did "little to fit the public health nurse for her work," particularly as an educator.[64] Without specialized training, the "unprepared" nurse "falls all too easily into the habit of doing what she is told without much thought as to what her special role is in the community programme." One of the first things that a public health student must be taught is how to adjust to working outside the orderly, well-equipped hospital setting and to deal with a different caseload. For this, graduates "require additional instruction along many lines: nutrition as a factor of health rather than in disease; in mental hygiene with special emphasis on habit formation and behaviour; in social casework, in order to have an understanding of problems met in homes; in prevention and educational work, emphasizing the care of well children." Mirroring the RF's preference for a generalized public health service, Kerr argued that the well-trained public health nurse must understand the "the broad underlying principles of the public health movement and of public health nursing as a phase of this movement." In Kerr's opinion, however, learning how to teach during home visits, in a manner that was "unobtrusive and acceptable," was the most important skill that the public health nursing student must learn: this incidental health teaching "is often of greater importance than the bedside nursing itself."[65] Accordingly, Kerr insisted that Lyle and her classmates become accomplished public speakers and masters of parliamentary procedure.

Kerr kindled her students' professional enthusiasm "not only to be teachers of health but to be interpreters of the goals of nursing." Margaret Kerr, in Creelman's view, provided her students with the fundamentals to become the voices of nursing "wherever their place of work or field of speciality."[66] In the years to come, Kerr's portrait of public health nursing's unique educative role and essential contribution to health care provided the intellectual loom for Creelman to re-weave nursing's professional identity in her own career performance and nursing's on-going transformation.

Chronicling Creelman's daily activities in these years is challenging. Unfortunately, it was only in her final year that she decided to begin a diary – a habit that she would continue intermittently for the rest of her life. But the VGH and UBC yearbooks and photographic records illuminate her involvement in residence life at VGH and in the UBC Nurses Undergraduate Society (NUS); both were important vehicles in socializing young women and in helping them to develop a shared professional identity. During their training at VGH, all the nursing students lived in residence either in Laurel House or in the temporary residence for nurses at West House. Like its counterparts across the country it was built as a home for nurses in the public sphere; designed to extend the domestic sphere into the public one, it in fact fostered gender and professional solidarities.[67] The residence experience of this small nucleus of UBC students fostered its own group identity. They entered the program during the summer when no other students were admitted, and their rotation through the hospital departments, determined by the UBC faculty, differed from that of the regular nursing students. UBC students were awarded preferential treatment in their clinical experience – a distinction that did not go unnoticed by their fellow VGH nursing classmates. While her contemporaries recalled that many aspects of a student nurse's life were less than ideal, they forged enduring friendships by sharing their experiences on the ward at the end of the day, quizzing each other for examinations, and creatively circumventing the restrictive practices of having to report into residence by 10:00 p.m. They also composed colourful songs and skits about their clinical instructors and medical staff as a release from their regimented nursing school environment. VGH yearbooks suggest that Creelman's serious scholastic bent and social reserve constrained her involvement in the lighter side of student life in VGH's nursing residence. In contrast to the witty, personal poems describing her UBC classmates, her fellow VGH student nurses chose to highlight her academic prowess in their 1936 yearbook.[68] Her stern intellect, intimidating at times to colleagues and close friends, would be a barrier to social intimacy throughout her life.

Creelman excelled in the nursing program during her final year, earning an 88 per cent average on her January 1936 examinations; it is not thus surprising that she found her interview with Mabel Gray "very nice."[69] Yet, despite her academic achievements, self-doubts lingered below her outward confidence. She often expressed criticism of her performance in her diary, as in a terse entry reading: "Taught lesson. I think my language is poor."[70] In another entry, she reproached herself for procrastinating in starting her thesis. Astutely, she had selected a comparative study of tuberculosis in the Canadian provinces as her subject. It was highly topical at the time and an issue for which she could obtain information from her stepbrother, Dr Prescott Creelman, a well-respected tuberculosis specialist. Shared professional interests became an important bridge in re-establishing connections, and fostering a deep and genuine affection, between Lyle and Prescott.

Before beginning her field placements in her final year, Creelman carefully noted a public health nurse's creed in her daily diary: "Faith, hope, charity and the greatest of these is tact."[71] In all likelihood, she had to remind herself of that creed on many occasions to temper her dissatisfaction with some of her placements.

Dr Henry Esson Young used field placements as a basis for recruiting future staff. During his tenure as provincial health officer, he arranged that all public health student nurses spend four weeks within a rural health unit staff[72] and received confidential reports on the "suitability of graduates for rural public health work" within the rapidly expanding provincial nursing services.[73] In terms of future employment, it was therefore a great let-down for Lyle when, on being introduced to Young during her first placement, he told her that "they placed university students first" but was "very general & did not give away anything."[74]

Despite the fear of contracting tuberculosis that made some UBC nursing students reluctant candidates, the two-month clinical placements at the provincial sanatorium at Tranquille stood out "as a pleasant dream" – a welcome relief from the long working hours and regimented social life of VGH. One of her contemporaries' recollections resonate with Creelman's own photographic record of Tranquille – the only surviving photos of her student nursing days. "Our pleasures there were many and mixed – to wit – hiking in the purple hills, bathing patients only twice a week; late leaves every night spent swimming or canoeing in the moonlight; watching the patients successfully satisfied gastronomically without any effort on our part; lounging in a 'cure chair' under the apple tree with the music of the robins to delight our ears and the coloured hills to delight our eyes ... with bonfires and eats to end the perfect day."[75] The idyllic pastoral portrayal of life at the sanatorium belied the very real problem of tuberculosis among student nurses; the rate for student nurses was seven times greater than that for student teachers.[76]

Creelman's time at the Saanich Health Unit on Vancouver Island, where school and home visits were interspersed with social calls for tea or games of ping-pong, received a mixed evaluation from the young public health student nurse: "I don't think the P.H. Nurses here justify their existence – but we may change our minds by the end of two weeks."[77] Similarly, her visit to the Spencer Clinic and Mental Hospital proved a disappointment because she was shown only the refractory patients, those who did not respond to normal treatment.[78] For the most part, Creelman enjoyed her time in February 1936 working in Coombs, a small community on Vancouver Island, with Isabel Chodat.[79] However, when Chodat took the day off to recover from a near-fatal mishap with her car on the icy country roads, her replacement failed to meet Creelman's high expectations. After she gave a bed bath to a patient without putting on an apron or washing her hands afterwards, Creelman was thankful not to have to work with her again.[80] Attracted by the relative independence and caseload variety of rural public health nursing, she nevertheless left Coombs "more and more set on getting a district of my own."[81]

Later that month, Creelman began a series of urban field placements. She characterized her week with Vancouver's Family Welfare Bureau as "dumb" – especially after her supervisor forgot her one morning.[82] In mid-March, she and a fellow classmate, Eleanor Graham, went to Essondale to begin their mental-health placement. Some UBC students regarded their clinical placements at Essondale during these years, when tranquillizer medications were not yet in use and treatment was limited to custodial care, as simply "gruesome."[83] Creelman had a very different reaction. She found the challenge more to her liking and left thinking, "I shall never forget the mental case ... with the dirty mouth. What a terrible thing pride is."[84] In April, Creelman found her VON assignment under the supervision of Electra MacLennan[85] a stimulating break from student routines and confidently concluded that she would be able to handle similar night-duty cases on her own.[86]

Her reaction to a particular field placement reflected her personality. She delighted in rotations that provided new and challenging work environments but was easily irritated by those that wasted her time. More generally, her dissatisfaction reflected the lack of integration between theory and practice in the UBC/VGH nursing program, which would not be addressed until after she graduated. While her reports from her field rotations were "very good," she received some criticism at Essondale for "being reserved and hard to get acquainted with."

At UBC, Creelman successfully juggled a wide range of student and community activities with the heavy academic program. Among other things, she was selected to serve as the hospital representative on the executive of the Nurses

Undergraduate Society. While the NUS organized social activities and sporting events for the nursing students, it also served, through its welfare activities, as a forum for Mabel Gray and Margaret Kerr to imbue their students with the professional ideals of service and sense of community responsibility.[87] Creelman's growing confidence within these professionally linked social activities was not always matched in her private social life. Socially reserved and older than many of her classmates, she frequently relied upon friends to arrange dates to dances. Her anxiety seldom dissipated once an escort had been found: "It looks as though Lorna [Makepeace] and I are going to make it [to the dance in February 1936]. Hope we have a good time and our escorts enjoy themselves."[88] Again in March, when she obtained a "blind date through the President of Science Club, to the graduation dance," she fretted: "Hope he won't be too disappointed in me."[89] What is more remarkable by contrast is her lack of concern that her nursing instructor, Margaret Kerr, drove the couple to that dance. Fortunately, the night and her date were a success: "He was very nice – young but a dandy dancer." The evening festivities continued well after the formal functions were over.[90] Having arrived home at 3:30 a.m., Creelman almost fell asleep in Dr Amyot's lecture the next day![91]

Yet in the spring of 1936, as she approached her final university and provincial registration examinations, she struggled to balance the mounting academic pressure with her desire to socialize with friends. The strain typically manifested itself in diary entries dealing with her unwanted weight gain: "Have broken diet badly all week ... Am going to try to be more moderate. Feel my old pain again quite a bit."[92] Her repeated vows – to reduce her weight to 150 pounds, in part to be more physically attractive – remained out of reach.

The need to pursue future employment added to the stress, distracting her attention from examination preparations. She approached Elizabeth Breeze, then in charge of school services in Vancouver, and left with some hope that "there might be a chance to get into the schools this year."[93] In the interim, she applied for the position of summer camp nurse at the Alexandra Fresh Air Camp at Crescent Beach, near White Rock, in the hope that it would lead to a more permanent position.[94] Discouraged to learn that a more experienced nurse was wanted and would be required earlier than she could be available, she consoled herself: "I'm just as glad as I feel there will be something turn up before September 1st when the camp would be over."[95] Two weeks later, however, arrangements had been made for another public health nurse, Hazel Dobson, to cover for the camp's nursing needs for the first six weeks until Creelman was available.[96] The easy-going Dobson assured her that "the responsibility is nothing to worry about." Creelman told only one of her classmates about the job; she wanted to keep her employment options open. Her spirits plunged – "I was in an argumentative mood" – upon hearing that another nurse had been recommended for the Richmond school position.[97] Despite this setback, by the end of the month, she had determined to approach Dr McIntosh and Dr Amyot to test the waters about applying for the Richmond job.

In the meantime, Creelman had ample reason to savour success amidst the social whirl of teas, banquets, and dances surrounding the dual graduation ceremonies at VGH and UBC in early May 1936. She had sailed through the examinations ranked as the top student for both UBC and VGH. She was one of six students at the VGH graduation ceremony to receive the Provincial Board of Health Award.[98] It was, however, the more informal get-togethers after graduation that proved most enjoyable. In one of these, the outgoing Margaret Kerr, remembered for her "abundant energy and zeal for life,"[99] joined her students following the president's tea for a rousing game of Black Jack, during which Kerr provided the musical accompaniment by singing A.A. Milne songs.[100] As one of her former students recalled, "Like many 'FSOMs,' as former students of Margaret Kerr were known, Creelman thought Kerr both an "inspiring and forceful teacher" and a "kind counsellor and friend."[101] Creelman often recorded how Kerr shared the hospitality of her home with her students or took them – on at least one occasion still clad in pyjamas[102] – for a spin in her much-beloved car.[103] "She taught us to enjoy our work but taught us the importance of recreation too"[104] – an outlook that Creelman emulated throughout her life. One of the longest-lasting personal connections that Creelman made during her UBC days was with Margaret Kerr.

Lyle Creelman's lifelong approach to nursing bore the imprint of her UBC years. One of Mabel Gray's and Margaret Kerr's brightest students, she would help to set national and international standards for nursing education in the decades following the Second World War. Throughout her career, Creelman shared her UBC instructor's belief that nursing students should receive a broad liberal educational experience comparable with that offered by other professions and that their education should not be driven by the hospitals' requirement for cheap labour. At UBC, Creelman received an elite education that was open to only a privileged few. Certainly, her early exposure to the social sciences at UBC broadened her academic appreciation of the socio-economic and cultural factors that shaped the delivery of nursing services. Both a more cosmopolitan education and years of experience, however, would be required to refine her understanding that international educational standards must acknowledge these profound socio-economic differences among the nations of the world.

Obtaining a degree in public health nursing shaped the subsequent career patterns and professional identities of Creelman and her fellow UBC graduates. Like the women who taught them, Creelman and her classmates would be active in nursing associations provincially, nationally, and internationally. Their professional paths would be inextricably interwoven with their personal friendships as each created legacies that clearly bore the imprint of their formative experience at UBC. For Creelman, the strong sense of professional identity, underpinned by a network of personal friendships, became a key strategy to creating personal and professional space within the provincial, national, and international health-care communities – all still within the purview of the male-dominated medical community. Community nursing would remain contested territory throughout Creelman's career; she too would come to understand the value of forging strong political alliances outside nursing's ranks to achieve nursing's goals and advance their careers.

But that was in the future. For now, she was eager to start her first job as the camp nurse at Crescent Beach and to see what the future would bring.

Chapter Two

New Beginnings, 1936–1939

As a public health nurse, Lyle Creelman could expect to deal with everything from tuberculosis and infectious diseases to maternal and child health clinics, armed only with "the revolutionary tool applauded by social reformers during the progressive era – education." Contemporaries argued that public health nursing presented more than the opportunity to spread the gospel of health: "It also offered the chance to fulfil women's highest career aspirations."[1] The reliance upon the nurse's intelligence and education carried the implicit expectation of greater professional autonomy and personal freedom among the UBC graduates who answered the call to service. Whether Creelman's first permanent appointment would satisfy her career aspirations remained to be seen. Expecting to utilize fully her new knowledge and skills to promote healthy living, the recent UBC graduate never anticipated the resistance that her progressive vision of the public health nurse's role would encounter on several fronts in the community. In the interim, she looked forward to a pleasant summer interlude while she searched for a permanent position.

Creelman held the position of nurse at the Alexandra Fresh Air Camp from June until 20 August 1936. Founded in 1916 as a summer refuge for children from the Alexandra Orphanage in Vancouver, the camp gave these children an opportunity to rebuild their health. In addition, it offered separate sessions "for underprivileged and pre-delinquent boys" and their parents designed to provide "a change in environment," where good parenting and proper nutrition practices could be demonstrated as "a way out of long-accustomed ruts of thinking" and as "a foundation for cultural beginnings and learning to appreciate the simple beauties and joys of living that are available to everyone regardless of circumstances."[2] As it turned out, however, the Crescent Beach residents' reluctance to associate with the Alexandra campers belied the idealistic belief that bringing the classes into contact with each other as neighbours would reduce class-based and cultural prejudices. Naivety underlay the missionary zeal with which middle-class activism cast the public health nurse as a "travelling evangelist" in the cause of good health.

Despite Dobson's assurance to Creelman that "the responsibility is nothing to worry about,"[3] waiting on the Union Station platform that first morning to accompany the first families to the camp "gave [her] cold feet. Some of them thought [she] was a tired mother."[4] Quite quickly, she took in stride the challenge of settling each new "tribe" and dealing with the regular changes to camp routines.[5] Creelman's own reaction ranged from impatience with a "foolish mother," who seemed unwilling to accept the camp nurse's parental guidance, to compassion for others forced to return to their impoverished dwellings as a result of their child's illness. Whether expected to or not, Creelman paid some of these families a home visit on her day off, which provided her with a first-hand view of how "terrible housing conditions" compromised a family's well-being.[6] Educating mothers could at best mitigate these unhealthy living conditions. Although brief, Creelman's time at Crescent Beach was the first step on a long journey that would allow her to look beyond middle-class perceptions and appreciate more fully the complex interplay of social economic factors as determinants of health. In the short term, the summer provided a welcome interlude from the regimented life of student nurse without the responsibilities of a district nursing position. But that was about to change.

In late August, Creelman accepted the position as the provincial public health nurse in Revelstoke in southeastern British Columbia. Nestled between the spectacular Selkirk and Monashee Mountains, Revelstoke was known in the early 1900s as "the capital of Canada's Alps." It was founded in the 1880s when the Canadian Pacific Railway (CPR) was built through the area, and the appointment of a public health nurse attested to the town's steady economic progress, which continued well into the 1940s.

On the occasion of Creelman's appointment to Revelstoke, Dr Henry Esson Young wrote to congratulate her on her academic success, to welcome her "to the guild" of public health nurses, and to offer a few words of support to one of those "fighting on the lines." Young expressed his pride in the work of the province's public health nurses, who "have established themselves firmly amongst the people." Adding that "we have never been asked to remove a nurse or close a centre," he simultaneously set high expectations for the recent graduate: "This is a good tradition to come into and judging by your record and your attention to your work you will carry on the work to our satisfaction and to the people's satisfaction."[7]

The direction of provincial health care had been the subject of a lively debate at the time of Creelman's graduation. A reference to the "fight being over" in

Young's letter most likely concerned the prolonged efforts to get approval for the Metropolitan Health Committee of Greater Vancouver, formed in 1936. That initiative was part of a larger ongoing battle being waged throughout the province to wrest control of the appointment of public health nurses from local school boards. Given the high political stakes, Young wanted to ensure that provincially appointed public health nurses were well qualified and that they understood the importance of their role as his chosen health crusaders. In short, Creelman was expected to be the state's messenger not only by teaching healthy living but also by acting as a personal model of the social decorum and good-health habits expected of an educated middle-class woman of that day.

Creelman's relationship with both Young and the local public officials began on an uncertain footing. In April 1936, when Creelman had approached Dr J.W. McIntosh, senior medical officer for the newly formed Metropolitan Health Committee, and Dr Grégoire Amyot, then the provincial health officer and adviser on hospital services, about a possible posting at Richmond, "they seemed rather encouraging."[8] Accordingly, she had written Dr Young about the Richmond position. Her hopes grew when she heard that "Dr Amyot has his eye on me for a position he hopes to open in a Normal School."[9] But Creelman's initial excitement upon receiving a telegram in late June asking her to arrange a meeting back in town quickly dissipated. Young wanted her to go Revelstoke, not Richmond. Although she "didn't feel very elated over it, she felt unable to "tactfully refuse" and so tried to convince herself that "it was the best thing for me."[10] As the weeks passed, Creelman regretted her hasty decision, especially after the current public health nurse, Agnes Thom, came to visit: "Thom told me about Revelstoke. Thinks I should write Dr Young & ask for a change on account of mother. Made me feel rather discouraged about it."[11] Given the sustained pressure from friends to request another assignment and her mother's obvious distress at being left alone in Vancouver, she became increasingly disheartened.[12]

Towards the end of July, she gathered up her courage to tell Dr Young that she preferred to wait for an opening in the Vancouver area. Although he had appeared cordial during their phone conversation, saying "It was up to her," Dr Amyot quickly called to inform her that Young was furious with her about-face. Determined to earn Amyot's and Young's respect to advance her career, she agreed to take the Revelstoke position.[13] Although Lyle felt "very sorry for her [mother's] sake,"[14] she had few alternatives; her mother was financially dependent upon her daughter's income, and employment opportunities during the Depression, even for public health nurses, were eagerly snapped up. A salary of $107.25 per month compared very favourably to her former salary as a teacher of only $90.00 per month.[15] Changed family circumstances – her father's death and illness in the home – had already forced Lyle to re-evaluate her personal and professional aspirations pragmatically. That same pragmatism would guide the difficult career choices still ahead. Young's subsequent letter calling her "angelic"[16] did little to dispel her disquiet as the time to take up her new post in Revelstoke approached. But his more positive attitude towards her was encouraging. It was her first introduction to the personal problems and politics involved in forging a successful career. What she would make of the Revelstoke appointment became quickly apparent.

Keeping step with the established practice, Lyle Creelman detailed her efforts to improve the nursing services during her first five months on the job in the March 1937 *Public Health Nurse's Bulletin*. Although regarded as the "father of public health nursing in British Columbia," Young never appointed a nurse to his administrative staff in a supervisory capacity, preferring instead to maintain direct contact through letters with the individual nurses and nursing committees throughout the province.[17] Recognizing the isolation that rural public health nurses often faced, Young had launched the *Public Health Nurses' Bulletin* and requested his nursing staff to contribute accounts of "their trials and tribulations, giving or asking for advice."[18]

After her arrival in Revelstoke at the end of August 1936, Creelman quickly took stock of the deficits of her predecessors' practice and methodically expanded the existing public health program. Even while recalling a UBC instructor's sage advice to "go slowly and be satisfied to reach a single objective at a time,"[19] she determined to push ahead with her public health agenda. Creelman's article in the *Bulletin* provides a carefully constructed, positive snapshot of her work and the reception that she received within the community. The reality was far more complex and fascinating.

Revelstoke did not offer the wide range of public health nursing activities experienced by her UBC classmates in more remote rural settings during the 1930s. Bedside nursing or home confinements were not part of her job, in part because Revelstoke had its own hospital run by the Canadian Red Cross. Moreover, as her predecessor had observed, "we are more fortunate here than other communities, in that few of our families are on city or Provincial relief. We are a railway town and medical care is provided for C.P.R. families."[20] The bulk of Creelman's work in Revelstoke centred on school services, which included preparing reports on each student's physical condition and general cleanliness and teaching the health-education programs for the town's elementary and high schools.[21] Schoolchildren, long considered society's most prized possessions, were the prime targets for social reform.

But Creelman quickly sought to expand these traditional duties of weighing and measuring by shifting the focus of her school work towards prevention.

Previously, health lessons within Revelstoke schools coincided with the monthly class inspection; after Creelman's arrival, health instruction was given bimonthly in every class. Her article in the *Bulletin* claimed that her program avoided "shaming" students into adopting good personal hygiene habits by encouraging them to keep their classroom clean through monthly competitions, with a prize being awarded to the classroom demonstrating the greatest improvement. Her public health programs were designed to foster good citizenship and proper parenting skills. She introduced home-nursing instruction for girls, first-aid courses for senior elementary students, and the first Canadian Junior Red Cross branch in Revelstoke. Her article suggests that she derived considerable satisfaction and community approval from her public health teaching. In referring to the home-nursing classes, the students' mothers often remarked to her, " 'We had nothing like that when we went to school and I am certainly glad my girl has such an opportunity to learn. Thus one is amply rewarded for any extra time given in these classes.' "[22] An educator by disposition, Creelman relished the opportunity to inculcate the gospel of public health in the wider community. Her approach as a health educator reflected the prevailing view that the child's character was akin to "a growing plant that needs to be pruned and supported, but always trained in the direction it needed to go" – through guidance, not punishment.[23]

Similarly, Creelman's article emphasized the unique role that public health nurses performed as a vital link within the local community connecting teacher, student, and parent: "Many a misunderstanding is cleared by the home visit, with the result that the parent realizes the best is being done for his child." During her first six months, she made 397 home visits to school-age children, in part because these visits also presented opportunities to observe and treat health problems in those of preschool age, already targeted for greater attention in her future program planning. But there was another reason as well. As she told her fellow public health nurses, her "chief delight" came from her maternal health and child-care work. Already, each Saturday morning, she visited new mothers in town and encouraged rural mothers to sign up for neonatal letters.[24] Creelman asserted that the mothers "soon look[ed] forward to the Saturday morning visits with nurse with her scales, which tell how much baby has gained. Usually the mother has a question regarding the health and care of the baby." She invariably left homes feeling "that some service has been given."[25]

Like her fellow provincial public health nurses, Creelman sought an expanded role for nursing; by making health care less threatening and accessible, public health nurses cultivated the trust required to eradicate or to control home-based diseases. Enthusiastically, she shared her future plans to have a monthly weighing station for infant and preschool children: "All public-health workers realize the need for service to this group, for it is here that a good foundation is laid for future health. Even if these do not appear very popular at first I shall not be discouraged, because I believe that in time more and more mothers will avail themselves of this opportunity of visiting the station monthly to have their babies weighed and checked for defects and to obtain literature and advice regarding diet, habit formation, and the countless everyday problems which worry and perplex the young mother." She would proceed slowly, however, to avoid having the social stigma of the "unfit mother" becoming attached to women attending these clinics. Creelman's actions make it clear that she subscribed to Mabel Gray's teaching that "our energy should be directed towards providing for the child such conditions – in the home, in the school and his play and playmates – as will help in the up-building of a good citizen."[26] Her public health initiatives provided a respectable veneer for the greater social control inherent in expanding the public domain into the private domain. Like her public health nursing counterparts throughout the province, Creelman was expected to reinforce gendered behavioural patterns assigned to women as caregivers. Creelman, however, genuinely saw herself as an agent of change engaged in spreading the "gospel of health to improve the lives of mother and children."[27]

Creelman's determination to provide maternal health-care services, "even if these do not appear very popular," is telling, reflecting as it did the larger anxiety over Canada's high rate of maternal mortality and the declining Anglo-Saxon birth rate[28] – a trend that initially continued, even as all aspects of maternal health care increasingly came under physicians' control. As Wendy Mitchinson and others have pointed out, the extension of maternal services within the wider community was not without racial and class overtones.[29] It was not uncommon for provincial health nurses to encounter resentment from parents, who disliked being instructed on how to be better parents.[30] Nor should this come as a surprise. Public health nurses often adopted an authoritarian stance, championing a highly regimented approach to childrearing that scheduled feeding, sleeping, toilet-training, and play routines and advocated that parents withhold overt expressions of affection, such as cuddling or kissing.[31] They in turn were often "stunned to find that their pre-natal advice was not wanted because they represented 'new-fangled ideas' which the local women found foreign."[32] Scientific principles were not a substitute for maternal instincts – a greater appreciation on Creelman's part of both the mother's and the child's psychological needs still lay in the future.

Equally, she would have to tread lightly to carve out a niche not already occupied by private physicians, who viewed public health nurses as economic rivals in tough economic times, or community philanthropic groups. Public health nurses often had to make a special effort to court the cooperation of the local medical community. In contrast to her classmates, Creelman did not publically record any overt opposition to her proposed preschool program from within the medical community.[33] Nonetheless, she avoided making plans to offer prenatal clinics, choosing instead to gear her efforts toward early detection of problems that then could be referred to the physician.

Her own quiet confidence and drive were already discernible. Creelman understood the value of publishing as a vehicle to gain acceptance for her public health initiatives and to raise her professional profile in Revelstoke. Ambitious to advance her career, she astutely concluded her article in the *Public Health Nurses' Bulletin* with an acknowledgment of Dr Young, "without whose kindly advice and encouragement my way would have been less easy," and an invitation to share her "dream" that all the schools in the rural areas surrounding Revelstoke would one day have public health nurses.[34] The themes and ideas of Creelman's articles in the local newspaper, the *Revelstoke Review*, bear the clear imprint of the views of her instructors at UBC/VGH and Young's guidance. Significantly, the subtitle of her first article echoed Young's philosophy: "It is cheaper and easier to prevent than to cure."[35] Equally important, it reveals that the eager graduate was learning to navigate local politics and customs. Chaffing at the idea that public health nurses' main duties should be the weighing and measuring of children, she seized every opportunity to publicize the social value of these nurses' role in preventing disease and promoting overall health within the modern health-care system. She wrote regular articles encouraging parents to have their children protected against diphtheria and smallpox and explaining the purpose of the monthly weighing station sponsored by the Imperial Order Daughters of the Empire (IODE). The articles, directed at changing community attitudes and past practices, reveal another side of story.

Both professionally and personally, the transition from the classroom to the field had been more difficult than Creelman publically acknowledged. Her private diaries record her initial struggle both to gain acceptance for her professional views and to make friends within Revelstoke. On arriving at her boarding house there on 30 August 1936, she wrote, "Shed a few tears after I went to bed but feel better about it now. Have a very nice room."[36] Subsequent diary entries attested that her sense of loneliness lingered over the next several months, exacerbated by many unexpected professional setbacks that had to be sorted out before she could institute change.

She found her predecessor's record system incomplete and a jumble:[37] "Felt terribly blue today. Can't find any records of infants."[38] Outside the office, she struggled to gain the community's support for public health activities that contravened their understanding of her role. Unprepared for the initial resistance

to her plans for the immunization program that she encountered at her first
meeting with the local school board, she "felt squashed" and complained, "They
certainly aren't very far seeing. Think that the school work is all important."[39]
She displayed a condescending attitude towards parents "who are so ignorant
of modern public health" that 45 per cent of the children still had not been
immunized against smallpox in Revelstoke.[40] Creelman, like other health-care
professionals, assumed that the benefits of immunization were so obvious
that well-informed parents would immediately accept them.[41] She responded
by writing articles advocating an expanded role for public health nursing:
"School nursing is one branch of public health but there is the need for some
interest in the health of the pre-school child."[42] In the meantime, she continued to feel "rather lonesome" and complained, "I'm only meant to plug away
at school work."[43] Many evenings she still cried herself to sleep.[44] Initially, she
was discouraged by her inability to use her new scientific knowledge and skills
as quickly or completely as she had, naively, anticipated. As the public health
nurse in Revelstoke, she had to adjust what she had been taught at UBC to
the realities of small-town life, where voluntarism and traditional views on the
role of the school nurse shaped community attitudes towards health care. By
the end of September, however, she had taken her new professional duties more
in stride. Following the advice of her UBC instructors, she eventually learned to
involve the community in her preschool programs, drawing on the assistance of
the IODE to become more than simply the school nurse.[45] By the end of her first
six months in Revelstoke, for example, she had made 119 home visits to infants
and preschoolers; in contrast, her predecessor had not made any during 1935.[46]
It simply took time to be accepted within the community. Patience was never
Lyle Creelman's long suit; it was acquired over time.

Creelman's experience typified that of many other provincial public health
nurses; many found their actions and judgment constrained by the local school
board, physicians, and town officials, and all struggled to address their communities' needs with far too few resources to meet either their own ambitious
goals or those set by Young. Like other recent graduates of the UBC program,
Creelman gradually realized that she had to market herself as a member of the
community to sell her new approaches to public health. In the years to come,
the setting would change, but both local politics and inadequate resources
would continue to constrain the public health nurse's role.

Isolated from friends and family, Creelman found the personal adjustment to life within the small rural community difficult, particularly since her
position carried a high degree of social accountability. Community leaders
assumed that she would be pleased to accept the "invitation" to teach Sunday
school, to attend the Young People's Society, and to serve on the Missionary

Committee of the local United Church. Much of her leisure time was spent in taking tea in local homes or playing bridge at fundraisers – all activities considered socially acceptable for a single woman who was expected to be a role model of healthy living and good citizenship for the community. Moreover, Creelman probably never imagined that the local newspaper would keep track of her social activities, weekend visitors, and excursions out of town.[47] Evenings out at the Young People's Society banquet left her still yearning to "go out someplace where I could be myself."[48] Perhaps, in part, she felt that the social constraints compromised her opportunities to date. While other single friends found matches, she remained on the outside wondering, "Why [do] I never attract anyone?" Forlornly, she concluded, "I might as well resign myself to being an old maid."[49] Throughout October, however, her spirits improved. She abandoned working in the evenings to play badminton with other young people and began receiving more invitations to parties. By November, she was out practically every evening, often well after midnight.[50] But even then the need to maintain decorum tempered her enjoyment on these social outings. Once, when she was scooped up at the boarding house to attend a friend's surprise birthday party, Creelman "had a dandy time" playing cockade, enjoying the joking mood around the table before hitching a ride home on the running board of a friend's car in the early hours of the morning.[51] The next day, she was consumed with worry that she had been foolish. While she missed the Vancouver social scene, she determined "to make the best of it"[52] and, through a concerted effort, adjusted to the social rhythms of small-town life.[53]

Creelman's year at Revelstoke expanded her horizons. On the personal front, the adaptation required of "fitting into a new community" and creating new friendships would become an integral part of an itinerant career dedicated to international nursing. Professionally, her appointment and year there provided an early indication that, whatever her expectations of greater professional autonomy as a public health nurse, physicians and public health officials would have the final word. Her public health work in Revelstoke had to be adapted to local health needs and cultural expectations and be cognizant of the ongoing bureaucratic rivalry between the local school board and the provincial government over control of health-care delivery. She began to understand the importance of involving the diverse elements of the community to advance her public health agenda, and the need to forge strategic alliances to expedite that process. Accordingly, she successfully cultivated closer connections with volunteer community organizations to expand the delivery of maternal health services to meet the needs of rural women around Revelstoke. While her views were certainly informed by middle-class values and the accepted gender norms prevalent in interwar Canada society, Lyle Creelman saw the public health nurse less as an agent of "cultural imperialism" than as a passionate teacher of health.[54] Over time, she would refine her own views on the role of public health nursing. But her belief that the nursing role within the school services needed to be re-evaluated to utilize more effectively the public health nurse's specialized knowledge only grew stronger over the years.

In the fall of 1937, new challenges awaited back in Vancouver; she had been appointed to the Richmond Unit in the Metropolitan Health Committee of Greater Vancouver under the directorship of Elizabeth Breeze. She was to be paid $1,700 per annum but had to supply her own car.[55] Richmond, where many families were on welfare, would present nursing challenges different from those that Creelman experienced in Revelstoke. First, though, she left for the east coast, stopping in New York and Boston on the way to join her mother, who had travelled ahead to the Maritimes in April. Five years later, her most vivid memory of that New York trip remained spotting Columbia University from the roof of the Rockefeller Tower; quietly, she vowed to study there one day.[56] A little over a year after the trip, that dream would come true. Once she joined her mother in Halifax, she enjoyed visiting relatives in Portapique and Upper Stewiacke before spending time in Prince Edward Island with her stepbrother, Prescott, and his family. She would never forget the feelings of shared kinship that she experienced on that visit. It would be the first of many trips to strengthen family connections with Prescott's family and rediscover her Maritime roots.

Lyle Creelman returned to Vancouver to find that her appointment had made headlines: "Metropolitan Board Robs Province of Best Nurses." According to this newspaper report, "Dr Young took strong exception to the fact that he had not been notified." The matter was passed off as "nothing more than a storm in a teacup."[57] That her appointment warranted commentary at all, however, speaks to the rivalry engendered by the staff raiding between the provincial nursing service and the Metropolitan Health Committee.

In October 1936 the Metropolitan Health Committee had begun operations with an overall budget of $36,080, of which $13,309 was provided by the Rockefeller Foundation, $13,309 by the province, and the remaining $9,462 by municipal governments.[58] Interested in finding long-term rather than short-term solutions to problems in society, the RF worked through governmental agencies rather than providing direct support on a project basis. At the time of Creelman's appointment, the committee was the first Canadian urban health unit to adopt a progressive, generalized approach to public health that amalgamated several specialized nursing services under one administrative roof, allowing one nurse to provide all these services to the families under her care.[59] It had two separate departments for the school system: the School Medical

Service supervised the physical needs of the pupils, and a new Child Welfare and Mental Hygiene Department took care of the emotional, social, and psychological needs of schoolchildren.[60] Dr Stewart Murray, well qualified in paediatrics, psychiatry, and public health, was appointed the first senior health officer of the Metropolitan Health Committee of Greater Vancouver. The first director of the Mental Hygiene Department, Dr C.H. Gundry, however, was not appointed until 21 December 1938.[61]

Creelman was one of three public health nurses in Unit 2, located in the Richmond area where she had gone to school and later taught. The medical-services program, "entirely one of prevention and education and no curative services included,"[62] was an excellent fit for Creelman's temperament and career aspirations. Yet, in practice, delineating the role of public health nurses within the two departments responsible for school services proved challenging. Visits to schools, follow-up home visits, and the mandatory visits to check any student who was absent from school for more than three days continued to occupy most of her day. But preliminary steps were taken to initiate child health centres and tuberculosis home visiting[63] and to provide a rudimentary mental-health program.[64] She had barely settled into her new position when her life was suddenly turned upside-down.

Only eight months after joining Unit 2, she was chosen to direct the nursing services of the Metropolitan Health Committee following the sudden death of Elizabeth Breeze in April 1938. Creelman's promotion was both unexpected and initially unwanted. Following Breeze, who had started the school nursing service in Vancouver in 1911 and was heralded for her "unfailing tact and patience,"[65] would not be an easy task for the straightforward and relatively inexperienced Creelman.[66] Reluctantly, she acceded to Dr Young's and Dr Murray's demands that she take the job, but she wisely insisted on first being given a year's study leave at Teacher College,[67] an option made possible through a Rockefeller Foundation fellowship. Reserved exclusively for preparing nurses for senior positions in administration or education, RF fellowships were central to the RF's vision of building public health leadership to improve population health. For the moment, Lyle put aside her reservations.

For Lyle Creelman, the year in New York represented adventure, escape, and opportunity. While she was away from family and work colleagues, her fellowship year allowed Lyle to develop her own world view and make different choices about her social life as single woman. As the world inched closer to war in 1938–9, international affairs provided a hot topic of discussion among Columbia University's student body. Yet, on another level, the daily life of campus co-eds remained largely insulated from all of this. For Creelman herself, student life as a Rockefeller fellow at TC presented new personal opportunities as well as improved professional prospects. While at TC, then considered the premier university for postgraduate nursing studies, she benefited both from the cosmopolitan nature of its student body and her encounters with some of the most innovative nurse-educators of her generation, including Canadian Isabel Maitland Stewart, the director of the Department of Nursing at TC from 1925 to 1948. A key figure within a closely knit group of North American nursing leaders, Stewart was regarded as the pre-eminent international nursing educator in the interwar era, and her overriding interest in curriculum development earned her the nickname "Miss Curriculum."[68] In fact, her approach to curriculum development served as a blueprint for generations of nursing educators, including Lyle Creelman.

A proponent of the collegiate school of nursing, Stewart believed that nursing education deserved the same support accorded other public services.[69] Envisioning nursing education as a lifelong process, Stewart told her students, "It is not a case of education *or* service but education for service."[70] She always contended that nursing education should be "less complacent and more defiant of hoary and old educational abuses and traditions."[71] Stewart stressed that nursing education should be appropriate to the times and adapted to the needs of the nursing profession.[72] Like Mabel Gray and Margaret Kerr at UBC, she abhorred the authoritarian educational model controlled by physicians and predicated upon the rote learning and unquestioning compliance with doctor's orders that had characterized hospital-based apprentice-nursing schools. The regimented educational environment of those schools, in Stewart's opinion, failed to develop the character of the individual or produce "resourceful workers." Promoting dependence instead of self-mastery, it also failed to provide individual guidance and self-direction.[73] Accordingly, Stewart championed the right of nurses to become self-governing and promoted open debates and consensus-building behaviour among nurses with the goal of democratizing the occupation. Her concept of "adjustment" as the primary goal of nursing education was refined through her work with the National League on Nursing Education (NLNE).[74]

Stewart had determined that a complete overhaul of the NLNE's 1927 basic curriculum was required to strengthen the level of nursing education before an effective graduate program could be built. But she sought equally to use the exercise to inculcate a more democratic approach to curriculum planning; nursing schools, working in collaboration with allied medical professions and the community, would construct their own curriculum by drawing upon relevant materials provided by the Nursing League but adapt them to their own needs and stage of development.[75] To accomplish this, the curriculum study posed penetrating questions that challenged the very essence of nursing education's underlying philosophy, goals, core values, and capacity to evolve to meet future needs. The individual nurse's development assumed centre stage but was still accompanied by an overriding sense of social responsibility and a continued emphasis on the traits required to function within a democratic society. Only such an approach to nursing education, Stewart believed, would produce nurses capable of independently assessing and adapting to the changing demands placed upon them throughout their nursing careers. But she added an important caveat to this guiding principle. Adaptation would occur only if nurses could also "identify with the welfare of the social group and serve its needs."[76] Stewart taught that nursing must embrace the goals and aspirations of many different individuals and cultures in order to move away from the authoritarian model. Her views reflected her long-standing interest in international affairs and involvement with international nursing, including serving as the chair of the Committee on Education of the International Council of Nurses (ICN) from 1925 to 1947,[77] and were, in turn, refined by her extensive contacts with foreign students at Teachers College.

At times Creelman privately complained that Stewart's lectures on trends in nursing bordered on boring. Eventually, however, she built on Stewart's legacy in advancing nursing professional autonomy and raising educational standards and carried it forward to a new generation of nurses around the world. Both the underlying concept of "adjustment" and the actual process of curriculum building, whereby the end users were intimately involved in its development to ensure compliance and suitability, provided fundamental building blocks for Creelman's future approach to international nursing. Creelman, like Stewart, came to believe that only an approach to nursing education based upon a sound scientific foundation could strengthen the profession's stature and authority within the medical community and equip nurses to meet societies' changing health needs. The opportunity and necessity to fully test and refine the knowledge absorbed at Teachers College quite simply required a broader canvas than that offered by directing the nursing services within the Metropolitan Health Committee. Those challenges remained ahead.

Another faculty member, Virginia Henderson, co-author of the revised *Textbook of the Principles and Practices of Nursing*, would influence nursing practice, education, and research worldwide over the next several decades.[78] While its antecedents reached back to her involvement in drafting the 1937 revisions of the NLNE's basic curriculum,[79] Henderson's famous definition of nursing as a distinct profession separate from medicine was first enunciated when she was asked to revise Canadian Bertha Harmer's nursing text. "The unique function of the nurse," Henderson declared, "is to assist the individual sick or well, in the performance of those activities contributing to health or its recovery (or to peaceful death) that he would perform unaided if he had the necessary strength will or knowledge. And to do this in such a way as to help him gain independence as rapidly as possible."[80] Henderson's concept of "the nurse as a substitute for what the patient lacks to make him 'complete,' 'whole,' or 'independent,' by the lack of physical strength, will, or knowledge," was incorporated into an ICN pamphlet on basic nursing published in 1961.[81] With its direct approach, easily understood and concise language, and emphasis on the nurse–patient relationship, Henderson's definition would serve as a guide for Creelman and her WHO staff, who would regularly publicize and promote it throughout the world.

For the moment, academic courses and public health fieldwork captured Creelman's interest. She took a wide spectrum of courses from some of the leading figures in their respective fields, including Mary Swartz Rose, a pioneer in nutrition education, and Dr Haven Emerson, the elder statesman of public health in the first half of the twentieth century.[82] In addition to the prescribed courses in child guidance, Creelman audited the Psychology of Family Relations, a very popular course taught by the prominent family-life educator Dr Ernest G. Osborne. In all likelihood, Creelman, like her TC contemporises, flocked to the course because of its innovative format; Osborne "refined educational procedures to facilitate self discovery in his students."[83] Each student defined her own modus operandi on the journey to "self understanding" and "self disclosure," which Osborne believed were crucial constructs underpinning the role of the family-life educator.[84] He argued that nurses were ideally suited for a parent-guidance function and should be specifically prepared for it.[85] The nurse's primary function in advising parents was not "that of serving as a conveyer of information." Rather, "the nurse was to assist parents to think through their problems, after considering their concerns, rather than lecturing them into temporary compliance."[86] Osborne's classes on the Art of Being a Woman and the Role of the Father were among the few mentioned in Creelman's private diaries. Increasingly, her views on the public health nurse's role – as one of guidance and advocacy and centred on the family rather than the individual patient – reflected Osborne philosophy.

At Teachers College, the education of students was based on the notion that lessons conveyed in classroom lectures, wherein nursing was conceptualized as holistic, comprehensive care including physical, social, and mental health as well as the teaching of healthy living habits within the community, were put into practice during the students' public health field placements. Based upon her first-hand observations of the Metropolitan Health Committee and private conversations with Drs Murray and Young, Mary Elizabeth Tennant, one of the assistant directors of the International Health Division (IHD) of the RF,[87] carefully orchestrated Creelman's schedule to provide a wide range of field experiences focusing on administration.[88] Accordingly, Creelman's fieldwork in the East Harlem Nursing and Health Services (EHNHS) was especially designed to allow her to be free on Mondays and Tuesdays to visit other health agencies, and, further, all her TC's field placements wound up in April 1939. This permitted time for an extensive tour of other public health centres and nursing-education programs both in the United States and in Canada beginning in May.[89]

Creelman got her first glimpse of the precarious working and housing conditions of black and immigrant women during the 1930s when, on 10 February, she started her field assignment with the EHNHS. By 1930, the New York City neighbourhood of Harlem had the largest and most diverse urban black community in the United States. Although predominantly African American, there were also southern Italians and Sicilians, Puerto Ricans, Cubans, and Africans, and the result was a dynamic cultural mix that, as far as Creelman was concerned, created a dramatically different practice setting and required considerable adjustment. After a brief period of observation, she would typically be assigned responsibility for a two-block area, encompassing about 2,500 people. Field experiences included prenatal clinics and classes, maternity and postnatal care, and infant and preschool care, as well as general family care carried out in cooperation with nutritionists and social workers.[90] The EHNHS typified the RF's preferred approach of training public health workers through comprehensive field experience within a designated teaching centre, as opposed to arranging separate field placements within specialized agencies.

Funded by the RF since 1938, the EHNHS's community-based services formed part of a larger project with the City Health Department in which five of the districts worked in close cooperation with the New York Medical College.[91] It was described as "a department store of health and welfare" conveniently located in one room and easily accessible to the population it was designed to serve.[92] The concept of a community-health centre providing health care on a neighbourhood basis and its institutionalization in organizational forms provided the core for a widespread movement that emerged in the second and third decades of the twentieth century before dissipating after the Second World War.[93] Designed to meet the needs of the urban poor and immigrant community whose living conditions were adverse to health, it was predicated upon the pious, but often unrealized, aim of involving the local population in the health-care program.

Despite her initial eagerness to get started, Creelman's private reaction to fieldwork in the EHNHS was qualified. Her diary entries indicated periods when she was "fed up" with her work there, without further explanation. Official assessments, suggesting that the work brought new challenges and frustrations, offer insight into the character of the student. Creelman was assessed not only on her skill, knowledge, leadership, and teaching ability, but on her personality and reaction to supervision as well. The report on her stint with the EHNHS sent to Tennant noted that Creelman was "eager for field experience & felt a definite obligation to obtain as much information as possible for future use in a position for which she felt [that] she is inadequately prepared on basis of experience." As a result, she initially spent too much time trying to tabulate all the information she gained for future use. Eventually "she relaxed somewhat and became more interested in activities." Her superiors characterized her as a "tense, reserved person with a conspicuously professional attitude" who adjusted "satisfactorily on the intellectual level" but who experienced "difficulty in establishing easy relationships with people." Significantly, her supervisors also observed that it was "less difficult for her to approach her peers than the families in the district." Differences in social class, ethnicity, and race between the nurse and her patients in Harlem – so unlike Revelstoke and even Richmond – would have been considerable. "Miss C," the report noted, "is a perfectionist in her attitude towards herself and others and seemed disturbed when an occasional error was brought to her attention." Overall, her superiors portrayed her as "an intelligent, reliable person, whose awareness of her own limitations should make it possible for her to make effective adjustments."[94] Their portrait bears striking similarities to earlier field evaluations at UBC. Though keenly intelligent and dedicated, she was socially reserved and demonstrated little patience either for her own errors or for those of colleagues who were not equally professional in their outlook.

Outside class, Creelman sampled a wide range of cultural and sports events new to her, sometimes even convincing classmates to skip classes to attend plays. She loved the club nightlife of New York, renowned as the hub for jazz. Many evenings, she joined members of the "Canadian group" or the "Oxford Group" from International House at Duke Ellington's jazz concerts or uptown at the best jazz clubs like the Onyx Club, where Stuff Smith, the Three Deuces, Jimmy Ryans, and the Famous Door reigned. Although she found New York's performing arts scene exhilarating, she still poked fun at her lack of cultural sophistication. When she found herself disappointed by Wagner's *Siegfried*, she wrote, "Not high brow enough to appreciate it."[95] This was a woman who found equal pleasure cheering loudly at baseball or basketball games and watching the former Olympian Sonia Henie perform the same daring jumps as male skaters in the elaborately staged ice show at Madison Square Gardens. During the year, she exhibited a passion for the performing arts and architecture and an insatiable curiosity about other cultures that would continue to provide an emotional refuge from her chosen path as an expatriate career woman.

But New York's vibrant array of performing arts is only one reason why student life at TC proved so agreeable to Creelman. She experienced a kind of freedom, and encountered a world, unlike anything she had known in her earlier student days. Symbolically, she welcomed in 1939 with friends at the International House dance; afterwards the group greeted the dawn of the new day in Times Square. She and fellow UBC graduate Electra MacLennan had a standing date for supper every Wednesday night. Her diaries indicate her delight that "there were lots of partners" at the Tuesday evening "regular dance."[96] Even when there were no new men or fewer partners, she generally "had a fairly good time" at the house dances.[97] She also had many fond memories of the fun she shared with the Indian, Czechoslovak, and Puerto Rican doctors and her special Norwegian friend, Jack Jardine, a member of the Oxford Group. Jardine frequently escorted her to dances, dinners at the International House, art exhibits and the theatre, and meetings of the Oxford Group, all of which provided both social and intellectual companionship. The "grand time" of formal dances in mid-April, however, paled against an earlier "unforgettable" outing. Enthralled by the moment, Lyle and Jack had a great time "skipping through the streets of Harlem at 2 am on a February night."[98] At the end of term, she would be sad to say goodbye to the "Canadian boys" and the Oxford Group, especially Jack. But before they parted, they were all determined to experience the major cultural event of 1939 – New York's World Fair.

Timed officially to celebrate the 150th anniversary of the Constitution and the presidential inauguration of George Washington in New York, the fair was really designed as an antidote to the Depression and growing international uncertainty. Dedicated to "building the world of tomorrow," a world set in the still distant 1960s, the fair heralded a return to social and economic prosperity and was predicated upon the belief that science and technology could re-engineer the very basis of human society. Creelman's fascination with the World Fair reflected her acceptance of the progressive viewpoint that championed democratic collectivism and rational planning as a solution to society's ills. The social-reform movements that had shaped her educational experience both at UBC and at TC embodied the beliefs espoused by these disciples of Henry Ford and Frederick Taylor; they were convinced that scientific management and expanding production would eliminate class conflict.

Creelman was captivated by the fair's streamlined, futuristic architecture. Like millions of its other visitors, she was caught up in the romantic atmosphere carefully orchestrated in the utopian exhibitions and demonstrations of the "World of Tomorrow" – especially two of its most popular diorama exhibits. Democracity, housed in the Perisphere, portrayed "the perfectly integrated garden city of tomorrow"[99] where pleasant suburbs for nuclear families radiated from a thriving core. While touring it, Creelman was treated to an audiovisual presentation narrated by the popular newscaster H.V. Kalternborn, which "culminated in images of farmers, industrial workers, engineers, bankers and professionals holding hands and bursting into song."[100] In the Futurama exhibit at the General Motors pavilion, she and her friends were seated in individual chairs with their own loudspeakers that moved across a 36,000-square-foot model of an idealized United States in 1960 liberated by the automobile. They were whisked above cities replete with futuristic homes, bridges, dams, and surrounding landscapes as well as spacious highways that permitted cars to reach 100 miles an hour while pedestrians were transported on elevated walkways.

Unsurprisingly, her diary remains silent on the politics underpinning the fair's exhibits. Marco Duranti has argued that "the exposition's innocence and optimism were out of step with the realities of its own days. Its progressive utopias and nostalgic longings were intentional acts of defiance, calculated to create an imaginative dreamscape where the traumatic consequences of technological progress could be defused ... [But it] could not escape the spectre of war that descended on its grounds."[101] Creelman's own experience as a graduate student at Teachers College reflected a similar paradox. Just as the fair offered Americans a welcome antidote to economic depression and international tension, Teachers College gave Creelman greater personal freedom and a respite from her future administrative responsibilities. Neither Americans nor Creelman, however, could elude the shadow of war much longer. As it turned out, the war would complicate the new administrative challenges that awaited Creelman in Vancouver. For the moment, she was busy finalizing summer travel and study plans before returning to work in September.

Creelman graduated from Teachers College with an MA in public health administration and supervision in the spring of 1939. Looking back several years later on her decision to attend TC, Creelman remained convinced that "if I had to do it over I would go to TC. It was grand year."[102] At TC as at UBC, she was influenced by a small cadre of closely connected, progressive, and influential nursing leaders. Yet, despite Teachers College's reputation and Creelman's adherence throughout her career to its guiding philosophy of nursing education, she always maintained that her UBC training was more rigorous. It should be kept in mind, too, that because of the close personal and professional contacts between members of the UBC faculty and Teachers College, Creelman already had some exposure to the new trends and approaches inaugurated by TC's Division of Nursing Education. For Creelman, the Columbia interlude built upon the foundations laid by the nursing faculty at UBC and VGH. The closely knit group of North American nursing leaders were an integral part of the transatlantic nursing network that provided continuity between the two educational experiences.

The RF was a key player within this network.[103] Moreover, the RF connection permeated both Creelman's educational experiences and her early work within the Metropolitan Health Committee. Obtaining a degree from Teachers College on an RF fellowship gave Creelman entry into an elite group of nursing leaders who would shape the direction of nursing at home and abroad for decades to come. Friendships forged there continued and provided important links with Canadian nursing leaders; for example, Electra MacLennan, often a willing companion on theatre outings, would have a distinguished career as a nurse educator and serve as the president of the Canadian Nurses Association (1962) and a member of the International Council of Nurses (1962–9). As Creelman's international nursing career unfolded, other professional connections made as a Rockefeller scholar proved equally useful. Just as Tennant had opened doors for Creelman within the medical community during her summer field visits, the RF's nursing leaders and fellows would prove valuable allies. The Rockefeller Foundation continued support for local health services in British Columbia, including the Metropolitan Health Committee and UBC's·School of Nursing,[104] allowed Tennant during future visits to Vancouver to evaluate first-hand how well Creelman put into practice the knowledge gained during her study year abroad.

Before leaving TC in May 1939, Creelman visited public health agencies in Boston and New York, including the Henry Street Visiting Nurses Association, the cradle of modern public health and one of the most influential public health agencies in the country. At the end of May, Creelman had one last meeting with Tennant to discuss what aspects of public health should be observed at each of the planned field visits over the next several weeks to other "innovative" Rockefeller-funded public health facilities in Canada and the United States.[105] In Washington, the major tourist attractions, the Smithsonian and Mount Vernon, were sandwiched between visits to the American Red Cross, public health facilities affiliated with the Eastern Health District of Baltimore City, and Johns Hopkins Hospital.[106] Creelman found the fifteen-hour trip to Cleveland on 4 June and the heat and humidity during her five-day stay to observe the University of Illinois nursing-education program and its community health programs simply exhausting. In mid-June, after picking up her car in Windsor, she headed for Toronto, where she was scheduled to spend almost a month.

The Rockefeller Foundation, which held the Toronto Department of Public Health, the Connaught Laboratories, and the University of Toronto's School of Hygiene in high regard, regularly sent fellowship students to the city for practical experience.[107] The School of Nursing at the University of Toronto was the

RF's "lighthouse school," a model for emerging public health nursing programs worldwide. It was chosen as the preferred site for RF nursing fellows "because of its innovative programs and because students from varying racial backgrounds who could not be accommodated in programs in the United States were accepted into its programs."[108] The Toronto nursing leadership was well known and respected by both the RF and Teachers College; Edith Kathleen Russell's efforts to establish nursing education on an independent footing at the University of Toronto would not have been possible without the strong financial backing of the Rockefeller Foundation.[109] At the university, Creelman was again exposed to other Canadian nursing educators, such as Russell, who fervently sought to secure the same educational opportunities for nurses afforded other professional groups, both to gain "better pay" and "more rewarding occupation" and to provide the basis "of knowledge and culture" that would prepare nurses to meet the new challenges inherent in an increasingly complex health-care system.[110] Connections with these Toronto nursing leaders such as Jean Wilson, Ethel M. Cryderman, Jean Gunn, and others would become an important future strand in the professional network crucial to advancing both nursing's interests and Creelman's own career aspirations.[111]

The assistant director of the School of Nursing at the University of Toronto, Florence Emory, had tailored an intensive round of field visits for several public health nurses holding RF fellowships that summer[112] to the Department of Health, pre-school clinics, maternal health clinics in the Parkdale district, the Blue Mountain Camp for Crippled Children north of Toronto, the Bolton Fresh Air Camp, the Weston Sanatorium, and the High Park Fresh Air School. Russell routinely discussed the customization of each fellow's program with Tennant. Creelman's attendance at the meeting of the Executive Committee of the Toronto Department of Public Health and her meetings with senior officials to "discuss administrative problems"[113] substantiates that her program was individually tailored to her future role with Vancouver's Metropolitan Health Committee. Afterwards, en route to vacation in the Maritimes, Creelman visited the Eastern Ontario Health Unit (EOHU), centred in Alexandria, before arriving in Ottawa early enough on 18 July to visit with Gertrude Hall of the Victorian Order of Nurses (VON). Established as the first county health unit in late 1934, a five-year pilot project funded by special grants from the Rockefeller Foundation and the province of Ontario, the EOHU had dramatically reduced infant mortality.

The months on the road after leaving TC marked a transition from student life towards a more appropriate demeanour and lifestyle that accompanied admission to leadership and civic responsibility. Increasingly family and professional activities took centre stage. A weary Creelman arrived at Prescott's

PEI home late on the evening of 23 July. Even there, reconnecting with family and relatives went hand-in-hand with work-related visits. Prescott Creelman, who had been the medical superintendent of the PEI Provincial Sanatorium since 1930, escorted his stepsister to clinics and sanatoriums under his administration. But years later her most pleasant memories of the trip were of games of tennis, attending church, swims, and beach bonfires at night. All provided opportunities to become better acquainted with her stepbrother and other members of the Creelman family. For a woman who, despite having a large extended family, had spent her early years as an only child, discovering family roots and ties remained an important legacy of her year-long study leave.

On 2 August, Creelman set out from Charlottetown to begin the arduous seventeen-day drive home, picking up TC classmates Dot Clarke and Dot Wilson en route. With the exception of the torrid heat during the trip through the Badlands, and the occasional difficulty of finding an automobile camping ground, the journey was an enjoyable one, including as it did shopping in Chicago; purchasing Indian souvenirs in Ennis, Montana, the quintessential western town; bathing in the Mammoth Hot Springs in Yellowstone Park,[114] Wyoming; and seeing the Old Faithful geyser in California, before heading North to Vancouver. Undaunted by long days behind the wheel, Creelman seemed to take in stride the uncertainties of bad roads, with little assurance of assistance in case of breakdown, or the terrifying narrow switchbacks through the steep mountain passes – all in era before either more reliable cars or interstate highways civilized transcontinental treks. It was typical of Creelman. Her adventurous, independent spirit and insatiable quest for new experiences ensured that she would remain an ardent traveller throughout her life. Captivated by the lure of travel, she seized every opportunity to live history and to deepen her understanding of world cultures.

The road trip also allowed time for Creelman to make the final transition from the carefree days as a graduate student to her increased responsibilities as a senior nursing administrator. Several years later, recalling her study leave, she confided somewhat guiltily in her diary, "I considered it as my last fling and perhaps from an educational point of view did not gain as much as I should have otherwise."[115] Her self-recrimination was simply too harsh. It would take time and a wider opportunity to apply the new knowledge gained during her study leave before a more balanced assessment would be possible. In many ways, her cross-country odyssey encapsulated her year away from Vancouver. The year 1939 had been a time of great personal and professional growth.

Creelman's desire for a "last fling" speaks to her concern about her new role, one that would test both the nursing knowledge and the leadership skills so recently acquired. Whatever her self-doubts about her abilities to become the director of nursing services before she departed for Columbia University, she could not have predicted how profoundly the outbreak of war would complicate the leadership challenges that awaited her in Vancouver. The outbreak of war on 3 September 1939 set in motion a train of events that altered the course of millions of lives. On the home front, the rising tide of patriotism and racial intolerance created demands on the administration of the nursing services for the Greater Vancouver area that no amount of training could have anticipated. Later, from the ashes of war came renewed hope for peace and security; the call for service overseas to build a better post-war world opened new doors on the professional front for Canadians from every walk of life, including Lyle Creelman.

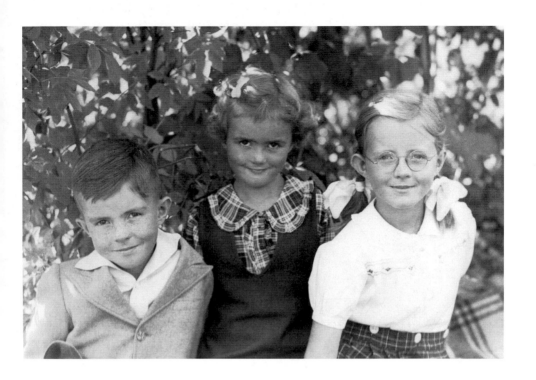

Lyle (right, with glasses) as a schoolgirl, probably shortly after moving to British Columbia

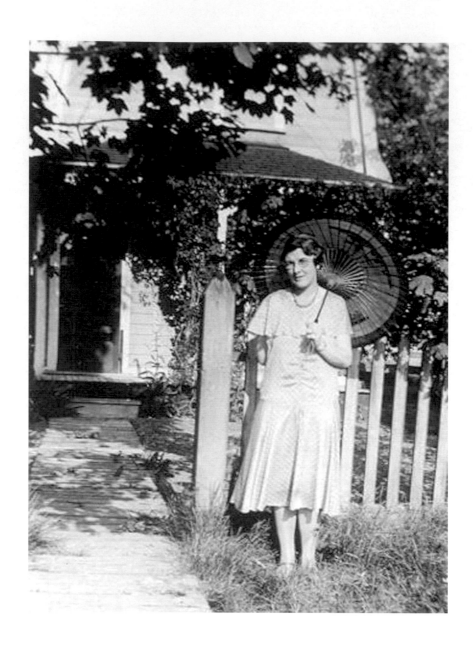

Lyle as a young woman in Steveston, British Columbia

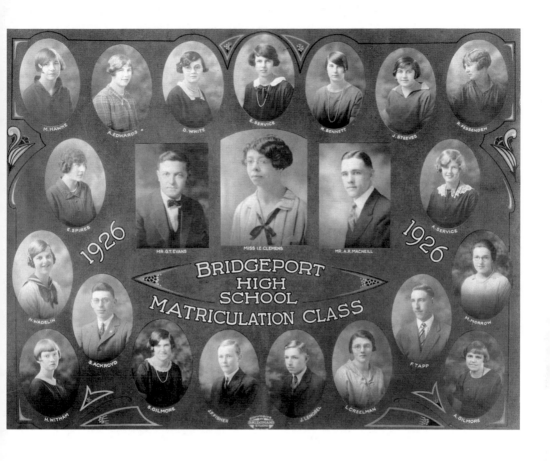

1926 Graduation photo from Bridgeport High School (Lyle bottom right)

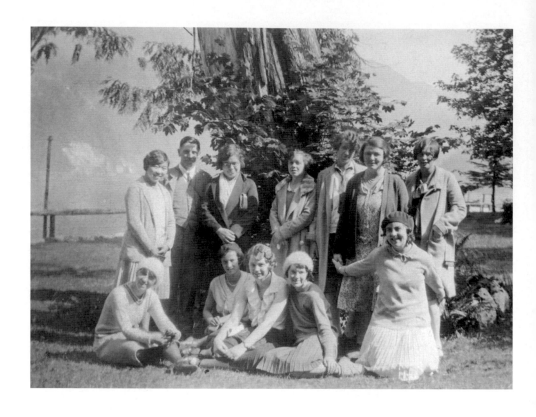

Lyle's first teaching appointment was to the staff of the Lord Byng Public School in Steveston, where she would continue to teach until the summer of 1932 (Lyle third from right).

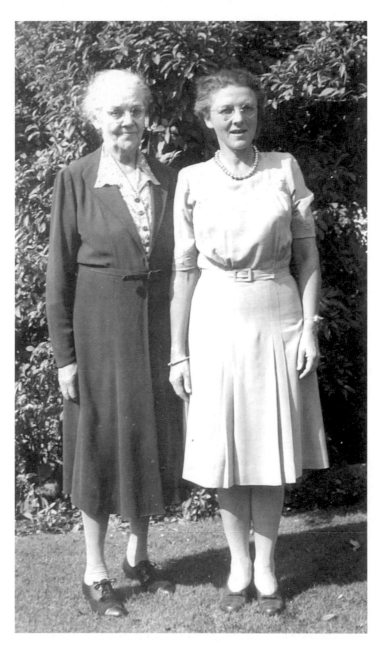

Lyle and her mother Laura

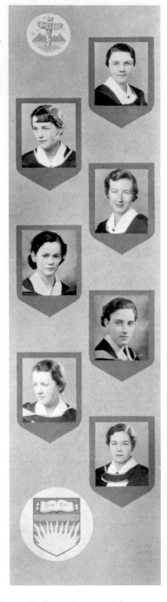

Lyle Creelman

Eleanor Scott Graham
New Westminster
Public Health
Badminton

Lorna Makepeace

Frances V. McQuarrie
Vancouver
Teaching and Supervision
Vice-President, N. U. S.
Alpha Delta Pi

Madeline M. Putman
Creston
Public Health
Alpha Omicron Pi

Ethel Jean Rolston
Vancouver
Teaching and Supervision
President of Nurses' Under-
graduate Society
Alpha Phi

Vivian Williams
New Westminster
Public Health
Badminton Club

The 1936 *Totem*: Lyle (top right), Eleanor Scott Graham, Lorna Makepeace, and Frances McQuarrie would remain lifelong friends and supportive colleagues.

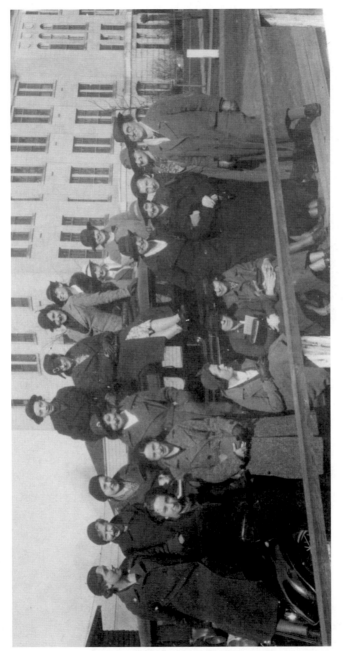

Lyle and her fellow nursing students with Margaret Kerr and her "beloved" car

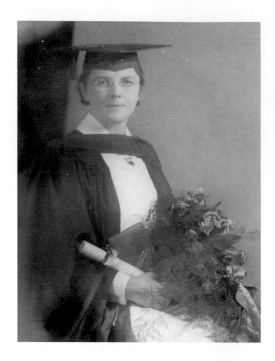

In 1936, Lyle obtained a BASc(N) from the University of British Columbia.

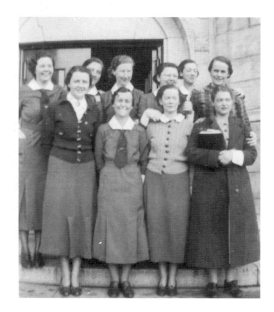

Lyle (third from right, rear) with her fellow public health nursing students, 1936

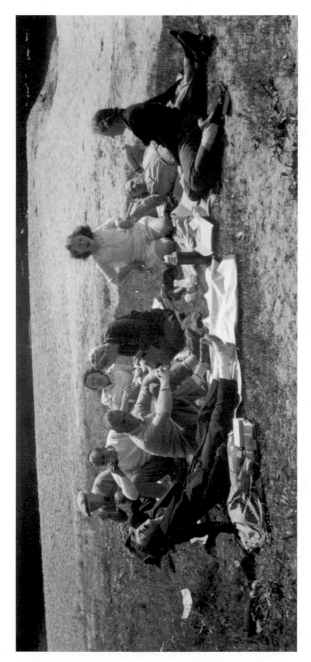

In the spring of 1943, Lyle learned to ride a bike well enough to join the Photographic Society's weekend excursions.

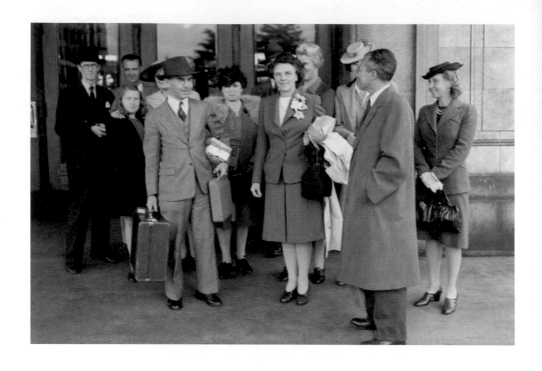

Twenty-eight of Lyle's friends and staff, loaded with parting gifts, bid Lyle an emotional farewell on 25 April 1943 (Dick Pullen carrying Lyle's suitcase).

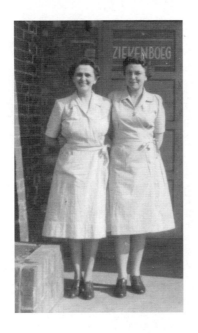

In 1945, awaiting their first UNRRA assignments in London, Stephanie Skeoch (left) and Lyle volunteered to assist with the care of the Dutch children being sent to Coventry, England, where the youngsters were to recover from their years of wartime malnutrition under Nazi occupation.

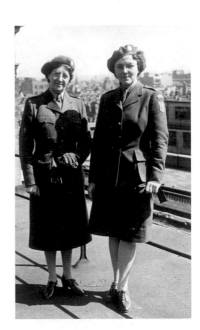

Muriel Doherty (left), matron of the Belsen Hospital and Lyle in London shortly before leaving for Germany in 1945

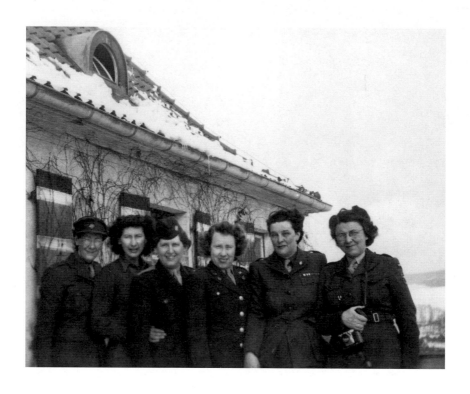

Lyle (right) and her UNNRA nursing field supervisors

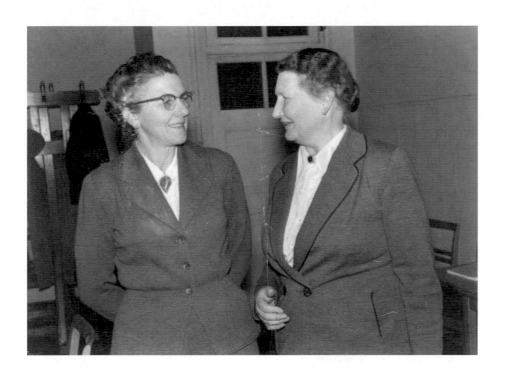

Lyle (left) and Olive Baggallay

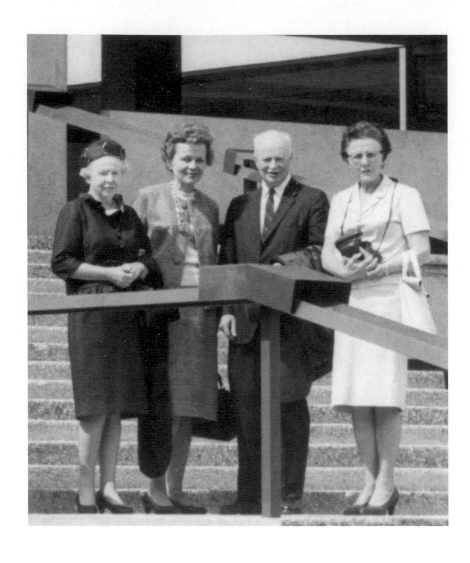

Lyle (right) and Brock Chisholm, first director general of the WHO, in front of WHO's Geneva Headquarters

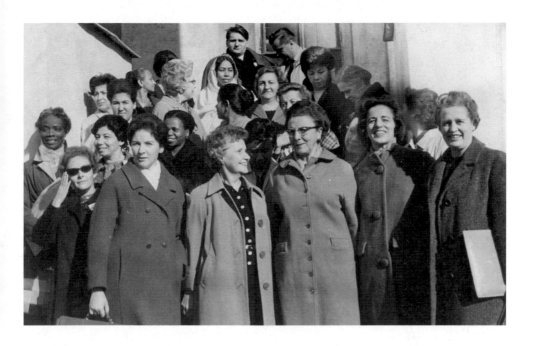

WHO Travelling Seminar, March 1966, USSR, in which Canadian Helen Mussallem (second from right, next to Lyle) acted as the WHO consultant.

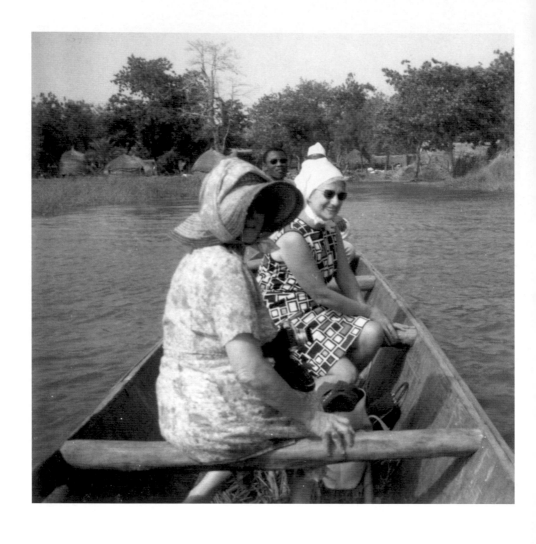

Lyle (with hat, foreground) on duty travel to Africa in the 1960s

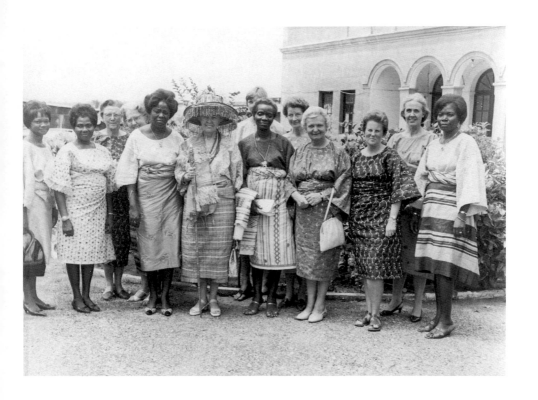

In 1968, Lyle (third from left) returned to the Faculty of Nursing in Ibadan, Nigeria, to attend the inaugural graduation ceremonies. During this visit Virginia Arnold (in hat), who had retired as associate director for medical and natural sciences of the Rockefeller Foundation the previous year, was made an honorary chief.

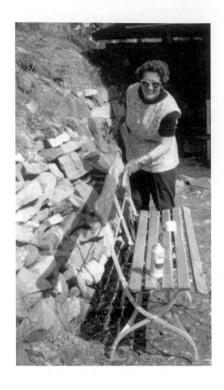

Lyle's Secret Service: Eleanor Kunderman

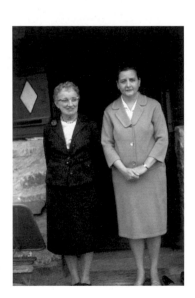

Lyle's Secret Service: SEARO Regional Nursing
Advisors Francis Lilywhite and Dorothy Hall

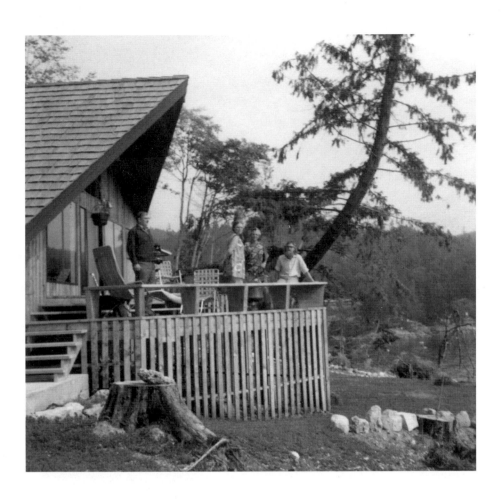

Building Cedar Chalet on Bowen Island, 1971, proved immensely important in easing Lyle's transition from the cosmopolitan life of Geneva to the intimacy of a small island community.

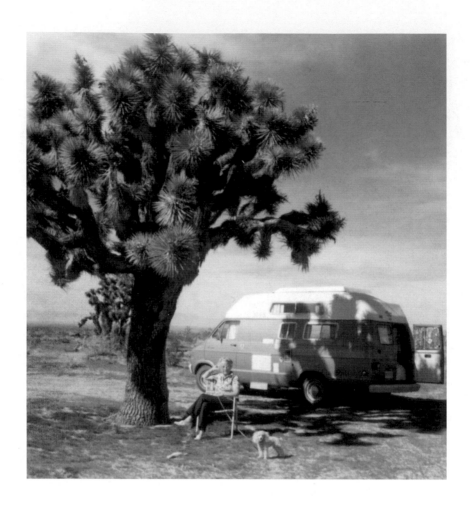

A new travel chapter opened for Lyle in August 1972, when she purchased a mini camper van, the perfect second vehicle for wilderness adventures to the Navajo desert.

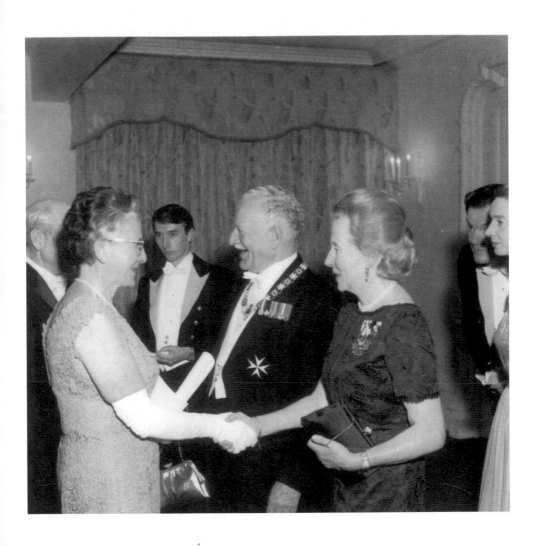

Governor General Daniel Roland Michener presented Lyle with the Canadian Centennial Medal in 1967.

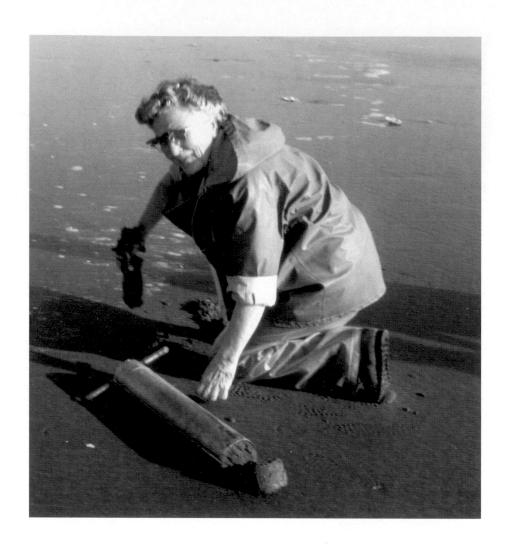

Always an ardent outdoor enthusiast, Lyle enjoyed digging for clams along Bowen Island's shoreline.

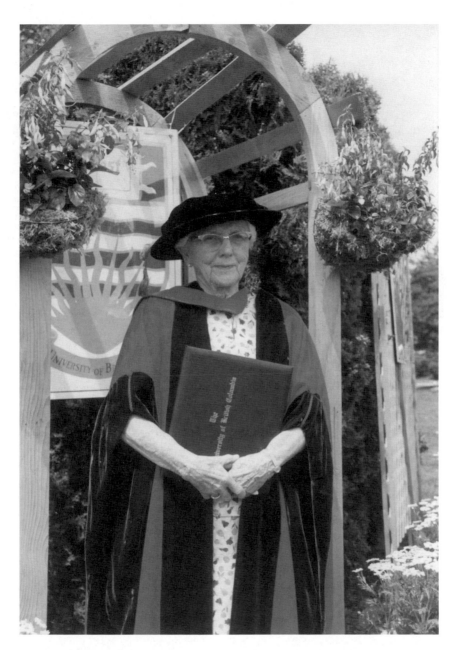

Lyle received an honorary doctorate from the University of British Columbia in 1992.

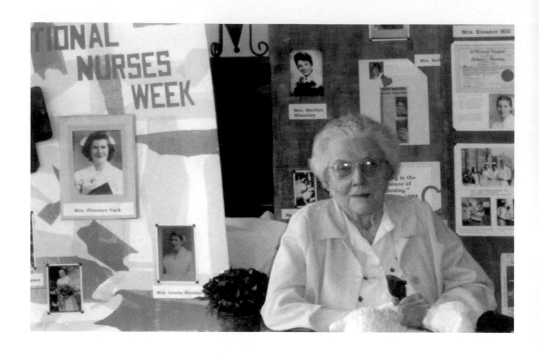

Lyle celebrating Nursing Week in 2002 at Hollyburn House

The Shadow of War, 1939–1944

As the threat of war cast its dark shadow over Canadian society, Lyle Creelman was busy with last-minute preparations before her return to work. Awaking at 6:30 a.m. on 3 September to prepare for her first day at the office, she turned on the radio to hear the news that Germany had invaded Poland. Canada declared war on Germany seven days later. Few Canadians, including Creelman, fully grasped the unimaginable human suffering that would be unleashed or the level of economic and human resources that the Allies would need to mobilize to defeat Hitler. The war shattered millions of lives and reshaped the country's history; by the end of the conflict, 22,000 Japanese Canadians would be interned in British Columbia by the Canadian government. In the case of Creelman herself, as she reflected on international events, she could not have anticipated how the war would complicate her new responsibilities for reforming and expanding Vancouver's public-health nursing services to meet expanded wartime responsibilities as more and more nurses volunteered for military service. Nor could she have foreseen how the war would alter the course of her own life.

Sporting a new hat carefully selected before her first meeting with Dr Murray, Creelman camouflaged her lingering self-doubts beneath a public visage exuding self-confidence. That meeting went a long way to quiet her nervousness. She was both flattered and amused by Murray's noticeable anxiety that Dr Young might be trying to "pull a fast one on him" by enticing Creelman back to the Provincial Nursing Service.[1] She was relieved to learn that Aletha MacLellan, a veteran of the Vancouver public-health system since 1911, would continue as the acting director of public-health nursing until her retirement in September 1941.[2] In the interim, Creelman was the titular head but acted as supervisor of school nursing.

Creelman, like other Canadians, was sheltered from the grim realities of war for many months. Her days were soon filled with routine staff meetings, supervising the physical examination of teachers at the start of Normal School, and organizing home-nursing groups through the VGH that were to begin in mid-October. Despite her own disgust with her performance teaching infant care during the first class,[3] by the end of the course she would be praised for her efforts.[4] Hectic days meant that many evenings would be spent either completing paperwork, preparing speeches, or attending work-related events.

When she graduated, Creelman had joined the VGH and UBC nursing alumni associations. Shortly after her return to Vancouver, she was appointed assistant treasurer at the October monthly meeting of the Science Girls Club (SGC) and treasurer the following January. She became heavily involved in the SGS just as the recent graduates began to challenge its mandate. Attesting to new professional aspirations among recent alumni and wartime patriotism, heated discussions on policies at the SGC meetings[5] continued through the winter until a new constitution was hammered out in March 1940. According to its 1940 constitution, the SGC was intended to furnish "social, cultural, and professional inspiration" for UBC nursing alumni and "to provide a vehicle for philanthropic work within the community."[6]

Recent graduates urged the SGC to "contribute something to nursing, such as a form of a refresher course or course in supervision" modelled on a plan similar to that of the Collegiate Institute of the United States. When Grace Fairley proposed canvassing other university alumnae groups, Creelman was appointed "chief investigator" for the project.[7] By the January meeting, Lyle Creelman's committee had developed and sent out questionnaires to twenty-one university-based nursing-education programs.[8] While the minutes provide no indication that further action was taken, the exercise proved useful for Creelman's work in planning a refresher course at the Metropolitan Health Committee. Similarly, Creelman urged that the group officially write to the Registered Nurses Association of British Columbia "offering their assistance in special duties relating to war."[9] Many nurses, including Creelman, were anxious to make as meaningful a contribution to the war effort on the home front as the military nurses did on the front lines. More immediately, she wanted the club's assistance with the British war orphans and other refugees being relocated to Canada, including British Columbia.[10]

After taking over as the director of public-health nursing in the Metropolitan Health Committee in the fall of 1941, Creelman stepped down from the SGC treasurer position but remained supportive of the club's fundraising efforts on behalf of British civilian nurses and other social activities.[11] As the provincial nursing organizations took the lead in credentialization and labour and political activities, the social function of the alumni associations acquired more prominence. Creelman's own focus increasingly shifted towards provincial and national nursing associations as the most effective vehicles to advance nursing's interests. Yet membership in the Science Girls Club had a lasting impact. Women such as Geraldine Langton, Eleanor Graham, Lorna Makepeace, Frances McQuarrie, and Anne Beech remained steadfast, lifelong friends and valued colleagues. For all of them, the SGC cemented the professional and personal networks formed during their shared experiences in nursing residence and UBC.

Meanwhile, Creelman's diligence had not gone unnoticed by her superiors. Dr Murray was well pleased with her efforts and fully expected that she would "instil a new attitude into the Metropolitan Nursing Services."[12] But that recognition had come at considerable personal cost. Signs of work-related stress punctuated her daily journals. She complained of the "difficulty to sit down and do some constructive thinking" and of the length of time required to recover "some of her old pep" after being off work with a cold.[13] She continued to chide herself for bringing work home at night, but little changed. The occasional bouts of loneliness persisted too. While she valued the fellowship shared at church and the evenings out with nursing friends, her sedate private life seemed incomplete, especially when compared with the previous year. In a diary entry on the first anniversary of her registration for the second term at Teachers College, she wrote: "Such a change from 1 yr ago ... A rather lonesome day."[14] Her innate perfectionism as well as her determination to be fully prepared for her future responsibilities precluded other options for the next year.

Later she summed up her first two years: "I worked very hard and was very tired."[15] By September 1940, she found lecturing and grading student teachers at Normal School increasingly arduous, especially as she spent additional hours after work[16] reviewing the new staff manuals for public-health nurses. She was also busy preparing a summer refresher course to be given in Vancouver and Victoria for both the Metropolitan Health Committee and provincial public-health nursing staff. Her increasing involvement in the provincial and national nursing associations added to this workload but at least offered Creelman a chance for the personal and professional growth that she had missed since her return from Teachers College. These associations provided important forums to network with other nursing leaders facing similar issues across the country. She therefore considered it "quite an honour" to be invited by Margaret Kerr to speak on mental hygiene at the CNA Convention in Calgary in June – especially because a stipend of $850 would be provided to cover her fare.[17] Creelman had worked diligently to prepare a well-crafted speech and was understandably disgruntled to discover that no time had been allowed for discussion afterwards.[18] Nonetheless, her election as secretary-treasurer of the Public Health Section of the CNA reflected her growing national profile.

By 1 September 1941, Creelman, eager to assume the directorship of the Metropolitan Health Committee, was relieved when the formalities surrounding the transition ended. She recorded her anxiety in her diary: "First Supervisors' meeting. Isobel Chodat [Creelman's new assistant] came to tea at Miss MacLellan's after. Stayed for supper. Glad that over but was not so bad."[19] Despite her initial fears "of feeling like a lost sheep,"[20] Creelman believed that serving as the supervisor of school nursing had provided a useful transition period before the assumption of her new post. It was a "good experience and helped to smooth over many ruffled feelings before I took over," she said, referring to the protests from more senior nurses that her appointment had provoked. It also allowed her time to assess the administrative changes that needed to be made. Having found that she was "trespassing when trying to supervise," she soon realized that the supervision of the schools was really the responsibility of the unit supervisor.[21] Within a few months, she had gained the majority of her staff's trust and loyalty and "enjoyed the work more than anything I have ever done."[22] Creelman's assessment of the transition was substantiated by Mary Elizabeth Tennant's confidential report on her visit to Vancouver in February 1942: "Miss C[reelman] has almost more than a full time job since taking over from Miss MacLellan in September but finds the work extremely interesting and enjoys it more than the previous 2 years … It was most fortunate for C[reelman] that Miss MacLellan could carry on for 2 years. It gave C[reelman] an opportunity to study the problems, and most of all to gain the full co-operation of her staff." Despite the increased workload, Creelman "liked it much better than [the] previous job."[23] Quite simply, she preferred to lead change.

According to Tennant's report, Creelman's "greatest problem has been with the TB division." The supervisor (Elliott) acted as a liaison officer with the chest clinic "and this has never been satisfactory." She "has never been able to identify with a generalized program." Although Creelman had attempted "to gain the Supervisor's full support in so far as it is possible," the situation was "coming to a head now and C[reelman] believes that there will be some changes for the better."[24] By April 1942, Elliott had relocated to the Central Office and the tension subsided for a period.[25] Creelman did not confide to Tennant that her extreme anxiety surrounding office politics manifested itself in a dramatic weight loss and the onset of an attack of tachycardia.[26]

From her various evaluations, it is clear that Tennant approved of the changes that Creelman had instituted: "[She] impresses one favourably. She is a thoughtful, intelligent person who has gradually developed her program and one gains the impression that she has done a constructive piece of work."[27] Her praise of Creelman's leadership was echoed by Dr Murray.[28] While Creelman retained overall administrative responsibility, she selected two other nursing supervisors to share the heavy wartime administrative burden. Isabel Chodat, who had just returned from a year at Teachers College as a Rockefeller Foundation fellow,[29] was appointed as the coordinator of nursing services. Her appointment reflected the continued consolidation of specialized nursing services into one generalized nursing service within the Metropolitan Health Committee to provide a comprehensive program of community-health care aimed at preventing disease and promoting health. Under the new system, Chodat was expected to coordinate nursing services with dieticians, social workers, dentists, Children's Aid workers, and physicians. The following year, Trenna Grace Hunter[30] was chosen to take charge of the public-health nursing students' program. Creelman, after encouraging her to complete her university training on the grounds that "there is much more of a future if you have your degree," arranged for her to take a four-month course in supervision and administration at McGill University in preparation for her new duties.[31] She was subsequently promoted to the full-time position of student adviser and soon was described by her superior "as a tower of strength."[32] Chodat and Hunter proved able administrators who helped to carry the increased workload as the war progressed and to improve the nursing unit's working relationship with UBC.

During Creelman's directorship, the Nursing Division's administrative structure melded the progressive RF-inspired models that she had seen in operation in the United States with aspects of the existing administrative set-up. More significantly, Tennant had recommended a similar administrative structure to Dr Murray during her 1939 visit. Tennant told Murray that "practically all of the progressive organizations consider it most important to have well-qualified supervisors who have a fairly good knowledge of public health in general, and perhaps a little more of some one subject." She further explained, "The plan is to eliminate specialized supervisors in so far as is possible, by having two qualified nurses as assistant to the director, one in charge of service and personnel and the other as educational director."[33] Creelman was quite prepared to devolve responsibility to well-qualified staff within clear parameters of reporting authority. While she adopted the RF administrative model of a director and two specialized supervisors, Creelman avoided ruffling her current staff's feathers by leaving intact the existing supervisory structure at the unit level. It is not surprising, then, that Tennant approved the direction that Creelman had taken since assuming the directorship. The changes, which allowed one public-health nurse to cover the work done previously by several specialists, were equally welcomed by provincial officials dealing with limited wartime budgets to meet growing demands for public-health services.[34]

Other administrative difficulties were not as easily addressed. The shortage of nurses, aggravated by high turnover resulting from nurses deciding to marry or to answer the call to military service, remained a fundamental barrier to expanding public-health programs throughout Creelman's tenure.[35] The nursing shortage was particularly acute among the significant Chinese and Japanese communities in Vancouver. In the 1941 *Medical Health Officer's Annual Report*, Creelman noted, "We have been particularly fortunate in having the services of a Chinese nurse and two Japanese TB nurses." Though she acknowledged these nurses' qualifications to participate in the wider work of the unit, "we feel that it is in this branch of the work that the nurse who understands the language and the customs of her people can be the most value."[36] Creelman's attempts to provide better nursing service for the Japanese and Chinese communities were constrained by the prevailing prejudice against Asian Canadians. Even after Japanese students were admitted to UBC and VGH, upon graduation they were directed to care for their own racial community and faced enormous racial prejudice in obtaining employment with equitable pay and fair working conditions. Creelman's statements illustrate the extent to which public-health care continued to be negotiated in the context of cultural assumptions, existing social supports, and barriers, which were just as significant as the medical technologies available.

Fear and resentment of the Japanese, combined with the long-standing discrimination against them that predated the outbreak of war, intensified when, only seven days after the attack on Pearl Harbor, the Japanese forces overran Hong Kong and killed or imprisoned most of the 2,000 Canadian soldiers defending the island. In the aftermath, the federal government passed an Order in Council authorizing the removal of "enemy aliens" within a 100-mile radius of the BC coast. On 4 March 1942, 22,000 Japanese Canadians were given twenty-four hours to pack one suitcase each before being interned in hastily constructed camps.

A temporary facility at Hastings Park Race Track in Vancouver was one of the areas where Japanese families waited, sometimes for months, to be relocated to the internment camps in the interior of British Columbia. Creelman arranged to have Trenna Hunter lent to the British Columbia Security Commission until 1944 to supervise the health care of the Japanese interned in Hastings Park.[37] On being asked by Creelman to undertake this responsibility, Hunter had replied, "If you think I can do it, I'll certainly give it a try."[38] Creelman, if not

Hunter, believed that Hunter possessed the maturity, adaptability, and composure required for this difficult and emotionally charged assignment.

Given responsibility for organizing a 150-bed general hospital and an
80-bed tuberculosis hospital in addition to supervising general public health
and attending to the living conditions of camp life,[39] Hunter later claimed that
this "fascinating" and "unique" experience was one of the most interesting of
her nursing career.[40] "My first glimpse of the Japanese," she wrote, "was looking into the housing building which was an old live stock building which had
just been vacated by the army ... Row upon row of the beds with the little
Japanese families being allotted one or two or three to accommodate the size of
the families. It just seemed to be a sea of people and confusion. However, we got
started with what we had to do to organize services for them."[41] With the help
of the Japanese and discarded hospital equipment, she created a hospital with
mobile walls that could be changed as patient needs shifted; fought to improve
the diet to reflect more traditional Japanese cuisine; and found nurses – even
training one Japanese nursing student so that she could graduate – to provide
comfort for the camp's unfortunate inhabitants. Hunter admitted, "We weren't
aware of many of the troubles that they were experiencing because I suppose
we were all too busy looking after the jobs we had to do."[42] Yet she believed
that "we mustn't have done too bad a job because at the end of the time ... [the
Japanese internees] presented me with a fountain pen and a very nice letter
from the committee for being understanding and helpful to them."[43] No matter
how hard Hunter and others tried to ameliorate the dreadful living conditions,
nothing they could do would compensate for the traumatic effect Hasting Parks
had on the Japanese.

Others agreed that Creelman had made the right choice in selecting Hunter.
During Tennant's visit to Vancouver in June 1942, she accompanied Creelman
to see the Hastings Park camp where 2,000 Japanese were still interned. Hunter
impressed Tennant as an "able efficient administrator" who had demonstrated
considerable initiative in setting up programs to train nurse's aides and provide first-aid courses to the Japanese women.[44] The surviving documents do not
provide any indication of Creelman's involvement with Hastings Park beyond
Hunter's appointment or this visit. More significantly, despite her own involvement with the Japanese fishing communities, both growing up in Steveston
and subsequently as a teacher, Creelman's diary remains strangely silent on
the plight of the Hastings Park residents. It was her former colleague in the
Richmond Unit, Eileen Williams, who would be the conscience of Canadian
nursing on this issue; she set out her views in a compassionate article written for the *Canadian Nurse* in 1941 describing her experiences at Lord Byng

Public School where 400 of the 500 students were Japanese.[45] It remains unclear whether Hunter and Creelman simply did not question the Mackenzie King government's decision at the time, or whether they realized that, whatever their personal feelings, their only option was to provide the best possible care for the Japanese internees under the circumstances.

Throughout her tenure Creelman continued to apply modern management techniques to improve supervisory and administrative operations and thereby expand the scope of public-health nursing services provided. Early on, she took steps to strengthen and to clarify the supervisory functions within her division.[46] While she believed that the supervisory staff had done an excellent job under increasingly difficult conditions, she was fully aware that, as long as four of her six unit supervisors had to carry heavy caseloads, proper attention could not be given to the administration and teaching, which she believed to be their primary and vital functions. She also struck a policy committee known as the Unit Representatives to provide staff nurses with greater input into the development of nursing policies while allowing her to gain their support in advance of implementing any new policies. The committee initially focused on staff training, choosing as its first topic the growth and development of the child from one to six years of age.[47] Ongoing staff education, a key construct of Creelman's progressive administrative approach, evolved by 1943 to include four meetings for all staff in addition to bimonthly meetings at the unit level. These initiatives resulted in the development of staff manuals dealing with child welfare, general policies, school nursing, and tuberculosis.[48] She regularly invited speakers from other health agencies and arranged annual refresher courses for her unit supervisors and those from the Provincial Nursing Service at the University of British Columbia. In addition, she introduced a separate orientation program for new staff members. Her actions reflected her strong belief that the public-health nurse's primary function – prevention of disease – could be strengthened only by clearly distinguishing nursing responsibilities from clerical functions and by providing ongoing professional development to keep the nurse up-to-date with the changing times.

As Creelman reminded the medical community in the 1942 *Medical Health Officer's Annual Report*, "education is still our chief weapon against Tuberculosis. Science has not found a drug for cure or immunization. It is the nurse who is the vital force in wielding this weapon."[49] Creelman had a clear reform agenda designed to reorient the public-health nurses' work away from traditional school services in favour of a heavier emphasis on health-education programs, especially for preschool children. She recommended that many routine activities currently being performed by the school nurse could be eliminated or reassigned to the classroom teacher.[50] Over the next two years,

Creelman expanded community-based public-health programs targeted to children, especially within Vancouver's high-risk populations. Her 1943 annual report championed the incorporation of nursery schools as part of the school system: "The health programme for this pre-school group will then be a more effective and co-ordinated effort towards the building of healthy citizens."[51] But, despite these efforts, the demand for children's services continued to outstrip the Nursing Division's ability to open enough new centres or to provide an adequate level of follow-up home visits within existing centres. Education and the family continued to be viewed as the main avenues for social progress.

Creelman repeated her plea for more staff, arguing that "the rapidly increasing school population, coupled with the poor living conditions in many quarters of the city, has put an additional burden on the nursing staff."[52] Once again she pointed to the causal effects of poverty and social dislocation on the incidence of disease that the public-health nurses witnessed on their daily visits and the need for more social-welfare services: "The number of cases for which each nurse is responsible is much too great ... The need for regulations, increased facilities for hospital, boarding and nursing home care, adequate social assistance for both the patient and his family – all these are felt more keenly by the nurse who is daily meeting the situations which point to them. In the face of the apparent unconcern of the authorities, the nurses are rapidly becoming discouraged." That was strong language for a senior public-health official – especially a nurse.

Equally, it was reflective of new societal values. In the wake of Depression conditions, the winds of political change were blowing through the provinces. In British Columbia, Premier Duff Pattullo had instituted a series of public works and social services, which eventually became known as the Little New Deal. Across Canada, new views of the welfare state appeared in the publications of the League for Social Reconstruction (1935) and in the reports of social reformers, such as Leonard Marsh's classic, *Report on Social Security for Canada* (1943). At the federal level, the King government increased the amount of federal relief assistance to the provinces, which had the constitutional authority to deal with the prevailing social problems, and deliberately incorporated deficit financing into its recovery strategy. In so doing, the federal government was following the theories of British economist John Maynard Keynes, who argued that, when faced with the failure of private enterprise to provide full employment, the state had to take the initiative to create jobs, even if it meant incurring substantial budgetary deficits.

For Creelman, funding and staff retention remained constant concerns. While many progressive reformers of the time urged a move away from volunteerism, she instead cultivated long-established community-based volunteer groups in order to gain their assistance in expanding the Metropolitan Health Committee's child health programs. She was careful to acknowledge the assistance of the IODE in providing an occupational therapist for the outpatient clinic. The TB Division, especially its social workers, also received high praise: "The regular conferences which have been held in the Units with the Social Workers have greatly aided in solving the many problems which nurses bring to those conferences."[53] Creelman strove to define nursing services in a manner that maximized the efficient use of nurses' specialized skills at current staff levels. She advocated a team approach that envisioned the public-health nurse as the focal point, coordinating patient health care with other health-care workers such as physiotherapists, social workers, and nutritionists. An innovative retention strategy, it was designed to reduce her staff's heavy workload while staking out nursing's professional enclave within the public-health community. Just as important, Creelman was beginning to glimpse and articulate the idea of family-centred health care.

Accordingly, Creelman actively supported overhauling the public-health students' field placements to align them more closely with her vision of family-centred care.[54] After the university increased the number of nursing students by 50 per cent during the 1942–3 academic year, the problem of finding suitable field placements for students became acute.[55] Creelman and Isabel Chodat met with Geraldine Langton and Mabel Gray at UBC to resolve the issue. (Creelman had close personal and professional ties with Langton.[56]) Given the close personal connections of key nursing personnel and the ongoing financial support of the Rockefeller Foundation for UBC's nursing program, the new direction taken is not surprising. It clearly bore the imprint of Creelman's and Chodat's experience as RF fellows. The new program incorporated the cardinal Rockefeller tenet that the public-health nurse should be introduced to the principles of public health within a generalized nursing service rather than through the work of any one agency and that her field placements should be connected to a university public-health-based program. Indeed, the idea of using a "special teaching district" had already been suggested during Mary Elizabeth Tennant's visit in 1939 while Lyle Creelman was still at TC. Tennant argued that "when students are sent to different centres and when supervised field practice is not carefully worked out so that there is a correlation of theory and practice they are often left with a confused idea of their work."[57] A new course, called Introduction to Family Services, was designed to allow the public-health nursing students a longer period of independent field experience under the supervision of the Metropolitan Health Committee and the Victorian Order of Nurses. Each student was expected to assess the "medical, behavioural, social and economic aspects" of the four families for which they were responsible over a nine-week period, in which the first half of each week was spent attending lectures and the second half working under supervision in the field.[58] Given the acute shortage of public-health nurses, Creelman clearly understood the importance of cultivating nursing students' long-term interest in public-health work. The innovative changes to field placements for UBC students closely reflected her own preference for providing a generalized field experience designed to integrate classroom teaching with hands-on experience, as well as the importance she attributed to the public-health nurse's role as a teacher.[59]

Instilling new attitudes within the Metropolitan Health Committee both provoked and reflected existing antagonisms within the wider British Columbia public-health community as different groups complained about the performance of the others. The immediate impetus to reform the fieldwork came from criticism voiced by Heather Kilpatrick, the first director of nursing for the provincial Department of Health (1940–4), and Dr Amyot. Dissatisfaction with the UBC nursing program, particularly its preparation of public-health nurses, had been brewing for some years in several camps. The need to address the shortage of field placements opened the door to overhauling the whole program. Glennis Zilm and Ethel Warbinek contend that the program under Mabel Gray had not responded to the younger faculty's demand that the public-health nursing curriculum "needed to be carried a big step. There were specialists coming in … many more clinics available that you could talk about."[60] Zilm and Warbinek correctly surmise that the growing dissatisfaction with Gray's lack of academic qualifications was a contributing factor to her precipitous departure in the summer of 1941. According to Tennant, Dr C.E. Dolman, who had been both the acting head of the Nursing and Health Department since 1936 as well as acting head of Bacteriology and Preventative Medicine, had wanted for some time to find "a well-qualified nurse" to replace Mabel Gray so that he could step down as head of the Department of Nursing.[61] Neither Tennant nor Dolman was prepared to support Margaret Kerr as Gray's replacement. Both agreed that "Miss Margaret Kerr is not satisfactory and that she should not have been kept on the staff all these years." Unfortunately, she never elaborated on why Kerr's performance proved disappointing. Again according to Tennant, Dolman had a similarly negative view of both Amyot's teaching of the public-health administration course and the leadership capabilities of Heather Kilpatrick as the provincial director of nursing. Amyot's portrait of Kilpatrick as being "negative" in her reaction to all new proposals[62] does not reconcile with others' views of her leadership capabilities. At a minimum, it does, however, expose the tensions surrounding the education of public-health nurses.

Differences among the senior public-health nurses quickly surfaced in June 1942 during a luncheon attended by Creelman, Chodat, Langton, and Mary

Henderson, who had replaced Effie Young as the instructor in public health on the UBC nursing faculty.[63] When the group complained about their difficulties with Amyot and Kilpatrick, "whom they feel have not been fair with their criticism" of the UBC program, Tennant adroitly sidestepped being drawn into the political fray. Instead, she told "them to get together and talk out their differences because it appears that they are all practically saying the same things and what is needed at the present time on the part of each one concerned is statesmanship." She reminded them, "[Your] problems are not great in comparison with the serious problems in the world today."[64] In the end, further initiatives to restructure UBC's nursing program would have to wait until someone could be found to replace Mabel Gray after her retirement.

Tennant's consultative approach to assisting nurses in other countries left an enduring imprint on Creelman. There is no doubt that Tennant's position within the Rockefeller Foundation and close personal contacts with many of British Columbia's senior public-health nurses gave her considerable influence over the development of public-health nursing services in line with the Rockefeller philosophy. At times, Tennant chose not to intervene but rather to mentor the elite group of RF nurses being groomed for leadership around the world.[65] During the interwar years, the RF's International Health Division played a decisive role on several levels in the lively traffic of ideas, people, and resources across borders in support of its worldwide initiatives to develop modern public-health departments and medical-education programs in Canada, Europe, Latin America, and Asia. RF nursing officers such as Tennant sought to provide opportunities for nurses to travel and exchange views about nursing. They may not, however, have been as fervent about spreading the RF/American version as the true gospel as their medical counterparts.[66] The belief that nurses benefited from cross-cultural exchanges of ideas but in the end had to find their own solutions appropriate to their situation – which Mary Elizabeth Tennant, among others, embodied – became a main principle of Creelman's leadership style.

Amidst this political turmoil, Creelman honed her administrative skills to navigate the local politics encasing wartime health care in British Columbia. Her annual reports always acknowledged the contribution of other voluntary community-service agencies and the support from the medical community – especially her superior, Dr Murray. She couched her plea for more staff in terms that would be attractive to the community's political leaders in wartime: "The service, which the public health nurse can give in this community, is of vital importance in maintaining the health of the civilian worker. The call to the armed service is very great but we now realize that there is very important service to be given on the home front."[67] At a time when the suffering of soldiers and civilians figured increasingly in her daily diary entries, that argument also offered private reassurance that her work on the home front contributed to winning the war. In summary, the vested interests of public and community stakeholders coalesced, allowing Creelman to align the delivery of nursing services within the Greater Vancouver area more closely with her understanding of progressive, generalized, community-based health services.

Since first inviting Creelman to speak at the CNA convention in 1940, Margaret Kerr had continued encouraging her to write articles for the *Canadian Nurse*. Creelman was happy to comply, and the articles she prepared for it probed the professional implications of current policies for public-health nursing. "Mental Hygiene in the Public Health Program,"[68] her first article, published in 1940, provides an important window on nursing's attitude towards the eugenics movement that was then shaping public views of – and policies in – public health throughout Canada and especially in British Columbia. The *Canadian Nurse* had run a series of articles exploring the main concerns expressed by the eugenics movement and championing nursing's expanded role in public hygiene dating back to the early 1920s.[69]

Tapping into popular anxieties, the eugenics movement spread like a prairie wildfire across Canada: "The average English Canadian was schooled to be as accepting of the notion of 'race improvement' as the idea that Canada was a Christian nation." The belief in "the primacy of heredity" and in the principle that "like begets like," together with underlying concerns about the "feeble-minded," the "morally depraved," the insane, the physically handicapped, and criminals, gave rise to fears of racial suicide that permeated the fabric of Canadian society during the interwar period. The main support for eugenics came from people within the respected ranks of the medical community who believed that "an understanding of heredity could improve *public* health."[70] And the views of the medical community carried weight. Advances in medical knowledge after the discovery and popularization of the "germ theory" had augmented the medical profession's authority at a time when state authorities had begun seeking its assistance to address the social problems brought on by urbanization, industrialism, mass immigration, and the perceived decline in Anglo-Saxon birth rates. They looked to the medical sciences "to provide more efficient methods of social control."[71] The medical community, for its part, was happy to oblige. Promoting the idea that the inequalities plaguing Canadian society had hereditary and individual, not social, causes, it lobbied the state to legislate a series of eugenic controls, such as immigration and marriage restrictions and the segregation, institutionalization, and sterilization of those with physical or mental disabilities or illness.

As for Creelman herself, she would have been familiar with the eugenic arguments for social reform. Her background as an educator and public-health nurse provided her with a dual focus while observing the "medicalization" of

British Columbia as it was manifested within the Vancouver school system. The segregation of mentally deficient children within the school system dating back to 1910 and the passage of British Columbia's Sexual Sterilizations Act in 1933[72] indicated the influence of eugenics ideology on British Columbia's public-health officials and educational authorities. As the provincial medical officer of health, Dr Young served on the British Columbia branch of the Canadian National Committee on Mental Hygiene (CNCMH). "The vast majority of delinquents and prostitutes," according to the CNCMH, "were driven to their evil deeds by their mental illnesses rather than due to social inequality, adverse environment, or other manifestations of what may be comprehensively termed the 'forces of circumstances.'"[73] By the time Creelman had entered the UBC nursing program, British Columbia had become the second province – Alberta was the first – to enact legislation permitting the sterilization of the mentally ill and retarded.

By 1940, the new generation of environmentalists had abandoned the crude eugenic theories of the 1920s – concerned with the incarceration and steriliza-tion of the defective – and instead were preoccupied with devising programs that would pre-empt the very emergence of "abnormality." Already exposed to "anticipatory guidance" approach at TC, Creelman worked with the psychiatrist appointed to Metropolitan Health Committee, Charles Hegler Gundry, who had completed his postgraduate studies at the Cleveland child-guidance clinic, renowned for "its use of schools and social agencies in trying to avert chronic delinquency."[74] Gundry's appointment marked a move away from the previous approach to mentally deficient children, centred on segregation, towards the concept of psychiatric intervention to prevent the onset of a child's delinquent behaviour.

Adherents of this approach, including Creelman, believed that children were not born bad but developed delinquent behaviour as a result of "emotional stress" triggered by "insecurity" and that, if left untreated, bad children became the mentally ill of the future.

Accordingly, Creelman's "Mental Hygiene in the Public Health Program" noted that there were two types of mental disease – "the organic and the functional" – and that the latter applied to two-thirds of the mental patients institutionalized. She then warned that, if minor problems were not identified and corrected before they gave rise to more serious ones, there would con-tinue to be "as many children in the average class in school who would later enter a mental hospital as there are children who would later enter university."[75] Advocating that greater emphasis be placed on education than on regulations, she aimed "to build up a program that will enable us to teach the principles of mental hygiene to a fairly large number of individuals in key positions."[76]

She argued that this would allow for earlier detection and treatment and, more important, increased opportunities for anticipatory guidance – that is, "applying prevention rather than early detection or treatment."[77]

Her portrait of the origins of mental illness, however, was not entirely disinterested from a professional vantage point. Like their medical counterparts, nurses were eager to exploit the opportunities presented by the mental-hygiene movement to enhance their professional status, and indeed in this effort they had the support of some members of the medical community.[78] The new behaviourist theories that correlated a child's early developmental environment with future mental health and economic productivity opened a wider professional role beyond testing and measuring.[79] Publicly, Creelman argued that the public-health nurse's special training and position on the front lines in the community made her the ideal worker to carry on this education campaign. Privately, Creelman, chaffing at nursing's failure to exert its jurisdiction, remained adamant that "social workers are not taking over the p.h.n'g. [public-health nursing] field in BC."![80] She pointed out that the Metropolitan Health Committee had a mental hygienist but no social workers for investigation or follow-up because "we want the nurses to do this work themselves."[81]

Creelman's article expressed progressive views on several issues, from venereal disease to childrearing. Creelman advocated viewing venereal disease as a health issue instead of a moral question. She also told her readers, "For so long we have been dogmatic with parents about habits of sleeping, resting, and bathing, [with the result] that we are finding it difficult to educate parents to the fact that general rules are general and do not necessarily apply to their child." Her progressive views, however, were not without limitations. Creelman never questioned that the public-health nurse's superior education and training made her well positioned to guide both parents' and teachers' handling of the child's "bad behaviour." While Creelman's call for mental hygiene to become "an integral part of the nursing service not a foreign body"[82] was laudably progressive for the era, it was naive for her to assume that a "few discreet suggestions" from an empathetic public-health nurse could help the mother of an unwanted or unplanned child "adopt a new attitude toward the baby and help her give it the love which is so necessary for the normal development of a child."[83] As McLaren argues, "One should not exaggerate the differences between the eugenicists and environmentalists; their tactics differed but their goals of 'efficient social management' "[84] were the same.

Just as interestingly, Creelman's article advocated a holistic definition of health "as something more than physical fitness or the mere absence of disease." Rather, personal health should be thought of as total health: it meant "a state of mental, physical and spiritual fitness and a harmonious adjustment of the individual to the social environment."[85] Less than a decade later, a similar definition would be embodied in the founding documents of the new World Health Organization. In Creelman's case, she expanded Western medicine's view of the body, which traditionally had been seen as merely a machine subject to measurements of normality and appropriate medical interventions to preserve or restore.

Creelman's views on leadership were a complex blend: traditional yet modern. She was a woman of her day; her notion of leadership stemmed from a profound sense of duty to serve. Her progressive professional views coexisted with the era's conservative societal expectations that the public-health nurse be "a fine mature person, capable of handling her own life."[86] Social respectability, in her view, was a prerequisite for acceptance within a medical community that continued to view nursing as an extension of woman's maternal and domestic sphere. Yet, in her next article, Creelman, emulating her medical counterparts, relied upon the public-health nurses' scientific expertise to establish their professional authority within a gendered medical hierarchy. That trend over the next decades, as we shall see, transformed how nurses' envisaged their leadership roles in civil societies.

In "What Is Public Health Nursing?" – published in 1941 – Creelman identified the distinctive role of the public-health nurse as a communication conduit between the medical community, the school, and the family: "She is the person who translates the language of the scientific workers into the language of the ordinary citizen; she carries this knowledge into their homes and assists them in applying it to their every day situation."[87] Again, Creelman's idyllic vision of the public-health nurse as an agent of social change was tempered by a degree of class prejudice. She warned that the public-health nurse, when faced with the "resistance of ignorance due to a low degree of intellectual equipment," or "resistance based upon tradition and custom" or "resistance based on the lack of a desire to know and believe," must conclude that "she is dealing with uneducatable material." Creelman contended that this was not an indication "of the lack of ability on the part of the nurse"; rather, the nurse was to be "commended" for "using her time and efforts for those who have a will to learn."[88] Like other public-health nurses of the era, Creelman could be condescending towards those who failed to take an opportunity for self-improvement.

Creelman staked out public-health nursing's unique professional requirements in a third article, this one co-authored with Margaret Kerr in January 1942, which summarized the results of the CNA Public Health Section's survey of the qualifications and preparation of public-health nurses. The ability "to teach by demonstration" instead of by more didactic methods, she argued, demanded "qualities that are called for by no other group in the nursing field" and therefore required specialized training and ongoing professional development to keep current with new medical fields, such as geriatrics.[89] The nationwide survey found that Canada compared favourably with other countries, but "it is still far from our goal of the desirable minimum qualification of a public health certificate for all nurses engaged in public health work."[90] Creelman's call for an elite cadre of well-qualified public-health nurses spoke to the contemporary concern that funding for or enrolment in nursing programs might decline as the wartime demands taxed the country's financial and human resources. Neither fear proved well founded. Enrolment numbers grew during the war and the federal government provided bursaries to prepare nurses for advanced positions in 1943.[91] Yet, despite these efforts, according to statistics reported in January 1942 in the *Canadian Nurse*, "40 per cent of the new appointments went to unqualified public health nurses."[92]

Defining occupational space remained a crucial part of professional image making. Creelman's three wartime articles in the *Canadian Nurse* strove to legitimize the expanded scope of public-health nursing. All were early expressions of her lifelong concern that public-health nurses' jurisdiction would continue to be invaded by social workers and psychiatric workers unless a specialized body of knowledge and a distinctive scope of practice were established. Although her strategies would change as her career progressed, she would remain a staunch defender of public-health nursing's jurisdiction against any interlopers. Once again, there was an inherent tension in nursing leaders' support for social welfare and mental health services and their fierce support for strict professional barriers. As important, these early articles, in their emphasis on nursing's contributions to a more cost-efficient delivery of public-health services in a socially acceptable manner, testified to her growing political acumen. Her perception of the unique caring role of the public-health nurse built upon and was in part the logical extension of her own previous teaching experience, premised upon the nurturing tutor–pupil relationship geared to developing the healthy, socially responsible, and productive citizen of tomorrow. The public-health nurses' entry into private homes for follow-up school visits, or new baby clinics and preschool visits, allowed state surveillance of the inner working of family life without the appearance of too much coercion – an important factor for a liberal-democratic state.[93] In all of these early articles, the individual or the individual family unit remained the focal construct of society, which may have weakened Creelman's ability to comprehend fully the underlying structural problems that constrained access to medical care.[94] Already a nursing role predicated upon the notion of interpreter and advocate was creeping in to replace an earlier agency role that was state-directed and aimed at social control. In the not too distant future, Creelman would challenge the notion that public-health nurses should serve as the state's social police.

Creelman served as secretary-treasurer of the CNA in 1940–2 and then stepped up to the Executive Committee when she became chair of the Public Health Section, replacing Margaret Kerr, in May 1942. Attending CNA meetings allowed Creelman to compare public health work in other cities and to obtain an insider's view on nursing's post-war direction. For the moment she remained "very satisfied with our own organization [in Vancouver]. It has grand possibilities."[95] Prospects at the national level seemed promising as well. After attending the CNA's executive meeting in Montreal during October 1942, Creelman recorded that it had been "most interesting and history-making for Canadian nurses." She remained unsure "of what form our directive control [on a national level] will take but something is coming."[96] She would bide her time before making any career decisions.

At the time of Creelman's appointment to the CNA's Executive Committee, nursing leaders were grappling with the need to play a constructive role in the total war effort while "guard[ing] the professional advance already made."[97] Specifically, nursing leaders grew increasingly worried that the wartime shortage of nurses would result in a lowering of professional standards. Increasingly, Voluntary Aid Detachment nurses (VAD) had filled out the nursing ranks within military hospitals; soon nurses' aides were being hired across Canada to staff the growing number of hospitals. While the CNA had acceded to Ottawa's demands for accelerated nursing courses, the Executive Committee minutes urging that "educational standards must be kept in mind if this plan is put into effect" indicated that its support remained guarded.[98]

Despite Creelman's reservations about following Kerr as chair – "I doubt if I can carry on as successfully as Margaret"[99] – the position better suited her temperament. Here, as elsewhere, she preferred to address the major issues facing nursing than observe from the sidelines. In predictable fashion, Creelman offered pragmatic advice to the CNA Executive, suggesting, for example, how to increase the supply of nurses by making it more financially affordable for married or inactive nurses to receive temporary nursing permits. She also supported liberalizing the registration process within each of the provinces for military service, though she favoured restricting the process to applicants from the United States or from countries within the British Empire "whose schools of nursing have essentially the same requirements."[100] When the British Columbia Public Health Section brought forward a recommendation to introduce correspondence courses in public health, the issue was sidetracked. With "lack of time for discussion," it was referred to the Provisional Council of University Representatives, a precursor to the Canadian Association of University Nursing Schools, without recommendation. The choice was not accidental. UBC had been a founding member of the council in 1942, and UBC faculty, including Evelyn Mallory and Ruth Morrison, were among its early members. The referral enhanced the reputation of the fledgling body and reaffirmed nursing's right to establish its own educational standards. Creelman left the 1942 Montreal convention convinced that it had been a "worthwhile" experience and that the work of the Public Health Section had been "good."[101]

As chair of the Public Health Section, Creelman explored the future requirements of public-health nursing in a series of articles written for the *Canadian Nurse* in 1943.[102] In "What of the Future?" she emphasized public-health nurses' contribution to the wartime economy by reducing the loss of working hours due to preventable illness and, to buttress her case, noted their future role under a national scheme of health insurance: "Never has it been more essential," she wrote, "that we establish minimum requirements for employment in the field of public health nursing" – a certificate or degree in public-health nursing.[103] Educational issues preoccupied the older generation of the leadership, but the rank-and-file, who had endured the tough economic times of the "Dirty Thirties," focused on workplace issues rather than political matters.[104] As wartime work expanded employment opportunities, Creelman believed it imperative that public-health nursing be as attractive as other professions then opening up to women. Accordingly, the Public Health Section under Creelman's direction initiated a study of salaries paid to public-health nurses throughout Canada. She had no doubt that the study would find that "where the salaries are low there is a proportionately low percentage of qualified personal employed."[105] Creelman warned that employers would have to be convinced that the additional costs of higher salaries of well-trained public-health nurses would be "more than repaid by improved quality of services offered the community."[106] Creelman understood the necessity of dealing with issues important to the rank-and-file; she would fight that battle on the provincial level as well.

According to her diary, Lyle Creelman's first meeting with the Registered Nurses Association of British Columbia (RNABC) on 15 May 1941 proved "a rather stormy introductory" to the "wrangling" that could sidetrack productive discussion at nursing meetings.[107] Elected vice-president of the RNABC in 1942, Creelman moved automatically to the presidency when Margaret Kerr resigned to assume the editorship of the *Canadian Nurse* in May 1944. She approached her work in the provincial association, as in other areas of her professional life, in a business-like fashion. Contemplating her appointment as president of the

Vancouver chapter and first vice-president of the provincial association, she confessed that, despite the infighting and increased work involved, she "much preferred to be active in the organization than just an ordinary member."[108]

Creelman joined the Executive Council of the RNABC at a time when the CNA was passing down many pressing matters to the provincial associations. While some of these issues stemmed from wartime conditions, others portended more fundamental challenges for post-war nursing and the delivery of health care in Canada. Reviewing nurses' requests for reinstatement on the basis of temporary war-emergency permits and dealing with collective bargaining and superannuation demanded the RNABC's attention. All added to Creelman's already heavy workload. Particularly troublesome, and delicate, was the issue of unions. The desire to have nursing regarded as a profession translated nationwide into nursing leaders' concern to avoid association with working-class unions. The nursing leadership feared that unionization would fracture its membership.[109] This distrust of unions is clearly evidenced in the minutes of the RNABC, which had formed a committee to investigate socio-economic matters in 1943. As early as 1942, some nurses at VGH had begun to explore the possibility of unionizing. But, as late as the spring of 1944, the RNABC was urging its members to delay further action on an individual basis;[110] instead, following the lead of the CNA, it approved collective bargaining but argued that the national and provincial associations should be the bargaining agents for nurses.

The wartime shortage of nurses improved the RNABC's bargaining position. The hospital's previous practice – of relying on private-duty nurses hired on contract to provide private patient care, thus avoiding the costs of permanent staff – became a liability and nurses demanded better working conditions. Lyle Creelman played an active role in securing a more favourable agreement on salary schedules with the British Columbia Hospital Association.[111] This laid the groundwork for an aggressive post-war labour-relations program beginning in 1946 that saw significant gains, including increases in salaries and vacation time, the forty-hour week, yearly pay increases, and provisions for a greater voice in policy.[112]

Provincial health-insurance programs had been debated for some time and, despite opposition from the medical community, in British Columbia the concept won considerable support in a 1937 public referendum. In 1940 the province's coalition government laid the legislative foundation for the introduction of the 1949 BC Hospital Service program based upon individual contributions.[113] Lyle Creelman was appointed to a joint committee to consider any nursing questions arising from the program. Private-duty nursing had been in transition during the 1930s as more complex medical treatments called for hospitalization and more specialized nursing care; the conversion of nurses from independent contractors to employees was not smooth. Nurses resisted the move into hospital positions, and hospitals long accustomed to receiving low-cost nursing service via students had difficulty accepting graduate nurses as full-fledged employees. Unwilling to address nurses' concerns for poor working conditions and demands for higher salaries, hospitals looked to nurses' aides to solve their staffing issues. Noteworthy as well during this time were the RNABC's efforts to improve communications with industrial nurses by organizing a subcommittee of the public-health committee. As Creelman explained in the *Canadian Nurse*, bringing these more specialized nurses, "who might have otherwise feel isolated, into contact with other activities of generalized public health nursing" was "an excellent move."[114] Defining and defending professional space, while avoiding schisms between nursing groups, remained a lifelong concern for Creelman.

Creelman was also called upon to convene the provincial committee charged with recommending nurses for work overseas with United Nations Relief and Rehabilitation Administration (UNRRA), the temporary international agency that included among its many responsibilities the care of the millions of displaced persons awaiting repatriation or resettlement and the initial civilian relief of the war-torn liberated countries. Canadian nurses were recruited primarily from two sources: domestically, under the auspices of the CNA through its provincial associations; and overseas, from among the military nurses who were already on the scene. In 1944 the CNA had established the Committee on Post-war Planning for Assistance Abroad under the chairmanship of a highly respected Canadian nurse, Ethel Johns. During that year, the committee met directly with two UNRRA representatives at Washington headquarters to discuss Canadian recruiting.[115] Both these representatives were Canadian: Mary Craig McGeachy, director of the Welfare Division, and Lillian Johnson, acting chief nurse. Johnson, believing that nursing within UNRRA's displaced-persons operations would be groundbreaking work, deliberately set the recruiting bar high to attract recruits only from the upper echelon of Canadian nursing. Canadian UNRRA nurses were required to "have a sympathetic understanding of and respect for the customs, conditions and values of the people among whom they work; there must be no prejudice as to colour, race or creed. Co-operation is the keynote stressed."[116] Only Canadian nurses who had at least a bachelor's degree from a college or university of recognized standing or its equivalent and had supervisory experience in a variety of nursing fields were encouraged to apply. The nurses chosen constituted a female educational elite who were professionally and temperamentally predisposed to seize the opportunity of pioneering new frontiers in international nursing. Over time, Heather

Kilpatrick, Frances McQuarrie, Mary Henderson, and Lyle Creelman – all from the RNABC's Executive Council – would answer the call to serve overseas.

After her return from TC, Creelman's social life had settled back into its former sedate rhythm involving church, family, and nursing friends, with limited opportunities to meet eligible bachelors. Attempting to enlarge her social circle, she joined a local photography club. Photography had always fascinated her as a possible hobby. But, as she confided in her diary, she enjoyed the Photographic Society because it was "one group that are predominantly male & not all female."[117] A trip, after the CNA convention in Montreal in 1942, to visit her stepbrother Prescott in Charlottetown had offered a glimmer of summer romance when she was introduced to a young physician, Dr French. During the day Creelman thrilled at the physical challenge of learning to sail in French's company; some evenings they joined in the fellowship of family and friends at beach suppers or walked the beach, sharing the splendid ocean sunsets together. As her flight lifted off from the island, she was sad to leave and wondered "if my enjoyment of the Island on this trip were associated with the person or persons met. If they were not there would the island have been so beautiful?"[118] Over the next few days, as she wound her way back across the country, she reassured herself that "the tug at the heart" in a few months would "be forgotten & all will be well."[119] Shortly after returning home, there was further evidence that her matrimonial prospects were improving.

On several occasions, Lyle and her nursing friends visited a fortune teller or had their tea leaves read, primarily to forecast romantic connections. Despite the fortune teller's assurance that she was to be married before her next birthday, she left for CNA meetings in January 1943 feeling "bit disgruntled with life." Deep down, she "hated to think of having to work and earn my own living until I'm 60 & then to be retired. There isn't one unmarried and successful nurse I know that I envy. Must get my fortune told again to get some cheer up."[120] Reconciling aspirations for a career posed challenges for Creelman's generation of women, who were socialized to prioritize their duties as a mother and wife. Their jobs were expected to take second place next to marriage and childbearing. In the end, it was a bike, rather than a fortune teller's forecast, that opened the door to romance.

In the spring of 1943, Lyle Creelman learned to ride a bike well enough that she could join the Photographic Society's weekend excursions. In mid-April a new member, Dick Pullen, joined the weekend bike group, quickly earning the nickname "Dirt-Road Dick."[121] Pullen, already an employee of the BC Telephone Company for ten years, would remain with the company, rising to the position of director of public relations, until his retirement in 1963. Noted for his dry humour and public-speaking abilities, Pullen was an active member of Vancouver's social and services clubs, such as the Canadian Club, the

Gyro Club, and the Public Relations Society of British Columbia.[122] By the end of May, the "indomitable five" – Lyle, Dick, and three other members of the group – regularly left at 5 a.m. on a hundred-mile ride, stopping for lunch on an outcrop of rocks perched high above the Fraser River. "Dick and I," Lyle proudly recorded, "were the only ones who got home under our own steam."[123] The weekly pattern was soon set. Lyle and Dick enjoyed many picnic suppers during the week and joined the others for longer weekend tours, but increasingly the couple broke away to ride alone even then.

With Lyle and Dick increasingly becoming a couple within the group, the annual cycling holiday at the end of August provided them with a chance to clarify their relationship. Although she promised herself to jot down her emotions in her journal upon her return, by the time she got around to making the entry well over a month later she found that "this was hard to do. I think re-reading the facts will serve to recall accompanying emotions & feelings. It was undoubtedly the most pleasant holiday I have had."[124] After the holidays, Lyle and Dick continued their mid-week "rendezvous" for picnic suppers and frequently attended concerts or town hall meetings together.

That same summer, Lyle travelled to PEI again to visit Prescott's family. Having met Dick made it easier for her to deal with the news that Dr French was seeing someone else; she confided to her diary, "I have recovered from the crush I thought I had. A bit of a sissy anyway."[125] She spent her vacation making professional visits and enjoying conversations and walks with family and friends. This summer interlude provided Lyle with a greater sense of family and belonging. It was reassuring for her to find "that family were genuinely glad to see me and meant it when they said to come again soon next summer if I could."[126] Time away from the office also gave her a chance to ponder her personal and professional future; both appeared to be at a significant crossroads.

Believing that she would have to make a change relatively soon if she wanted a more senior nursing position, she was clearly mulling over her career prospects and the personal costs that would be involved in advancing her career in a new direction: "It is too bad that more nurses do not realize the amount of work that our leaders do for the cause of nursing. I wonder if the effort is worth it – does such a career bring satisfaction or not?"[127] Clearly interested in her own career prospects, Creelman speculated whether a teaching position would open up for her if Margaret Kerr got the job as editor of the *Canadian Nurse*. The question would become more salient as she visited with other nursing friends across the country who were assuming new and exciting positions. Gertrude Hall, whom she had got to know at the CNA convention, was going to be the director of the Public Health Nursing Division in Winnipeg; a former classmate at TC, Viola (Viv) Leadlay, was taking charge of the new public-health courses established by a federal grant at the University of Manitoba. Creelman's selection of future posts, however, was constrained by more than a desire to remain in Vancouver, close to her aging mother and Dick Pullen. As she had confided to her diary earlier, "Have been my own boss in nursing too long to work under another nurse."[128]

Returning to Vancouver by train, Creelman was feeling considerably healthier in spirit and body than the previous year. A diary entry earlier that summer had provided at least part of the explanation: "Think the good times I have been having, and am looking forward to, on the weekend with the cycling group has a lot to do with this feeling."[129] She was content to be returning home; Dick Pullen, she knew, would be there to meet her at the station. She believed that "there was evidence to suggest that Dick was going to take this affair seriously." Lyle, however, had still to determine if she was interested or not. This she would not do until she got to know him better.[130] She made a conscious decision to keep to herself on the cross-country train trip, using the time to relax and return mentally prepared for the year ahead. To other passengers, she knew she must have seemed a "very lonely person," but in truth "she couldn't be bothered unless the person looks particularly interesting."[131] Both personally and professionally, Creelman would bide her time until the right offer came along. The question that remained unanswered in her mind was which offer would take precedence if a choice had to be made.

At the CNA meeting held in Montreal in November 1943, Kathleen Russell delivered a letter from Dr Fred W. Routley, the executive director, to Creelman offering her the position as the first national director of nursing for the Canadian Red Cross. She was enticed enough by the offer to stop in Toronto on her way back to discuss it with Russell, Jean Browne, director of the Canadian junior Red Cross, and Routley. Without making any commitment, she returned to Vancouver to raise the matter with Dr Murray. Several factors contributed to her decision to refuse the offer. She preferred "to play [her cards] and wait for Health Insurance" – a decision she justified at the time by claiming that there was still a lot of work for her to do in Vancouver before "I would feel satisfied to leave."[132] There were other nursing positions that she hoped might open up. The CNA had been asked to think of a nursing director in anticipation that a federally funded national health-insurance scheme might gain approval, and Margaret Kerr's pending appointment as the editor of the *Canadian Nurse* opened other equally exciting possibilities at UBC. Helen McArthur, who followed Creelman as chair of the CNA's Public Health Section, eventually accepted the Red Cross post, ensuring that their paths would continue to cross in the future.

For the time being, Creelman happily settled back into her normal work routine; by now, her relationship with Dick Pullen provided greater emotional balance between her professional and private worlds. Her journal entries no longer looked back to happier times at Columbia University. Instead, after celebrating her best-ever New Year's Eve, she recalled the pleasant memories that had filled 1943. "Certainly many things have happened that I would not have dreamed of last year. Many features cannot even be put down in this diary."[133] And yet she still wondered whether her relationship with Dick would lead to marriage or "at its end will I be back on my own lonely way again."[134] She reconciled herself to accepting the continued ambiguity of their relationship on the grounds that she had "personally been much happier & more contented & have been in better health."[135]

It would be another six months before Creelman finally had time to record "the interesting highlights of her off-duty time." The many "grand" cross-country skiing and hiking outings from the ski cabin rented with friends and their families in Mount Seymour Provincial Park received special attention. For Creelman, these winter getaways were a time when the emotional warmth of being surrounded by friends and their children was complemented by the physical exhilaration of embarking on new outdoor adventures. By the end of the season, she delighted in gliding silently, as if dancing, over the snow-covered trails through old-growth forests perfectly framed against the majestic BC mountains. When the snow melted, she and Dick braved the mosquitoes as they hiked from the cabin to picnic and swim at Mystery Lake, where they were rewarded with spectacular views of Greater Vancouver. Lyle later recalled "the level of exhilarations one feels after climbing to the Peak and surveying the country far below," even though they got "lost coming down and had to hike back up." They didn't reach the cabin until midnight.[136] The rugged outdoor life would always continue to furnish an oasis from the cares of the work world.

Even though the beginning of 1944 saw her more settled professionally and contented personally, Creelman's decision to accept an offer from UNRRA that spring changed everything. It was not until mid-August, however, that her tentative appointment as chief nurse of Albania, part of the Balkan Mission, was confirmed. Before she reported to Washington in mid-September, there had been time for one final "wonderful holiday" with the cycling group, during which she and Dick visited Revelstoke while the others went to Banff. Remembering those final days of summer, she wrote, "It was grand to have such a happy memory of beautiful places and pleasant times to bring away with me."[137]

Several factors had come into play to lead Creelman to send off her application to UNRRA and apparently place on hold any prospects for marriage or a career change within Canada if and when universal health care came into place. During the last three years, she had overseen significant changes in the administrative structure and delivery of nursing services provided under the umbrella of the Metropolitan Health Committee. By 1944, however, her work there had settled into a more routine pattern. The chance to serve abroad afforded an opportunity to view health care and nursing issues from an international context while widening the prospect of leadership opportunities afterwards. Public-health nurses, especially ones as senior as Creelman, had been precluded from serving overseas with the military.[138] Becoming a soldier of peace offered a chance, previously denied, to combine adventure and humanitarian service. She also hoped that the distance from Canada would clarify, at least in her own mind, the long-term prospect of continued happiness with Dick. Over the next several months, she would try to put some perspective on their relationship but candidly confided in her diary, "Rather doubt I ever could think that offered the opportunity I would give up the career." She hoped that "Dick will feel that way when I return. It would have to be that or nothing – don't think I could continue as before not knowing how serious he is. It doesn't seem to be in my makeup to carry on from day to day." Lyle was already becoming emotionally defensive: "It will be interesting to see how feelings change. I mustn't allow myself to care too much in case some other girl came into his life."[139] For Creelman, nursing was not an alternative form of women's work until marriage. She saw nursing as a modern scientific career requiring years of college training; it could not easily be set aside without a loss of self-identity. So she personified the quandary that educated women of her generation faced; she hoped to have both a rewarding career and a meaningful, modern marriage in which intellectual companionship would be an integral part. She was far too independently minded for it to be any other way.

After a frantic round of packing, farewell teas, and cocktail parties, Dick Pullen and her mother accompanied Lyle to the train station. Twenty-eight of her friends and staff, loaded with parting gifts, bid Lyle an emotional farewell. It was "hard leaving but [I] didn't shed any tears at the station."[140] She had said her private goodbyes the evening before; Lyle Creelman was and would remain a very private lady. Under the veneer of apparent diffidence, an ambitious career woman resided – one who remained determined to set her own course.

As she set out on the journey to Washington, Creelman had much to think about. She may have thought she had a good idea of what awaited her in her new assignment, but if so, she was mistaken. While the radio had brought graphic accounts of the war into the homes of Canadians, it could never capture the scale of human suffering that Creelman was about to witness first-hand. The decision to serve abroad with UNRRA would profoundly alter the trajectory of her professional and personal life.

Chapter Four

Soldier of Peace, 1944–1946

The end of the Second World War on the European front was celebrated on 8 May 1945. The peace that followed, however, did not convey the same meaning for every country or, indeed, for many individuals within those countries. The upheaval that war had wrought on countless lives simply continued. National borders had been transformed and allegiances reshaped, but there was a host of questions about who would orchestrate the transition to peacetime and how it would be done.

Creelman, like other Canadian UNRRA nurses, was just as eager to serve as a soldier to win the peace in the pioneering post-war international organization, UNRRA, as her fellow Canadian military nurses had been to win the war. Well before Creelman reached her UNRRA post, twenty-six nations joined in a "Declaration of the United Nations" in 1942 pledging them to continue a joint war effort and not to make peace separately. On 9 November 1943, a year and half before the surrender of Germany, representatives from forty-four nations travelled to Washington to sign the UNRRA agreement. UNRRA, once it came into being in November 1943, represented a promise to the victims of war that, once the conflict ended, medicines and clothing and other emergency supplies would be quickly sent to rebuild shattered lives. Equally important, the massive relief campaign would act to prime the economies in the war-devastated countries as a bridge to restoring the peacetime multilateral trade system. Eventually, UNRRA would deliver $4 billion in aid to over twenty countries on a scale that surpassed even the movement of munitions by Allied forces during the war. A related task, important but controversial, was to provide shelter and health care for the millions awaiting repatriation or, as it unexpectedly turned out, resettlement. Significantly for Creelman's work with UNRRA, it provided camps for over one million who refused to return to their countries of origin, which increasingly had been incorporated into the Soviet Union's sphere of influence.

Motivated by a mixture of adventurism, idealism, and economic opportunity, Lyle Creelman joined UNRRA to do her part in establishing the basis for a new world order that would offer the security and prosperity absent after the Great War. The opportunity to travel and to experience nursing overseas, denied senior public health nurses during the war, added to the humanitarian enticement for her to venture abroad with UNRRA. Creelman and her fellow Canadian nurses also welcomed work with UNRRA since it offered a marked improvement in wartime salaries. UNRRA's entry-level salary range, between $2,400 and $2,800 annually, was approximately double what a public health nurse in Canada could make.[1] In Creelman's case, her original salary of $5,000 was raised by another $1,000 shortly after her arrival in Washington, making it even more attractive.[2] Besides, despite the wartime increases in salary and the shortage of nurses within Canada, there was no guarantee that the post-war work world would not be marked by the same unemployment or underemployment of the interwar years. Employment with UNRRA, then, offered both economic rewards and expanded professional horizons.

Still, UNRRA's three-tiered salary scale produced widespread discontent among staff in the field, exacerbating ethnic and class divisions.[3] As a Class I employee under direct contract with the organization whose salary level compared more than favourably with what she formerly earned, Creelman held a privileged place within UNRRA's administrative set-up. Despite the attractive salaries offered Canadian nurses, Creelman knew that the CNA continued to protest the terms of employment and working conditions for nurses serving overseas with UNRRA.[4] When UNRRA established its salary schedules, the salary floor was set using the applicant's current salary, with UNRRA paying a differential of up to an additional $200 per annum more. In practice, since Canadian nurses' salaries were significantly lower than those of their American counterparts, UNRRA actually paid differentials as high as $600. Even though the Canadian nurses had been made aware of salary discrepancies with American nurses, and without exception they would have been content to proceed with their UNRRA appointments regardless, the CNA aggressively petitioned both Ottawa and UNRRA on behalf of its members for pay equity with American nurses. The leadership within the CNA believed that "the principle of such discrimination is wrong and that our Association should not be content to let our nurses work under such conditions."[5] Even after Canadian UNRRA nurses, including Creelman, had entered the field, the CNA continued to protest the salary discrepancy. Canadian UNRRA nurses may have been international civil servants but their national association had no hesitation about lobbying on their behalf.[6]

UNRRA purported to create a new international civil service, based upon gender equality and a strictly neutral international perspective. Yet, while

UNRRA expected Creelman to behave as an international civil servant, the CNA right from the beginning had a clear political agenda for its nurses. The *Canadian Nurse* warned prospective UNRRA volunteers that "work abroad ... is no easy thing. Many sacrifices are called for and there are dangers and discomforts which must be faced with continuous courage and determination. The privilege of foreign service also imposes obligations. Overseas nurses have the responsibility of representing Canadian nurses to the peoples of other countries."[7] Accordingly, the CNA jealously guarded the professional status of its nurses abroad. When the controversial decision was made to allow American public health nurses to retain rank badges on their uniforms, the CNA took steps to ensure that Canadian nurses were accorded the same privileges of officer rank, which it knew meant everything in a military settings: "They feel that the situation might conceivably arise wherein American nurses would wear the insignia of their rank, while Canadian nurses – wearing the same uniform, but without insignia denoting any rank – would be considered inferior, and their use of officers' messes, etc. would be open to question. We definitely do not wish to have our Canadian nurses placed at this disadvantage."[8] The concern surrounding uniforms and rank badges should be read against the recent wartime experience, when Canadian nurses who held officer rank were accorded privileges that their non-commissioned British nursing sisters were denied. The CNA may have cautioned its nurses on the need to be impartial civil servants, but, as a national professional organization, it clearly had aspirations for international recognition. The questions of pay equity, uniforms, and grade levels relative to other UNRRA staff remained unresolved when Lyle Creelman entered the field to begin her UNRRA work. Yet, in the end, all these paled against the personal and professional challenges awaiting Creelman; the perspectives of those in the field were not necessarily those of the nursing leadership.

It remained to be seen whether either UNRRA or its new breed of international civil servant would meet the organization's idealistic expectations when tested. Nothing the CNA could have said would have prepared UNRRA nurses for the level of professional and personal adaptation required. Creelman discovered that international relief work, while rewarding, was more challenging, perilous, and sometimes life-changing than she ever could have predicted. She never expected to have to negotiate minefields of administrative rivalry, nationalist politics, gender issues, and professional authority while working on the front lines with UNRRA.

The social legitimacy of the Health Division, in contrast to that of the Welfare Division, was never questioned by the higher administrative echelons of UNRRA. But neither were nurses' contributions properly valued. Despite its avowed gender equality, UNRRA continued to perpetuate a gendered hierarchy at all levels of its administration.[9] The chaotic and constantly changing administrative environment in which UNRRA's Nursing Division operated – culminating in it being deprived of its independent status and placed under the Medical Division as UNRRA prepared to wind down – was symptomatic of the ineptitude that characterized UNRRA's entire internecine administrative history. Despite UNRRA's stated neutrality, the provision of nursing services was political.

Creelman's naivety as an international civil servant was soon challenged by the harsh reality of working for an untried, ill-defined, temporary organization operating on the uncertain boundaries of war and peace. UNRRA did not have a well-established blueprint of operation; its relief and rehabilitation require-ments could be accurately assessed only after the guns of war were silenced, and it had few precedents or guidelines to draw upon for guidance. Administrative structure and policy directives emerged gradually as the organization gained experience in the field and as the military situation permitted. Field directives governing the care and repatriation of those displaced from their countries of origin became enmeshed in politics of Zionism and the Cold War. Moreover, UNRRA was a child of compromise and concession right from its inception, making its mandate more difficult to implement than anticipated. Under the terms of the agreement setting it up, it could operate only under the military control of the Allied government whose forces occupied that particular area. Furthermore, the decision to delegate the provision of civilian relief to the military during the initial phase of European liberation effectively sidelined UNRRA. Creelman, like other UNRRA field personnel, was left to cope with the aftermath of the politics that threatened to paralyze medical procurement during the military period. Finally, the agreement's failure to define with clarity the financial arrangements or scope of the work until operations were under way sowed the seeds of future discord among member governments and fos-tered confusion within the field. As a consequence of these factors – Creelman would learn first-hand – power relationships, leadership, and decision-making were transitory, complex, and personal.

But the frustrations experienced by Creelman would be tempered by her belief that UNRRA's health work was making a difference. With the outbreak of the Second World War, international public health work virtually ceased until the formation of UNRRA. At a time when there was a global shortage of the personnel, medical supplies, equipment, transport, and facilities essential to the maintenance of health care, UNRRA formed a much-needed conduit between the pre-war international health organizations, such as the health-care arms of the League of Nations, and the post-war World Health Organization. The mandate of UNRRA's Health Division went well beyond epidemic con-trol; it included sections that dealt with nutrition, sanitation, tuberculosis, and laboratories. Even though the rehabilitation of Nazi nurses was not part of UNRRA's mandate, the issue ignited controversy from which Creelman could not remain aloof. In fact, given the shortage of trained nurses within UNRRA's displaced-persons operations, German nurses rounded out the staff in UNRRA hospitals and took care of displaced persons from the camps admitted to civilian hospitals. Nursing and living within a large multinational UNRRA team in an enemy-occupied country, where, at least initially, fraternization with German civilians was prohibited, intensified and complicated attempts to define professional and personal relationships in the field. For Creelman, it posed a supervisory challenge without precedent.

Even before reaching the field, Creelman battled against the administrative inefficiency, political intrigues, and sheer human pettiness and indifference that marred UNRRA's field operations. On 18 September 1944, four days after leaving Vancouver, Creelman arrived in Washington; within a week, she started questioning her decision to adventure abroad with UNRRA. Believing that her UNRRA appointment as chief nurse of Albania, reporting to Margaret Arnstein, the chief nurse of the Balkans, had been finalized, she soon learned that she was to be sent to Poland instead. Florence Udell, the chief nurse within UNRRA's London headquarters, had selected a British nurse for her original post. This was not unwelcome news. Creelman privately confided that she preferred being her own boss and was "very pleased with the [Polish] appointment as it is starting on something right from the beginning."[10] As it turned out, however, political considerations would preclude Creelman from serving in UNRRA's Polish mission.

Only a week later, the impatient Creelman was privately complaining: "Waiting here is very irksome."[11] Her arrival on 2 October 1944 at UNRRA's North American training centre at the University of Maryland did little to improve her mood. Once at the centre, where staff received additional training to familiarize them with UNRRA's mandate and administrative set-up as well as the high standards of conduct expected of them, Creelman came to understand why the *Washington Post* described its purpose as being to take "the slick out of the city slicker." Her first impressions of it "were not very favourable"; she found it "rather dirty."[12] Still, she knew and admired the dynamic Canadian, Harry Cassidy, who headed the centre. He had served as the director of social welfare and health in British Columbia from 1934 to 1939 before joining the Department of Sociology at the University of California at Berkeley. His administrative experience as well as his broad technical and historical knowledge of North American social welfare was unrivalled.[13]

Cassidy's lectures to the trainees emphasized the importance of an organization that sought to bring aid to a war-battered world, which had endured "global war and unparalleled destruction, starvation [and] disease." He made it clear in his lectures that UNRRA's goal was to head off some of the catastrophes that had followed the Great War. Reminding the new recruits that peace and prosperity were indivisible, he warned that chaos in Europe and Asia, as well as desperate poverty and rampant unemployment, stood "in the way of [the] creation of political machinery essential to a peaceful world." Warning the trainees that it was not enough for UNRRA "to be a soup kitchen," Cassidy imbued the future UNRRAIDS with the sense that they were part of a larger effort, uniting men and women from many different nations, backgrounds, and skills, to construct a future world with new social systems and international relations. Cassidy's view of what constituted relief and rehabilitation embraced the North American vision of social work, which centred on removing the socioeconomic causes of poverty and political instability. The essence of UNRRA was "to help people help themselves" through the supply of essential consumer goods and social services as well as medical care and repatriation.[14]

Not surprisingly, Cassidy's expansive views on UNRRA's role resonated with Creelman's own experience as a public health nurse. Having already identified poverty as the root of disease and unhealthy living in Vancouver, she expected government to develop preventative health and social policies to redress social-economic inequalities. For Creelman, "helping people to help themselves" meant moving beyond the focus of providing medical care and traditional interventions to emphasize measures that addressed the underlying determinants of health. In the years to come, her views would be both strengthened and clarified, even as they were being challenged.

While the orientation provided to UNRRA's staff at the Maryland training centre gave them an overall view of UNRRA's mandate, the political history of the receiving countries, and their role as impartial international civil servants in post-war recovery, many recruits, including Creelman, complained that it offered little of practical application.[15] While her assessment that the training period, while useful, would undoubtedly have been strengthened by the presence of more instructors at headquarters with field experience may have been correct, the roots of her dissatisfaction lay elsewhere. Creelman adjusted more easily to the "rough place," as she characterized the training centre, than to imposed periods of inactivity – especially after her fellow British Columbian nurses left for the field.[16] Restless by nature, and "more convinced than ever that London is where we need to be," she privately grumbled that she was being "wasted here." She chafed at being made to feel "quite the juvenile – quite a change for someone who is accustomed to being top-pin." In all likelihood, she remained unconvinced by her own rationalization that "everyone needs to be taken down some once in awhile."[17] Despite her protestations that she would refrain from questioning headquarters' decisions "until she knew more about the set up," Creelman regarded the orientation as inadequate and quickly came to the same conclusions about UNRRA's recruitment practices.

Fed up after only three weeks at the training centre, Creelman seized the opportunity to ensconce herself in Chief Nurse Lillian Johnson's Washington office, where the key nursing assignments would be negotiated with London. In Creelman's judgment, the American Association of Nurses had made a mistake in granting the United States Public Health Service (USPHS) and one nurse in particular, Johnson, the decisive voice in making UNRRA appointments.[18] She questioned the decision to take army cadet nurses into UNRRA: "Surely, if gone about in the right way, there are many experienced nurses who would apply. So much for UNRRA."[19] She also disapproved of the higher salaries paid American nurses but decided to reserve final judgment until she saw what salary scales were being used in London. Creelman's time in Washington provided an early indication of the personnel issues that would prove divisive in UNRRA's field operations.

Then, suddenly, Creelman received notice that she would set sail for London the following week. The transatlantic passage was uneventful. On 22 November, after "an experience not to be forgotten," Lyle Creelman debarked along with the Allied troops from the troop ship anchored in the Firth of Clyde, only to learn no arrangements had been made for her transfer from Glasgow to London. For the moment, her complaints about the preferential treatment granted USPHS nurses were temporarily assuaged – at least until her own prospects for an interesting UNRRA assignment appeared threatened once again.

Creelman's private record of her London sojourn paid particular attention to developments on the political front that were complicating UNRRA's effort to establish a Polish Mission. As the weeks passed, UNRRA's future work in Poland appeared increasingly uncertain. In January 1945 the Polish Committee of National Liberation, a coalition of leftist and communist factions known as the Lublin Committee, was recognized by the Soviet Union and was installed in Warsaw as the provisional government. Would UNRRA recognize the new regime or the constitutionally legitimate Wladyslaw Sikorski government-in-exile that had established a seat in London in September 1939? Before UNRRA could operate in any territory occupied by the Soviets, it had to come to terms with Moscow. UNRRA's failure to secure Russian approval for the Polish Mission left Creelman in limbo in London for several months and foreshadowed the deepening rift within the wartime alliance.

As these events unfolded, Creelman, realizing that her medical chief of mission, Dr Henry Holle, had nothing for her to do, either, until the Polish

Mission opened, grew restless and somewhat melancholy. Finding the "rainy and blowy" December days a source of homesickness, she determined "to keep busy to avoid giving away too much to the feeling."[20] Her melancholic mood also reflected the profound personal adjustment involved in living in wartime London. Wartime rationing was not nearly as disconcerting as the air raid sirens warning of approaching pilotless V-1 bombs or V-2 rockets that screeched through the London night skies. As the long nights of the London blackout continued, there were repeated episodes when she and the other UNRRA nurses were shaken by a V-2 landing close to their billet: "It was a very funny feeling. I knew that all was over, I started to tremble and just could not control myself." Afterwards, they drew all the beds into one room for the rest of the night, "thankful that it caused no loss of life." They hoped "never again to be in such close contact to one when it is exploding."[21] She supposed she would "learn to take them casually" but admitted she still "had inward shivers when they talk about them."[22] And so, despite the frustration and loneliness resulting from the prolonged delay in taking up her first UNRRA post, Creelman's time in London proved invaluable for her future assignment. Those months gave her, as she wrote, "some vague idea of what the people over here have gone through in the past five years."[23] Yet, in other ways, she remained a tourist. Her diary accounts of sightseeing, attending concerts, and shopping with other Canadian UNRRA nurses en route to their assignments, in a city that she characterized as overflowing with "with romance and tradition," appear surreal when contrasted with the wartime destruction of London. Her experiences there gave her only a preliminary glimpse of the grim conditions waiting in war-devastated countries.

Seeing Londoners' daily sacrifices augmented her sense of guilt at not contributing to UNRRA's work. She approached Florence Udell, UNRRA's chief nurse for the European Regional Office (ERO), to find something useful to do until the Polish Mission opened. Udell assigned her to assist with the care of the Dutch children being sent to Coventry, England, where the youngsters were to recover from their years of wartime malnutrition under Nazi occupation. Pending their arrival, Creelman began making professional contacts useful for her Polish UNRRA assignment. While visiting the Florence Nightingale International Foundation (the educational foundation of the International Council of Nurses), she received sound advice from its acting director, who had extensive experience in Europe between the wars, including with Polish nursing schools. She told Creelman, "Use good common sense and not to go in with fixed ideas of changing things too much and we would get along all right."[24]

Creelman also contacted a "Miss Mochnacka," attached to the Polish military and in charge of a six-month preliminary training program for Polish nurses at three military hospitals in Britain. After clearing her involvement with UNRRA, Creelman explored the possibility of helping to set up a permanent nursing school in England that could be transported to Poland when circumstances permitted. From 21 to 23 December, Creelman accompanied Mochnacka on a visit to Polish nursing personnel at the three military hospitals in the Scottish Highlands to assess how they might assist in the development of a nursing program. The majority of the medical staff of these hospitals had been part of Anders Army – formed of former political prisoners who had been recruited in Russia and who had fought alongside the British – and were all politically aligned with the Polish government-in-exile in London.[25] During the visit, Creelman quickly concluded that, with the Soviet Union's recognition of the Lublin Committee, there was little prospect that graduates of a permanent Polish school of nursing – if such a school were started – would be willing return to Poland. "It looks," she wrote, "as though Russia will control Poland and if so then the Polish group who are here would not return. What prospects for world peace!" Indeed, it seemed to Creelman that the shadow of the Cold War had already begun to dissipate the hope of peace and a meaningful UNRRA assignment. She had only begun to understand the ways in which nationalism and politics would undermine UNRRA's plans for the repatriation of the Polish people.

The trip visiting Polish hospitals over Christmas week offered a much needed diversion from the loneliness, uncertainty, and fear that pervaded her stay in London. But the serenity of traditional Polish Christmas celebrations – marked by the most "artistically decorated trees" Creelman had ever seen and centring on a Midnight Mass complete with magnificent choirs – was broken by the unwelcome sound of bombing nearby. For the moment, she was grateful that the imminent arrival of the Dutch children would offer escape from sounds of V-2s disturbing the London nights. She freely confessed to still being a "bit of a coward."[26]

On 9 January 1945 Creelman arrived at the Netherlands Government Children Committee Hostel at Baginton Fields near Coventry, where the evidence of the Blitz was again all too evident. Creelman found it "pathetic to walk down Cooperation Street and look at the temporary shops in which they are attempting to carry on." Events on the work front were equally disconcerting. The children did not arrive until February, and, once they did, Creelman's public demeanour camouflaged her private reservations about the quality of care given by both the Dutch and the transient UNRRA medical staff with whom she worked at Coventry. Articles she wrote for the *Canadian Nurse* positively recorded her time with the lively but mischievous children, who constantly let the air out of her bike tires.[27] In reality, she and Dr John

F. McCreary,[28] the Torontonian who headed the nutrition team sent to examine the children shortly after their arrival, were shocked by how little the Dutch staff knew about proper techniques of feeding children. She was appalled by the anti-Semitism that the Dutch group, predominantly Roman Catholics "who expected to run their own show," had exhibited towards the Jewish matron who withdrew shortly after their arrival.[29] Creelman complained that the priest was "poisoning the minds of the children against the English so that the children think English families are terrible and not fit for them to stay with."[30] Here, as elsewhere, religious strife and fierce national animosities would complicate attempts by UNRRAIDS, as the field staff were known, to be politically neutral while caring for and repatriating those displaced from their countries of origin. More extensive field experience would be required both to hone Creelman's political acumen to an international context and to enhance her cultural sensitivity to other countries' medical standards and practices.

There were many other "trials and tribulations" that Creelman encountered while caring for the children. She bristled at the condescending treatment that the nursing staff received from the Dutch medical personnel. They simply had an "altogether different idea of the duties of a nurse than we."[31] While Creelman made it clear to Dutch authorities that their expectation that the UNRRA nurse act as a housekeeper, chauffeur, and general clerical assistant did not fit her understanding of the nurse's role, she nevertheless waged an ongoing battle to maintain her professional authority. Six months after leaving Vancouver, it seemed that her decision to join UNRRA was a serious mistake. Her diary entry of 14 March captured her dark mood: "All the money that has been paid to me for doing nothing … Felt down yesterday. Had a good cry. The meal hour is terrible. Stand in line with all the sub-staff and then when you get to the table there is probably not a clean place to sit at. I asked … if nursing was profession on the continent. The way they ignore us here one would not think so." Coventry was an apt prelude to the struggle UNRRA nurses faced in the field for professional recognition.

Feeling guilty about her own inactivity, Creelman could not support any further efforts by the Canadian Nurses Association to rectify the continued discrepancies in salary levels between Canadian and American nurses; she believed that it "will stir up bad feeling and not get them anywhere."[32] Matters worsened. First, Creelman fell ill with jaundice, which the resident UNRRA doctor initially misdiagnosed. The almost weekly changing of the UNRRA medical guard did not improve matters, especially since Creelman detested the latest UNRRA replacement who arrived on 10 April: "Dr Kyper in charge for a week. She is a queer specimen. Rather untidy, homely, fat and not too pleasant a manner … Don't think she liked it when I said: I was going to London on Monday. Have an idea that she just said to herself that she would show me. I decided I would stay in bed until tomorrow and then be my own advisor."[33] In all likelihood, the Dutch doctor found the Canadian an equally difficult colleague.

Creelman returned to London on 19 April, still tired and weak but glad to be back in the hub of activity. She was looking for a new UNRRA assignment. Even if the Polish Mission opened up, she doubted that there would any real opportunity to contribute to the development of Polish nursing amidst the continued civil and political unrest.[34] Once again, she repeated the Washington pattern and carefully ensconced herself in Chief Nurse Florence Udell's office, where she pressed her case for any important nursing post that became available on the Continent. Creelman was chagrined to learn that once again her appointment would have to wait until the jockeying between Washington and London over key nursing assignments, including the determination of Lillian Johnson's and Margaret Arnstein's future roles, ended. She was "tired of waiting" and knew "that if I had to return to Wash[ington] to wait I would just resign and go home. They would just manufacture some clerk's job in Johnson's office for me. Had enough of that last fall." After a "frank talk about the whole thing" with Udell, she was somewhat more assured: "She would like me with D.P. [displaced persons] and could probably find a supervisory job or even better for me ... Johnson is coming over ... to be Chief Nurse for D.P.s in Germany. (Miss Udell and Rolf Struthers [a noted Canadian paediatrician] both say I could do a better job!)" It made Creelman "boil to think that she [Johnson] would be brought over here when I am sitting here doing nothing. That seems to be the way things are done in UNRRA." Her determination to bring the matter to a head was influenced by the letters from Canadian nurses that only strengthened her conviction that "there is so much doing at home I seriously doubt that this experience is worth it."[35]

But it was a letter from Dick Pullen that brought the final crushing blow. Despite all her attempts over the last several months to distance herself emotionally and put their relationship into perspective, the news that he was dating someone else devastated Creelman: "What this means I don't know. I am a ship on a vast ocean. I told myself I had to be prepared for this and further make myself believe it to be serious." A reserved, proud woman, she did not "let myself have any feelings about it when I read the letter in the office but shed a few tears for some nights afterwards." She spent most of the week attempting, somewhat unsuccessfully, to rationalize why they were ill-suited and never destined for marriage. "He's shorter than I, bald, he is maybe a bit dense, e.g. never sent me flowers or candy; used my car freely, he took advantages I should not have permitted, and he has not much education." In her heart, however, she knew that "they don't hold water. For every one of these trivial things

I can find good a point for which I love him." For now, she would "try to forget these & prepare myself for the news of his marriage." Creelman also knew that "she would not think about this so and it wouldn't be so hard to take if I were not alone here and having to restrict my activities so severely." After all, she noted, "it was just a slight to my ego. I am like the old maid who clutches at the last straw because she is afraid that she will remain unmarried."[36] Over time, by writing in her diary, she came to terms with her changed relationship with Dick: "Certainly if coming with UNRRA is going to cost me him it wasn't worth it. I remember trying to find this out before I left. He warned me so much about taking him seriously that I reasoned that maybe if I stayed he would drop me anyway. It was much better that I go away before that happened. However, one cannot tell what might have happened or what will happen." In the end, she accepted that "the only thing to do is to enjoy being here, get the most out of living and cultivate as many friendships as possible."[37]

Creelman held a complex blend of traditional and more modern feminist views. A respectable woman with conventional values, she still placed a high priority on marriage and family; "I just couldn't bear to live alone & I think that married life is the only way that one can have true happiness."[38] Besides the legal strictures supporting monogamy, there were many social and cultural factors that reinforced the institution of marriage in Creelman's era. While the advent of the Second World War would eventually loosen the mores and conventions of the time, extramarital sex remained taboo and birth control was often illegal or unavailable. Creelman's options for "true happiness," then, were constrained by this social environment as well as by her own conservative upbringing and perception of her social station. Yet she also saw herself as a highly trained professional woman whose expertise and skills should not be lost after marriage. Eminently practical, she soon wrote to Margaret Kerr asking her "be on the lookout for a job for me." The longer that she was absent from Canada, the more difficult it would be to return to the Metropolitan Health Committee; it would not, she thought, be fair to her successor, Trenna Hunter, for her to go back.[39] And unless her marriage prospects to Dick improved, in all likelihood, she would choose not to return to Vancouver permanently.[40]

Fortunately, life had become more interesting. By mid-June 1945, her perseverance and lobbying finally paid off. After much jockeying, Lillian Johnson remained in Washington and the former chief nurse of the Balkan Mission, Margaret Arnstein, resigned from UNRRA, leading to Creelman's reassignment as the chief nurse for the British Zone of Occupied Germany. She was both excited and nervous at the prospect of working with Sir Raphael (Ralph) Cilento, the Australian physician who was then the chief medical officer for the British Zone and would eventually become its director: "Quite inspired me.

A real Challenge. I hope I do not let Canada down ... I feel that this coming experience has all been worth waiting for and have a real feeling of adventure about it. Who knows it may bring great personal happiness. I am very lucky to have been on the spot."[41] Much more than luck had led to her appointment; she had deftly manoeuvred the political corridors, foregoing unwanted appointments and aggressively lobbying for an important post. There would be little time for contemplating personal relationships over the next year, with Dick or anyone else.[42]

Before her appointment to Germany came through, Creelman expressed some concern about her ability to do her UNRRA work "satisfactorily and be a credit to Canada";[43] nevertheless, she "had to confess that if there is a top job [chief nurse, Germany], I should like to have it."[44] Once appointed chief nurse, she used her remaining time in London to forge professional relationships with other organizations already at work in the field. Creelman carefully established boundaries that would avoid future jurisdictional squabbles. She met with the chief nurses of the Allied Control Commission to address their concerns that there was to be an UNRRA chief nurse attached to headquarters, especially since their responsibility for overseeing the de-Nazification of the national German nursing service included German nurses within UNRRA's hospitals. After discussing their relative functions, in which Creelman made it clear that she would be working with the displaced persons and not the German civilian population, she believed that "their fears were somewhat allayed."[45] Once in Germany, Creelman established a Nursing Advisory Committee to promote an effective working relationship with other international agencies that operated some UNRRA assembly centres, such as the British Red Cross, and with the chief nurses of the ACC, which controlled the employment of German nurses needed to care for the displaced persons admitted to civilian hospitals.[46] Creelman maintained that the committee helped prevent jurisdictional squabbles: the two chief nurses of the ACC "kept us informed also of developments in their own services – there was, in fact, a mutual interchange of information that was most valuable."[47]

Before leaving London, she had lunch with Elizabeth Brackett, now with the Rockefeller Foundation, whom she had first met while doing her field placement with the East Harlem Nursing and Health Services in New York. Later, she delayed her departure to the countryside for the weekend in order to meet with Olive Baggallay, former chief nurse of Greece, who was returning to the Florence Nightingale International Foundation. The newly appointed chief nurse of the British Zone took steps to see that her official position was recognized by both those in authority and those with whom she would have future dealings.

During this interlude, Creelman received advance warning of the chaos that had met the first UNRRA teams. Letters from UNRRA nurses recounted the looting and fighting among Polish and Russian displaced persons swarming to find food, shelter, and lost family members.[48] She also learned, from UNRRA's Dr A.P. Meikeljohn, of the horrors that awaited the first teams entering Belsen. The death camp, where typhus had been deliberately introduced by the Germans, had been built for eight thousand but was occupied by forty thousand when the Allies arrived. Creelman heard the horrific stories of sorting through the ten thousand unburied dead to identify those still alive and mounting death tolls that reached approximately one thousand per day. This was shocking enough, but it could not prepare Creelman for the challenges of working with concentration-camp survivors in UNRRA's assembly centres, as its camps were named to avoid any identification with their Nazi predecessors.[49] At this time, Germany was "a kaleidoscopic picture of humanity in chaotic disorganization."[50] The disruption of people, facilities, and government was extensive. The internal transportation system was crippled by Allied bombing, making the movement of relief personnel and supplies difficult, and there was little semblance of orderly civil government. In such circumstances, the political instincts necessary for dealing with bureaucratic annoyances, national animosities, and cultural obstacles – all inherent in the job of supervising a multinational nursing corps – could be acquired only on the spot.

But Creelman's personality was such that she preferred a tough new assignment to sitting around. Typically, once ensconced in Germany, she would turn down an opportunity in December 1945 to become the chief nurse of Poland. Expressing her strong feelings to her superiors about any reassignment at the time, she wrote, "I do not think that it would be fair to leave the job here, and in addition to that I am not convinced that there would not be a repetition of my last winter's experience of enforced idleness. There is a real nursing job to be done here."[51]

Creelman, like other UNNRA nurses, discovered that nursing with the enemy in Germany, where she was ultimately sent, provided a unique experience. Since the Allied Control Commission (ACC) had responsibility for de-Nazification and the restoration of the national nursing services in Occupied Germany, UNRRA's Nursing Division focused on providing health services for displaced persons housed within UNRRA's assembly centres and during their repatriation trips back home. Caring for the displaced persons, the majority of whom were survivors of the concentration and forced-labour camps, presented nursing challenges that few could have imagined beforehand.

Part of the ACC's job involved identifying Brown Nurses or Brown Shirts (because of their brown uniform), who had been trained in both political and nursing science and appointed to key government positions to disseminate Nazi propaganda to other German nurses. Allied nurses found it difficult to comprehend what had driven German nurses to condone – let alone participate in – mass killings in Nazi death camps. In attempting to explain German nurses' involvement in Nazi atrocities, the "darkest chapter of our German nursing history," the German nursing historian Hilde Steppe and others have singled out the cult of obedience to doctors inherent in the hierarchical German medical system.[52] Steppe decries the political naivety of nurses in the Nazi era, who "were under the illusion that they were remaining true to their professional ethic unaffected by social change."[53] Yet, after the war, Steppe found, "only a few nurses were condemned to death and were killed; others were sentenced to prison; and others in large numbers were acquitted." Strikingly, as far as she could discover, there was "no evidence of nurses being barred from practicing their profession."[54]

A 1947 article by Mabel G. Lawson in the *Canadian Nurse* provides a glimpse into how Canadian nurses portrayed their German counterparts' wartime role and the measures taken in the British Zone of Occupied Germany by those in charge of rehabilitating Germany's nursing services. It also provides a telling portrait of the political context in which Creelman was expected to define her working relations with both the ACC and the German nursing community. Lawson noted that she endeavoured to adhere to two guiding principles: "firstly, to help the German nurses to assume greater responsibility for their own affairs and to develop greater independence; secondly, to bring the various denominational and ancillary groups into closer professional relationship."[55] Both principles were intended to pave the way for the creation of a national nursing association as the preliminary step for renewed membership in the ICN. Canadian nurses were not provided with any description of the German nurses' participation in the Nazi programs of involuntary euthanasia, forced sterilization, and human experimentation. Instead, Canadian readers were reminded that "hitherto in Germany the nursing profession has had little to say in its own organization and nurses have not enjoyed the same privileges, or attained to the same status, as their colleagues in countries where nursing is regarded as a sister profession to that of medicine" and that many members of the nursing profession "were never party members and had no part in politics."[56] Like its American counterpart, the *Canadian Nurse* was more concerned with promoting international cooperation and solidarity within the international nursing sisterhood than with holding German nurses accountable.[57]

In the midst of the chaos prevailing in Germany, it did not help that the UNRRA nursing brigade within the British Zone was made up of twelve different nationalities without either common training or language to bind it together. Many of the difficulties that Creelman experienced were the legacy of attempting to build an international nursing brigade within an administrative structure that only gradually emerged and frequently changed. The history of UNRRA's work in post-war Europe can be divided into three discrete periods. During the initial period, in which the organization operated under the Supreme Headquarters Allied Expeditionary Force (SHAEF),[58] the temporary shelter and massive movement of those willing to return home and the care of the concentration-camp survivors proved the major challenges. In the eyes of many military commanders, UNRRA was just another unwanted layer in the command chain; their focus had been on winning the war and not planning relief at a time when there was a worldwide shortage of food, transport, and supplies. According to John Alexander Edmison, the Canadian given the daunting task of coordinating UNRRA's efforts with SHAEF UNRRA was "treated as the undeserving stepchild of the military, leaving it vulnerable to the charge of being hopelessly inefficient and an inadequate organization bogged down as one writer said, 'by red tape of 47 nations.'"[59] In its rush to meet the military authorities' demands for assistance, UNRRA dispatched small, ill-equipped teams to the field; others waited "frozen" until UNRRA supplies and vehicles sitting on the docks in London received enough priority to allow the teams to move forward.[60]

Once the military authorities relinquished control to UNRRA – a move marking the beginning of the second period – the organization attempted to refurbish its badly tarnished image. Its efforts in this direction were compromised by the growing controversy surrounding the treatment of Jewish displaced persons. This issue became highly politicized as "infiltrees" – Jewish refugees from outside Germany who were escaping persecution or seeking a better life – made their way into UNRRA's camps in the post-hostilities period and thus swelled the numbers seeking UNRRA aid. The organization was forced to expand its original definition of eligibility to cover these Jewish refugees, who technically had not been displaced from their homes during the war. Combined with the problem of those who refused to return to home countries in Eastern Europe under Soviet control, it became apparent that longer-term solutions would be required to deal with "hard-core" displaced persons. Public health and repatriation became much more politically complex problems than either UNRRA or Creelman originally anticipated.

The decision to merge the welfare and displaced-persons operations into the newly created Displaced Persons and Repatriation Division in April 1946 marked the beginning of the third administrative period as UNRRA prepared to wind down its operations. A series of tough new measures signalled a significant change in the protocol surrounding the care and repatriation of displaced persons and profoundly altered the working environment for UNRRA field staff and the living conditions for the displaced-persons communities throughout Germany. These changes reflected the desire of UNRRA's second director general, Fiorello La Guardia, to shift the organization's focus away from welfare work to repatriation. UNRRA's workers had been increasingly criticized for initiating programs that made the displaced persons "too comfortable" and so encouraged a sense of permanence within these communities.[61] Under the new July 1946 administrative orders, educational and vocational training or employment projects were to be "made available to displaced persons on a temporary basis pending their repatriation and are not to be of a character that they delay or prevent repatriation."[62] Coinciding with the council's renewed insistence on repatriation, finally, were a series of administrative directives issued in July 1946 that sought to eliminate any obstacles to repatriation in the camps, including the removal of anyone – not excepting UNRRA personnel – who had opposed repatriation. Simultaneously, several UNRRA teams were amalgamated into huge area units, in a move dictated by more than financial stringency. Divorcing its staff from their close association with any one camp or nationality was a prerequisite for implementing tougher regulations aimed at "encouraging" hard-core displaced persons to return home. The remaining displaced persons were moved from camp to camp, caught in the cruel vortex of Cold War politics that again uprooted families from their communities. Instead of rehabilitating broken spirits and families, UNRRAIDS were now expected to become agents of repatriation. The uncertainty both for UNRRA staff and for the remaining displaced persons persisted until UNRRA finally discontinued its operations in Europe on 30 June 1947. Lyle Creelman never expected to become a soldier of repatriation.

On 13 July 1945, Creelman and Cilento boarded the troop transport. At times in the months ahead, the stormy sea passage, through ocean lanes strewn with thousands of mines that had been broken loose by the storm then raging,[63] appeared no more difficult or dangerous than the task of organizing the nursing services within the British Zone.

Creelman's and Cilento's introduction to British Zone of Occupied Germany mirrored the administrative disarray rampant throughout UNRRA's German displaced-person operations during the early days in the field. Upon their arrival in Brussels, Cilento spent the better part of the first day searching for the UNRRA office, which had moved so frequently that no one knew where it was located. Disgusted, Creelman recorded simply, "A typical UNRRA show apparently."[64] Once the office was located, they were given the "special road maps" indicating the designated de-mined route that they were to follow from Brussels to Bad Oeynhausen in Germany, the headquarters for the 21st British Army Group.

The journey triggered a kaleidoscope of emotions as the Canadian nurse attempted to reconcile the seemingly conflicting and incongruous images of war-torn Europe. Given the food shortages and evidence of the grim fighting everywhere, Creelman felt uncomfortable when a waiter in tails served her breakfast in Holland. The strange sensation of trepidation that she experienced upon entering enemy territory was reinforced by the unbelievable devastation that she witnessed in towns like Bocholt, hardly "more than a mass of rubble."[65] She found it almost surreal that such beautiful agrarian countryside, where men, women, and children were harvesting the crops without the aid of machinery, had so recently been the scene of savage fighting.[66] At Nijmegen, on an early morning walk with Cilento, a very different emotion was triggered by the sight of the bridge that so many young Canadian soldiers had given their lives to defend.[67]

As they crossed the German frontier, they encountered a menacing sign: "You are now in Germany … You have been warned." The roadside was also heavily signed, warning that anyone seen walking more than twenty feet off the road would be shot! Shortly after one of their initial forays into the field, Creelman recorded that Cilento "was called out on the coals for being out with [Creelman] unarmed!" Afterwards he carried a revolver. No mention, however, was made of any security measures when she drove her own car throughout Germany unescorted. The German civilian population regarded the UNRRA staff with the same open hostility exhibited towards the conquering armies. Moreover, social tension and distrust were reinforced, at least initially, by the ban on fraternization with the German population. Amidst this human and administrative chaos, Creelman and Cilento had to establish their headquarters at Spenge, quickly appraise conditions in the field, and win the confidence of the military so that UNRRA could assume authority.

On arriving at the Hatert Camp, they met with UNRRA Director Schlee to sort out the medical personnel for Belsen. As Creelman viewed the barracks, which she thought clearly unfit to house UNRRA personnel awaiting final deployment to teams, she was disgusted that Schlee could think that it was a "good set-up – good discipline." The diary entry said it all: "Good God! Is that the kind of people we have at the Head of UNRRA."[68] Their working relationship was short-lived; Schlee was recalled to London in August and replaced by Brigadier Jackling, whom Creelman thought to be "very bumptious."[69]

Having "expected the worst" from the Belgian UNRRA nurses waiting at Hatert, she was agreeably surprised to find that only "one was definitely not fit, having only TB training and no state diploma"; the Belgian nurses were a much better group, in her opinion, than the French.[70] When interviewed years later about her UNRRA work, she admitted to being shocked by the poor calibre of European nurses, especially the French ones, some of whom had followed the army and were in fact prostitutes.[71] Her views in this regard were substantiated by others.[72] The visit was an early indication of the work ahead to overcome UNRRA's tarnished reputation during its early days in the field.[73]

Even before leaving London, Creelman had surmised that "[getting] along with Army personnel ... will be one of the keys to success."[74] Unlike her counterparts in the American Zone, Creelman developed effective working relations with both military and civilian authorities alike. She cultivated a close working relationship with Cilento during the difficult negotiations surrounding the transfer of responsibility for providing medical services to the displaced persons in the British Zone, and Belsen Hospital in particular, to UNRRA. Brigadier T.F. Kennedy, responsible for public health for the British Zone, opposed giving UNRRA control on the grounds that there were "insufficient Britishers to occupy the control positions."[75] But, as Creelman predicted, Cilento would obtain "their confidence and soon the D.P. program will be handed over to us. We really called their bluff. They didn't think we could do it."[76] On 27 November 1945 Cilento concluded an agreement – the first in the three zones (American, French, and British) – between UNRRA and the commander-in-chief and the military governor of the British Zone.[77] The two had proven an effective negotiating team. Creelman viewed Cilento as a "marvellous diplomat" and was "sure that no one else could handle the situation as he is doing."[78] Cilento included Creelman on his visit with military officials and allowed her complete discretion in assessing the nursing issues involved in making the transition of the displaced-persons operations to UNRRA.[79] He also made sure that Florence Udell knew that "Miss Creelman [was] most valuable"[80] during the negotiations.

The frequent picnic meals shared by the two during their travels provided an opportunity for quiet conversation that developed into a friendship based upon mutual respect. A measure of their friendship is that, while UNRRA nurses generally received a low priority in billeting, Cilento, after being appointed zone director, insisted that Creelman have accommodation in the director's house close to headquarters.

For her part, Creelman admired Cilento's vision of their work in Germany as laying the groundwork for the development of a more permanent world health organization.[81] She also respected Cilento's organizational skills and decisive nature. They shared other characteristics: both were ambitious and craved authority within their own sphere. Throughout his career, Cilento "had been the man at the top in the field. Facing now the greatest challenge of his professional life, he had no intention of being anything less."[82] The two were kindred spirits.

When Creelman and Cilento first arrived in the field, regional headquarters within the British Zone was still trying to fix the actual location of its teams. Once in the field, teams had often been reassigned by the military authorities. Locating and surveying the current nursing service in the four thousand camps located within approximately eight hundred assembly centres "was an adventure." Creelman and her staff often "felt almost the exhilaration of the great explorers" on their safe arrival back at headquarters in the late evening.[83] In the frenzied rush to get UNRRA teams into the field, too little consideration was given to individual nursing appointments or the need to supervise and support the nursing staff's work. It would be Creelman's responsibility to develop an administrative structure that allowed for the effective utilization the all-too-scarce nursing personnel and that supported their adjustment to the arduous working conditions. Their problems – workloads, shortages of supplies and transport – were acute. Ultimately, "some organization did come."[84] But before these issues could satisfactorily be sorted out, Creelman's attention was required to meet the immediate threat of epidemic disease among the displaced persons, whose health had been compromised by years of starvation and deprivation.

Lyle Creelman's steady hand would guide nursing within the British Zone right from the start. The hard work was balanced by a sense of new-found independence. Her administrative talents and skills were called upon in novel and creative ways to help her nursing staff face the formidable nursing challenges within a wide variety of conditions and practice settings that neither had fully anticipated. UNRRA nurses were expected to develop and supervise nursing programs well beyond their previous experience. Nursing practices had to be worked out by trial and error to accommodate the cultural and religious differences among the highly transitory camp population. Within the assembly centres, the team nurses supervised the sanitation of billets, living quarters, latrines, and grounds of the camps. They organized immunization clinics, isolation facilities, and the children's kitchens, while also preparing special diets and formula. They oversaw the nursing care given to the displaced-persons patients in civilian hospitals by the German nursing staff; arranged all the medical aspects for displaced persons during their repatriation; and, finally, gave basic instruction for nurses and nurses' aides from among the displaced-persons communities. Cultural difficulties complicated the day-to-day nursing routines, but perhaps the team nurses' greatest frustration was the lack of adequate transportation to carry out nursing visits to the widely dispersed and local hospitals.

Whatever their expectations of the physical hardship or professional adaptation that would be required, few nurses anticipated that they would have to work hard to gain their patients' trust. As Creelman later recounted, displaced persons were often reluctant to seek medical treatment since hospitals had gained a notorious reputation during the Hitler era.[85] Even such a simple act as offering separate care for new mothers during repatriation trips could leave the UNRRA nurse feeling like the adversary, not the healer. Mothers and fathers who had survived Hitler's concentration camps were reluctant to have a military-looking UNRRA nurse separate them from their spouses and babies yet again.[86] And all such nursing challenges were compounded when the treatment of the Jewish concentration-camp survivors became highly politicized in the wake of a scathing report by Earl G. Harrison. As General Dwight Eisenhower's special representative, Harrison had sharply criticized the army's treatment of the displaced Jewish people under UNRRA care.[87]

Belsen became synonymous with the public controversy surrounding the treatment of the Jewish concentration-camp survivors. One of Creelman's first tasks was to sort out the nursing personnel for Belsen Hospital – UNRRA's flagship hospital in the British Zone and the first one that UNRRA took over from the British military authorities. Creelman and Cilento hoped that "Belsen, if successful, can be an extremely good advertisement for UNRRA" and serve as an "excellent centre through which to stage all medical men and nurses sent to the zone." But nowhere were the tensions among the patients more strained or scrutinized than at Belsen Hospital, later renamed Glen Hughes Hospital. While Creelman acknowledged that nursing the survivors of the concentration camps required enormous compassion and adaptability, her priorities differed from those charged with their daily care.

Former inmates of Bergen-Belsen had been disinfected with DDT, scrubbed in a "human laundry," and evacuated from the typhus-ridden "Horror Camp" to a hospital organized in the barracks of the Panzer Training School. There they had come under the supervision of Matron Muriel Knox Doherty, a well-respected and experienced Australian nurse who "ran the hospital for the maimed in body and soul without orders."[88] Doherty complained about the lack of support she received from either headquarters or Chief Nurse Creelman: "The Head burst in today; her visits are never very satisfactory, always in too much of a hurry to give one a chance to discuss problems. Things must be pretty serious, I think, as UNRRA's plans have been changed and an agreement is to be signed with the Army next week."[89] Perhaps the personal tension reflected in part the inevitable differences in administrative responsibilities and priorities during the transition period – both UNRRA and Creelman still had to demonstrate their capacity to assume responsibility for the hospital. Doherty focused on the nursing needs of Belsen Hospital and, in Creelman's opinion, "worried too much about small details."[90] Conversely, Creelman was acutely aware that, in order to find additional staff for Belsen Hospital, she had to pull UNRRA nurses from the field and thereby leave teams understaffed until additional nurses arrived.[91] But, more fundamentally, Creelman believed that Belsen was adequately staffed. As she later told her fellow Canadian nurses, "This hospital had a greater number of nurses per patient and greater proportion of qualified nurses to unqualified nurses than any other hospital I visited in Germany."[92] Despite the considerable public pressure surrounding staffing at Belsen, as the number of patients decreased and UNRRA nurses left to take up other assignments, new nurses were not assigned to the hospital. Creelman had made her own assessment of the overall nursing requirements within the British Zone.[93]

While staffing levels remained a contentious issue throughout Belsen Hospital's history, the real root of the ongoing dispute between Doherty and Creelman was the decision to continue using the German nursing staff to care for Jewish patients. It had been a condition of the hospital's transfer to UNRRA that the German medical staff should be retained there and that UNRRA nurses would act only in a supervisory capacity. On one of her first visits to Belsen, Creelman recorded her impressions of the nursing care given in overcrowded and chaotic wards where "untidy, masses of clothing cluttered the beds ... Large numbers of flies were seen in the wards, in the kitchen, swarming over uncovered food and helpless patients."[94] She noted, "There has been no segregation of patients, T.B. mixed in with all the rest. The QA [Queen Alexandra's Royal Army Nursing Corps] have not done a very good job. Have shown little interest." Most of the work was done by the German and Latvian nurses, "who sleep in a large attic room over the one wing of the hospital. They are really prisoners and conditions are terrible for their living. If a little more consideration is shown to them I am sure they will respond and will carry on the nursing job with very little supervision from us."[95]

Later, Creelman could find "a word of praise for these German nurses, who gave excellent nursing care to the displaced persons under conditions which at times were most humiliating and most difficult." The very fact that Belsen was the first large UNRRA responsibility and the agreement dictated the retention of the German nursing staff.[96] Belsen earned, in Creelman's opinion, an undeserved notoriety for continuing to use German nurses to care for the concentration-camp survivors. Cognizant of the criticism levelled against UNRRA for using German nursing personnel to care for displaced persons, Creelman independently surveyed UNRRA personnel responsible for supervising the care of displaced persons in German civilian hospitals. Finding that "no instances have been mentioned that substantiate that the [displaced

persons] are not willing to go to German hospitals," she warned, "If it were necessary to establish hospitals staffed by [displaced-persons] the number of qualified nurses and nurses aides would be so few that the care it would be possible
to give would be far from adequate."[97] She never believed the claim made by
those who opposed the use of German nurses that there were sufficient qualified nurses among the displaced-persons community to take their place.

In contrast, Doherty never overcame her disdain for or mistrust of what she
regarded as the inattentive medical care of the German staff.[98] Essentially, she
could not reconcile herself to the German nurses, who had been trained "to
accept the shocking treatment meted out to the foreign slave workers imported
by the Nazis as part of this policy."[99] Every day on their rounds through the
wards, the Belsen nursing staff were reminded of Nazi cruelty whenever they
looked at the faces of their patients. All the staff spent a day at the trials of
Nazi war criminals and regularly saw members of the Belsen German nursing
staff carted off to prison for alleged Nazi activities. Nursing in this atmosphere
was more difficult for the hospital staff than Creelman realized. Moreover,
Creelman, like her counterparts in the American Zone,[100] was being encouraged by the chief nurses of the Allied Control Commission to rely more heavily
on the German nurses.[101] Doherty viewed the issue primarily from the patients'
perspective; the chief nurse did so through a pragmatic administrative lens
and as a nursing leader concerned to rehabilitate German nurses' professional
image.

Creelman also differed with her staff on the question of admissions to hospitals. UNRRA came under severe criticism for the excessive admissions among
the displaced persons.[102] Creelman told her fellow Canadian nurses that nearly
all hospitals had too many admissions on their books,[103] because many nurses
"whose sympathies were seized by stories of the sufferings of the DP's under
German rule, were easily persuaded to allow relatives and friends to remain in
the hospital with patients and at one time the percentage of 'patients' hospitalized was three times as great as could be justified on the statistics of bed provision for any ordinary, or indeed any poor community."[104] Doherty's letters from
Belsen indicate that she definitely figured among those nurses who used the
hospital as a family gathering centre.

On her first visit to Belsen, Creelman displayed greater sensitivity to the need
to balance good nursing standards with respect for individual cultural differences and appreciation of wartime tragedies, which had left deep psychological scars. Conditions within the maternity hospital, she confided to her diary,
were not nearly as deplorable as she had been led to believe: "The trouble is
that people expect modern standards. True the babies were in the same room
as their mothers, were wrapped in too many clothes but those are the custom

of the people. Also the Romanian woman Dr took the babies in her arms and loved them, but perhaps that is not as bad as we think … She was forced to kill some 5,000 babies at A – ? The terrible horror camp. After coming through such an experience one could hardly expect her to be normal."[105] Years later, Creelman recalled that it soon became apparent that there was a clash of professional views about maternal health care; the British nurses especially did not like the babies staying with the mothers, while many of these mothers, fearing separation from their babies, remained reluctant to come to the hospital for delivery for fear that this would happen.[106] Much valuable staff time was also absorbed in persuading visitors to stick to the visiting hours and stay away from the maternity wards.[107] As late as May 1946, Creelman indicated that "a great deal of time was spent at Glenn Hughes Hospital during the month to ascertain and help solve the problems of the Nursing Service."[108]

When Creelman first arrived in the field in mid-July 1945, several things needed to be done to overcome the sagging morale among her nurses and the predisposition of the military authorities and voluntary societies to view UNRRA as the untried newcomer. Creelman's immediate task was to get nursing supervisors into the field in order to standardize and support the level of nursing care being provided within the UNRRA assembly centres. The chief nurse, however, soon recognized that "each Assembly centre has its own problems and no one program can be set down. We can only work on general principles" – the most important one being that the team nurses would have to adapt to individual practice settings.[109] Creelman first appointed a district supervisor for each of the three districts within the British Zone and together they jointly selected the field supervisors who would be responsible for up to ten UNRRA teams.

Recognition of the benefits of a separate nursing supervisory echelon was achieved only after a hard-fought battle. Since many team leaders and nurses were not receptive to the idea of being supervised, Creelman knew that her choices for these supervisory positions would be crucial. One American, one Australian, and one English nurse were chosen as district supervisors. Four of the eleven initial field nursing supervisors, however, were Canadians: Lillian Rankin, Frances Pearl, Heather Gleason, and Jean Watt. In March 1946 Creelman promoted another well-qualified Canadian public health nurse, Edna Osborne, because of her "outstanding work" in a large assembly centre of eighteen thousand.[110]

In recruiting her field supervisors, Creelman selected those with a public health training background, which the Canadians – unlike many of the European nurses recruited – all had.[111] Moreover, the Canadian group had additional qualifications. Rankin, Pearl, and Watt had all been nursing sisters with the Canadian Army, Rankin was qualified in psychiatric nursing, and Osborne was a medical social worker.[112] Given the British military's initial concern to establish British control, Canadian nurses were probably more politically acceptable than their American or European counterparts. Equally, however, personalities played into Creelman's decisions. The British nurse who would replace her as chief nurse of the British Zone was passed over for a more important role. Creelman concluded that E.M. Thorne, who had not presented herself until Creelman was about to leave Iserlohn camp, "seems very nice and has done a reasonably good job; [but] she is not strong enough to move to another Corps to organize it."[113] Creelman admitted that "our ideal of mixing members of the team was really much too idealistic" but contended that she had tried to make the supervisory team "as representative as possible," so that, in the nursing conference meetings, "we can get many different views."[114] Nevertheless, the overwhelming Anglo-American composition of the supervisory echelon limited that possibility.

Creelman repeatedly paid special tribute to the accomplishments of the UNRRA field supervisors who were especially crucial in sorting out these problems of maladjustment or underutilization of nursing services that had plagued UNRRA's early days in the field.[115] Their appointments, she said, led to the better utilization of nursing staff and support for team nurses, "many of whom were not trained in public health or in the appreciation of a public health program."[116] Other UNRRA nurses' experience in both the British and American zones supported Creelman's assessment of the leadership provided by the field supervisors.[117] Creelman relied upon her supervisors to complete rapid surveys of the existing set-ups within UNRRA assembly centres, particularly the qualifications of the displaced persons "nurses," many whom she doubted were actually qualified as such.[118] Creelman's own feeling was that "the best way to improve health standards of the Displaced Persons is through the professional members of their own group," but she realized that training programs for nurses' aides would be required first. Thus, while it was her intent to retain as many "qualified D.P. nurses as possible," the operative word was "qualified."[119] Creelman maintained that the early placement of field supervisors allowed a quicker start to "the educational aspects of the program and the results have been very gratifying."[120]

Creelman met the field supervisors in person and made every effort to visit as many team nurses as possible. Her trips to the field permitted a better utilization of nursing staff within the British Zone and helped to improve the morale within the nursing brigade in spite of the hardships faced.[121] She also relied upon her supervisory echelon to evaluate every team nurse. By March 1946, Creelman had requested those team nurses who had failed to make the necessary adjustments to working in the field to resign.[122] But Creelman's concerns during these visits went beyond considering and balancing staffing levels. Time after time at nursing conferences held throughout the zone, she encouraged the early involvement of her staff in the planning of repatriation transports and especially for the concerted drive to encourage the Polish repatriations planned for early 1946. UNRRA nurses screened everyone to ensure that each was free of communicable diseases. A flight team, composed of an UNRRA nurse and two nurses' aides, accompanied the displaced persons on the journey home; other nurses joined the flying squads that assisted en route and manned the dispensaries at the UNRRA transit centres.[123] Since the nurses played key roles in the travel arrangements, Creelman maintained that nursing should have a voice in planning the health care of the displaced persons during their return journey.

At nursing conferences, she continually reminded UNRRA nurses to "assume their rightful place in the team as a large percentage of the nurses in this zone not only have their state registration but Public Health and additional qualifications."[124] The UNRRA nurse, according to Creelman, "does not work under the Doctor as is still the opinion of some Team Directors and lay people who do not have any knowledge of any other kind of nurse than one that does actual bedside nursing."[125] This was a constant concern for Creelman, who was quick to remove UNRRA nurses from situations that could be handled by nurses' aides or that underutilized their supervisory and public health skills. She transferred Heather Gleason from her position as the supervisor of a German hospital with a four hundred–bed capacity to a full-time field supervisory position when it turned out that the hospital would never have more than eighty patients from among the displaced-persons community. Margaret Inglis was transferred from her posting at Adelheide to Belsen because the Adelheide team director showed little interest in having her supervise the camp's activities from the public health point of view, instead of concentrating her efforts in the small hospital manned by Polish doctors. She transferred Jean Watt, despite reports that she had assimilated the apathetic attitude rife within her UNRRA team, because she concluded that a particular UNRRA team doctor "takes a very difficult attitude towards nursing and had no idea what it means to supervise."[126] Wherever possible, Creelman attempted to ease her nurses' transition by placing them where their specific special nursing skills could be put to best use and by insisting that they play the kind of supervisory role for which they had been recruited.

At a time when field visits were essential to improving morale, Creelman's superiors credited her with preventing "a great many resignations from the British Zone by making contact with the nurses in the nick of time."[127] Udell recommended that the system Creelman had implemented serve as a model elsewhere in Germany to address the problems of maladjustment and underutilization.[128] Her successor as chief nurse of the British Zone, E.M. Thorne, also praised her efforts: "When it was known that here was a Nursing Officer at Regional Headquarters and that she was available to the nurses, and was occupied in visiting them in their camps, interviewing their team Directors and Medical Officers, trying to help solve some of the problems that confronted them, I believed that the morale was considerably raised."[129] To be sure, while field supervision improved both morale and nursing services over time, it did not completely remedy the blurred lines of professional responsibility, especially between welfare officers and UNRRA nurses, that continued to mar relations between team members. Nevertheless, the history of the UNRRA Nursing Division in Germany suggests that Creelman had greater discretionary control than her counterparts in the American Zone.[130] Stable leadership provided by the chief nurses of the British Zone facilitated the earlier development of an effective supervisory function, and consequently resignations did not appear to be as frequent as they were in the American Zone.

In addition to two recruiting trips to Denmark and Holland, Creelman went to extraordinary measures to secure well-qualified nurses from within UNRRA. On one occasion, her request for two nurses triggered "a great deal of battling back and forth ... the battle for them had flared into one of administrative policy between the American and British zones."[131] At the same time, she remained adamant that her own raiding techniques would not be used to recruit nurses within the British Zone for UNRRA's China Mission,[132] though that did happen to a certain extent. Creelman deliberately handpicked Canadians for high-profile assignments, such as UNRRA's flagship hospital at Belsen or as trouble-shooters. She snapped up Norena Mackenzie, who did an "an excellent job" in cleaning up the unsatisfactory nursing situation in the hospital at Lübeck. A well-educated and experienced administrator, Mackenzie also had a proven track record in her two previous UNRRA assignments in Africa and Italy. Creelman's account avoided mentioning to her Canadian readers that neither she nor Mackenzie realized that the latter would uncover an appalling scandal – the UNRRA doctor was actually running a brothel! With the arrival of a new doctor, Mackenzie launched one of the first training programs for nurses' aides within the British Zone, even before the renovations at the hospital were complete.[133] Creelman repeated this recruitment pattern among the well-trained Danish nurses, "who appeared an interesting group" and who she believed would "give us good service this winter." She selected two of the most qualified Danish nurses for service with two teams run by the Salvation Army – the first appointments of this type that UNRRA made. Creelman

wanted to calm the troubled waters with the voluntary agencies upon which
UNRRA relied for personnel and relief and medical supplies.[134]

The application of modern management techniques learned at Teachers
College and refined during her directorship of the Metropolitan Health
Committee of Greater Vancouver, however, failed to address one of the most
serious issues that afflicted the operation of UNRRA's Nursing Division
in Germany. The chief nurse believed that improving the status of UNRRA
nurses was an essential part of restoring the nursing services in the war-torn
countries to a more modern footing and improving the status of the displaced-
persons nurses. But how could she argue the case for their professional recognition when it was denied within UNRRA's international nursing brigade?
UNRRA nurses held significantly lower positions in the organization's thirteen-
step grading system than other UNRRA workers, who frequently had far less
professional qualifications. The grading system was especially crucial since it
was used to determine salary levels and staff priority for transportation, housing, and other social amenities in the field. Once in the field, Creelman repeatedly lobbied Udell to press for a higher grade level for her UNRRA nurses.[135]
She expressed her outrage in a strongly worded letter to Florence Udell: "It is a
most preposterous situation that the nurses should be given only Grade 6 and
the Assistant Welfare Officer Grade 8 and the Principal Welfare Officer Grade
10. The latter is a higher grade than given to the Zone Chief Nurse."[136]

Creelman knew that UNRRA nurses' professional authority to determine the
nursing services was being contested in the field. She supported them in their
struggle to maintain their professional authority, believing it was crucial for
their survival in the field and to establish a foothold for nursing as a legitimate
profession within post-war Europe.

In both the American and British zones, there were complaints that the low
position of nurses on UNRRA's grading scale undermined their authority in the
field and contributed to low morale. In reviewing the nursing experience in the
British Zone, Chief Nurse Thorne wrote that the nurse on the team "was treated
as the most junior officer or as just the 'handmaiden' of the Doctor, without any
responsibility for planning a nursing service, as we know it today. Unless the
nurse was a strong-minded woman, the struggle was too big, and indeed quite
a few good nurses gave it up and returned to their countries, or remained and
accepted the situation, devoting their time to simple duties in M.I. [medical
investigation] Rooms under the direction of the doctors, which could have easily been performed by nursing aides."[137] When all was said and done, however,
the struggle for higher pay and grading levels for nurses met with only limited
success and did not come until late in the organization's history, primarily to
stave off the mass exodus of personnel seeking more permanent employment

once UNRRA was terminated. The ineffectiveness of Creelman and other nursing leaders within the UNRRA Nursing Division on salary and grading issues was symptomatic of the division's fettered authority within UNRRA's administrative policymaking circles. It also spoke to a continuation of the more conservative pre-war mindset towards nursing in Europe. Despite UNRRA's avowed gender equality, the upper echelons of power in the first post-war international organization remained a gendered space.

Other initiatives proved more successful. In contrast to the American Zone, a more extensive nursing education program within the British Zone began much earlier. Although intended primarily to train nurses and nurses' aides, chosen from among the displaced-persons community, to cover the nursing services required within the assembly centres, Creelman originally hoped that those graduating from the UNRRA nursing programs would continue their nursing education upon repatriation. As it became apparent that many displaced persons would never return to their country of origin, the Nursing Division shifted its efforts from giving refresher courses for those willing to repatriate to train nurses' aides to work with UNRRA's successor organization, the International Refugee Organization (IRO).[138] While greater administrative stability in the British Zone permitted an earlier start for the nursing-education program there than in the American Zone, its introduction was equally a reflection of the educational background and profound lifelong interest in teaching of its chief nurse. Creelman actively "head hunted" within the American Zone of Germany and other UNRRA missions for the Canadian nurse-educators whom she wanted to teach within the British Zone.[139]

Unable to obtain Frances McQuarrie, Creelman brought the well-respected nursing educator Norena Mackenzie to headquarters to oversee the development of nursing education within the British Zone.[140] In October 1945 Mackenzie was appointed as Creelman's deputy chief nurse, in which capacity she would continue to focus on the development of the nursing-education program for the British Zone while taking on the added responsibility of making improvements in the nursing services in some of the hospitals and sick bays.[141] Prior to her appointment, individual team nurses had often taken initiatives to give nursing instruction, despite the chaotic conditions. Although valuable, Creelman believed that these makeshift courses lacked uniformity. While the nursing leadership attempted to impose some level of standardized educational requirements, the rank-and-file camp nurses took a more pragmatic approach to prepare the displaced-persons nurses to assume complete responsibility for nursing services. In their leisure hours, team nurses began compiling nursing manuals that were "based entirely on practical experience of nursing within Germany's assembly centres, the composers having little or no reference materials."[142] Over time at zone nursing conferences, UNRRA nurse-educators, such as Mary Dunn, drew on their field experience to recommend changing the course guidelines for nurses' aides to remove those treatments never ordered by the European doctors and to include more emphasis on public health. Others also urged that nurses' aides be given instruction in dispensing simple medicines because they would be doing it with or without the training.[143] In the end, the official nursing courses still required modifications in light of actual field experience to be more culturally relevant and sustainable after UNRRA's nurses departed. Nurses on the front lines provided important feedback that refined Creelman's views. The collective experience of these nurses highlights the nascent sensitivity among UNRRA's nursing brigade to the pitfalls of applying foreign standards of nursing in cultural isolation.

The nursing-education programs suffered a better fate than other longer-term training programs within UNRRA's assembly centres that were cancelled on the grounds that they were discouraging repatriation. At least within the British Zone, nurses' aides courses were in fact opened for Polish students as a way of postponing or avoiding unwanted repatriation.[144] In more general terms, it is difficult to evaluate the long-term impact that UNRRA's medical-training programs had on restoring national nursing standards within the liberated countries to pre-war levels. Many who received nursing training would not return to their country of origin as originally expected but would instead take their skills as immigrants to other countries.

Creelman was especially proud, however, that the British Zone was the first zone to launch nursing-education courses; this was, in her opinion, "one of the most worthwhile of all the nursing activities."[145] From both UNRRA's and Creelman's perspectives, the benefit for the women enrolled in these educational programs went far beyond the nursing skills they gained. Creelman, like her successor, emphasized the rehabilitation benefits of the nursing-education programs.[146] The graduates emerged from the refresher course for nurses with a much altered attitude towards life; "they had developed community spirit, improved in manners and deportment and sense of responsibility."[147] She praised the efforts of nursing educators, "who sacrificed much personally to teach these girls, who have lived so long under abnormal conditions [without] some of the 'niceties' of everyday life which they have not known or forgotten."[148] Her goal as a nursing educator was to rehabilitate both the woman and the nurse in line with the accepted social norms of nursing as a respectable profession. Yet she also stressed that these nursing-education courses afforded opportunities both for improving the displaced women's moral and status within the displaced-persons community and for providing badly needed staff to care for their own people. Other UNRRA initiatives assisted nurses to regain the professional identity that they had lost when they were forced to abandon their homelands without any documentation. For example, Creelman supported the credentials program that would later be taken over by the International Council of Nurses; it provided a process for the thousands of nurses among the displaced-persons population, who lacked formal proof of their previous training or who had received training under UNRRA's program, to become internationally accredited.

UNRRA nursing educators' attitudes and objectives should be assessed within the organization's broader rehabilitation mandate of "helping people to help themselves" towards economic self-sufficiency and self-government after years of being subjected to Nazi tyranny. Memories of the political and social unrest fostering communism that followed the First World War still lingered. As with other UNRRA educational programs and experiments in camp self-government, nursing training and accreditation were seen by the leadership as important stages in the progression of individuals from concentration-camp victims to productive and democratically minded citizens. For UNRRA nurses in the field, by contrast, the emphasis was on something more mundane: acquiring the skills necessary to earn a living wage as a nurse became a survival strategy for displaced persons who were faced with an uncertain future of having to work within the unfriendly German economy until opportunities for immigration opened up.

Creelman's UNRRA appointment in the British Zone of Germany provided a broad scope for her considerable administrative talents. She gradually fashioned a more effective administrative structure for the delivery of nursing services within UNRRA's chaotic and internecine German field operations. Florence Udell repeatedly acknowledged Creelman's contribution to the development of a valuable nursing program in the British Zone and tried to persuade her to accept an assignment in UNRRA's China Mission.[149] The effective delegation of supervisory responsibilities, continuous trips to visit individual nurses in the field, carefully ensconced reliable lieutenants, and nursing conferences extended Creelman's administrative reach within UNRRA's highly transitory operations. Equally important, all three provided essential communication channels that began to refine her understanding of how to make the provision of nursing services more culturally appropriate and sustainable once the UNRRA nurses departed.

Creelman took great satisfaction in the fact that the Nursing Division was helping to improve the health of the displaced-persons population over time. After returning home, she defended UNRRA's record in this regard, noting in the *Toronto Daily Star* that the incidence of both typhus and typhoid was less than among the German civilian population and that the infant mortality rate was lower than in the homelands.[150] She also acknowledged the organization's weaknesses. While Creelman understood the importance of involving the displaced persons in public health work to encourage their return to independent living, she conceded, in an article written in 1947 for the *Canadian Nurse*, that it took time for UNRRA nurses to abandon the tendency of simply doing the job themselves. "As a health group, we were slow to make use of DP health committees. Perhaps because there were so few trained DP personnel. Many had suffered from so much deterioration of morale, and there were so many things that needed to be done immediately ... that it seemed easier – as it always does – to do it oneself. However, when there was time to think about it, committees were formed with gratifying success."[151] Work in the field began to refine her UNRRA nurses' professional understanding of what was required to convey nursing knowledge across cultural boundaries. Creelman set high expectations for her nurses but her success owes much to the UNRRA staff nurses themselves, many of whom led the way in adapting programs and nursing practices to the culture and training of those they had come to assist.[152]

By May 1946, as plans were being made to wind down UNRRA's operations, Creelman and her supervisors turned their attention to ensuring an orderly transition of nursing services for the "hard-core" displaced persons who would linger in UNRRA's assembly centres awaiting resettlement. The field supervisory level would be phased out and area team nurses would carry both supervisory and administrative duties for a much larger district. Supervisors briefed UNRRA nurses on their new responsibilities under the new administrative arrangements and the number of nurse's aides' courses and refresher courses was increased.

Creelman stressed the importance of regular meetings of team nurses to maintain morale during this period as camps were closed and teams consolidated. In preparation for the zone conference on the drawdown of personnel, she had drafted a plan that reduced the UNRRA nursing staff to fifty by October 1946. This plan was devised with two objectives in mind: to prepare, as quickly as possible, qualified nurses among the displaced-persons community to assume responsibility for the care of their own people, and to release UNRRA nurses recruited from countries that were all experiencing an acute shortage of nurses. It was unjustified, in Creelman's opinion, to retain personnel to do jobs that the displaced persons could perform themselves, "when our own countries have not sufficient personnel to staff hospitals and provide nursing personnel for other health purposes."[153] Creelman contended that the 260 qualified DP nurses and 260 nurses' aides, if properly supervised by UNRRA personnel, could provide an adequate level of nursing service. Recognizing that the transition would be challenging for the UNRRA nurses, she made it clear that two things needed to be done: encourage their colleagues "to cease thinking of themselves as [displaced persons]" and "give them responsibility."[154] She pointed out, however, that her scheme assumed that displaced persons would become UNRRA Class II employees; that expectation had been shattered by the field directive placing a freeze on further hiring of Class II employees. Dismayed by this development, she argued that "we cannot expect DP nurses to assume the responsibility we would like them [to] nor can we have the same control over them if they are not given the recognition required by making them Class II employees." This statement, she maintained, was based "on experience in the field throughout the past winter."[155] To have her argument carry the day, she knew that UNRRA officials needed to be convinced that the plan benefited the organization and not just the prospective employees.

Creelman, like many other UNRRAIDS, worried that her career options might narrow if she remained abroad much longer. So, in June 1946, she joined the exodus of personnel that was complicating the wind-down efforts. Her decision to leave coincided with that reached by Cilento; he was simply growing more and more out of step with UNRRA's tough line towards repatriation, especially to the London Poles who had fought with the Allies. Given her experience with the Polish community at Coventry, and later within Germany, Creelman empathized with those who did not want to or feared to return to Poland. It was one thing to offer food and provisions to those returning to Poland, it was quite another to force unwilling Poles to return home. Cilento's resignation in May most likely reinforced her decision.

Creelman had relied upon her growing network of professional transatlantic professional connections to gain an understanding of the political and social landscape that had shaped her UNRRA assignments. She took the advice offered before her departure; she did not approach her work with fixed ideas or attempt to make dramatic changes. "While she sometimes regretted the lack of uniformity in the three Corps Districts in carrying out the nursing responsibilities of UNRRA policy and questioned whether greater control should be exercised," she realized that greater uniformity and control was not feasible within a temporary international agency. It seemed "wiser to, in this type of program, permit this person to work in their own way rather than attempt too much unification which might only after a considerable period of time prove more efficient."[156] She relied upon her supervisory nurses to ensure the minimum level of uniformity necessary for the effective delivery of nursing services but adapted by drawing upon the experiences and advice of her nurses in the field. Her ability to develop and to manage an effective communication network with the field and other international agencies was crucial to her success. The establishment of the Nursing Advisory Committee, which included the principal nursing advisers of the Allied Control Commission, attested to her political acumen. Creelman had had a unique opportunity in serving as the chief nurse; she left UNRRA both a more experienced international administrator and a seasoned diplomat.

While Creelman's UNRRA service had provided her with an exceptional opportunity to work with nurses from other nations, it had also brought frustrations and challenges. In private conversation with Mary Tennant in New York en route home, Creelman was critical of some aspects of UNRRA's nursing service. She confided to Tennant that Florence Udell was "all right" but contended that English nursing methods were autocratic by comparison with those of the American and Canadian nurses. In discussing her decision not to accept the offer of further service with UNRRA in China, Creelman revealed that no information had been available about the work there. As a result, she concluded that the "health work in UNRRA had not tightened up." Claiming that "field personnel were never called in for conferences" and that "no esprit de corps had been established," she was reluctant to make a further commitment until March 1947. She made sure, however, that the RF chief nursing officer knew that she was seeking other options back in Canada but keeping the door open for international work with the future World Health Organization.[157] She trusted that Tennant would pass on more than her regards to Dr Wilbur A. Sawyer, the director of the RF's International Health Division who also headed the UNRRA Health Division.

For Creelman, the UNRRA years were a prologue to a professional odyssey that would continue long afterwards. The allure of international nursing, which offered challenging work and greater authority than could be readily achieved in either civilian or military nursing, remained. UNRRA would be a stepping stone to the international stage; she had helped pioneer new international initiatives to deal with the social-justice, humanitarian-relief, shelter, and resettlement issues that lingered long after UNRRA closed its doors. More immediately, it was the gateway to enhanced national prominence and an interesting new assignment. In personal terms, her decision to become a soldier of peace had been life changing. Although her contact with the displaced-persons population was more limited than that of the UNRRA team nurses, she nevertheless developed a deep respect for their ability to recreate their sense of personal and community identity. The faces of those lingering in UNRRA's assembly centres until permanent settlement could be found in "some hospitable land"[158] were clearly etched in her memories. Returning home with a new political lens through which to evaluate post-war Canadian society and with greater confidence to set her personal course, she joined other Canadian UNRRAIDS in seeking to liberalize Canadian post-war immigration policy, to promote a more accessible national health-care system, and to advance international peace efforts.[159]

By now, it had become abundantly clear to Creelman that international service could undermine important personal relationships. It was less clear, however, if an international nursing career could fill the void.

Chapter Five

Setting a New Course, 1946–1949

Creelman's time with UNRRA had offered challenging work that made a real difference in people's lives. With that experience now behind her, the transition from the frenzied activity of international nursing to the more sedentary pace of peacetime Canada was more difficult, both personally and professionally, than she anticipated.

During her time abroad, Creelman had become increasingly uncertain of what professional opportunities would open up or how her strained relationship with Dick Pullen would shape her future career decisions. She knew that it would be unfair to Trenna Hunter to return to her previous position. Accordingly, she put out feelers to secure international work, but, while waiting, she would have to find employment back in Canada. In retrospect, the interlude gave her time to refine her vision of modern public health nursing, sharpen her leadership skills, and expand her professional and personal connections within the North American nursing leadership. All that would prove crucial in the next stage of her career. But that still lay well in the future. In the interim she re-established her connections with Canada's nursing leaders with the goal of exploring immediate employment opportunities while keeping her name in front of those who would influence Canadian recruiting for the new world health agency. In particular, she renewed her involvement with the Canadian Nurses Association, serving as treasurer and the third vice-president.

After her return to British Columbia, Dr Murray requested that she supervise the nursing care provided for Vancouver's elderly within nursing homes and boarding houses. She found the overcrowded, ill-kept facilities disquieting.[1] Most important, the work was not challenging enough. She was therefore likely relieved to be asked to undertake another assignment, the first caseload analysis of public health nurses in British Columbia.

This assignment and her position on the CNA brought her to the attention of the Canadian Public Health Association (CPHA), then considering a joint study with the CNA to determine the scope of public health services and education required in future years.[2] The large number of military recruits who failed to pass the physical examination caused concern, as did the acute shortage of medical personnel; as these people joined the army, many areas of Canada were left without adequate public health services. The need to address personnel shortages and enhance Canadians' health provided the immediate impetus for a national study of public health practice, commonly referred to as the Baillie-Creelman Report, published in 1950.

The factors contributing to the CNA/CPHA's decision to convene the nation-wide study were in fact more complicated than suggested by the organizations' public pronouncements. Its creation and findings reflected the politics, both local and national, and the participants' individual agendas. From both Ottawa's and the medical community's vantage points, it was a propitious time for such a study. To address the electorate's growing concern that the country might slip back into recession, and to curb the rising political fortunes of the Co-operative Commonwealth Federation (which was offering similar welfare programs in its platform), the federal government began to consider a national health-insurance plan, among other social-welfare initiatives, to cushion the transition to a peacetime economy. If the Depression exposed Canada's lack of an adequate system of providing social assistance to the unemployed, the Second World War demonstrated the ability of the federal government to mobilize and regulate the economy for the future benefit of its citizens.[3] Universality, identified as perhaps the "strongest building block" of the new Canadian welfare state, was heralded as a social-leavening tool to foster "common citizenship across classes, ethnicities, and regions within the nation state."[4] Capturing the changing attitudes towards social policy that underpinned the emergence of the new welfare state, Prime Minister King told the House of Commons in the midst of the 1944 debate over family allowances that "the new order is not going to have things done as charity. What is to be done will be done as a matter of 'right.'"[5] Saskatchewan became the first province to institute a publicly financed health-care plan, and other provinces soon followed, leaving unanswered on what terms the federal government would provide the long-term financing required to sustain these new services.[6] There were also different positions on who would control any future health-insurance system. On the political front, the Baillie-Creelman Report would shore up local, as opposed to federal, jurisdiction over public health initiatives and carefully avoid endorsing particular national or compulsory health-insurance schemes.[7] As the report evidenced, the medical community, fearing regimentation and centralization, was not a devotee of the publicly funded, government-run national health-care system then being vigorously debated.

Well before the end of the war, the nursing leadership had begun work on post-war planning. The war years presented both challenges and opportunities for them. The CNA wanted to consolidate the wartime gains made as a result of nurses' contribution to the war effort and in UNRRA. In Canada, as in the United States, nursing leaders sought to use the war as a bridge to reforming nursing education and practice and to gaining a voice for nursing in the post-war reconstruction of the health-care system.[8] A nationwide study could provide the statistical ammunition to make their case for both. While public health nurses had been active participants in the long-standing debate over the direction of nursing education, that debate now assumed a new significance. Public health nursing was at an important crossroads. In Ottawa, discussions over veterans' long-term health care and, more important, a national insurance scheme that would extend hospital services to all portended significant changes for nursing practice and education, while the shift to hospital-centred patient care raised serious questions about the sustainability of community-health nursing. The advent of other health-care workers and public health clinics threatened the authority and autonomy of public health nurses' relationships with their clients within the community. Altruism and service, the core values underpinning public health nurses' role as agents of social change during the interwar years, had to be redefined to accommodate the new direction of post-war health care and the changed social attitudes that accompanied the rise of the welfare state. Creelman's election in 1947 to the Executive Committee of the CNA opened the door for leadership in advancing nursing's interests at this critical juncture.

Creelman was given a leave of absence from the Metropolitan Health Committee to undertake this CNA/CPHA assignment. Creelman knew that the past co-operation between the two groups had been qualified at best.[9] Her position as the third vice-president of the CNA ensured that body more than a strong voice in the preparatory committee's work. The CNA was adamant that this study not be considered a substitute for the broader survey of nursing for which it was attempting to secure financing.[10] A larger committee[11] defined its scope and methodology; Dr J.H. Baillie, then executive secretary to the CNA, and Lyle Creelman were chosen to conduct the field research and prepare the final report. Creelman acted as the secretary. The nursing representatives on the committee – all of whom would remain important contacts in the years to come – were Helen McArthur, director of Nursing Services of the Canadian Red Cross; Isobel Black, assistant superintendent, Victorian Order of Nurses

Canada; Helen Carpenter, lecturer at the School of Nursing, University of Toronto; and Florence Emory, associate director of the University of Toronto's School of Nursing.

The 1946 study was funded by a grant from the Kellogg Foundation of Battle Creek, Michigan, which had recently commissioned a similar survey of the quantity and types of health personnel required to meet the planned post-war expansion in hospital care within the United States. Genevieve Bixler, who had overseen the Kellogg survey in Michigan, became an important reference point for the CPHA committee's work.[12]

The "crucial link and negotiator between the Kellogg Foundation and nursing,"[13] however, was Mildred Tuttle, the foundation's director of nursing from 1944 to 1968. Responsible for the Kellogg Foundation's grant activities in the nursing field, Tuttle was instrumental in directing significant funds to Canadian projects and would become a valuable member of Creelman's extensive nursing network. She and Creelman shared similar professional and educational backgrounds. In 1938 both women had spent time in the East Harlem Nursing and Health Services project in New York City; both argued that nurses' training should be coupled with a generalized liberal education to prepare them for highly responsible roles, such as teaching, administration, and public health.[14] Tuttle's work with the Kellogg Foundation involved extensive travel in the United States, Latin America, and Canada, making her a rich source of information on nursing in those countries in the years to come.

Although Creelman's appointment began on 1 February 1948, it took several months to negotiate the study's scope and methodology before any field-work commenced. During this time, Creelman received a clear indication of how politics carefully circumscribed the selection and scope of field studies. The study committee identified representative urban and rural services in all provinces, with the exception of Newfoundland,[15] through consultation with the provincial subcommittees. Moreover, the field team was restricted to collecting information on practices of public health physicians and public health nurses; "the provincial health departments were studied only so far as the provincial policy affected the work of the physician and nurse in the urban and rural agencies."[16]

Despite all the advance preparation with the provincial subcommittees, Creelman still encountered considerable suspicion about the committee's work.[17] Many public health nurses "were jittery about this"[18] because they feared being individually evaluated. Some of the nurses interviewed undoubtedly found Creelman's direct manner and extensive nursing knowledge intimidating. Here as in UNRRA, setting the future direction of public health services would require negotiating a highly contested political terrain, often complicated by conflicting jurisdictional authorities, professional rivalries, and vested interests.

For the better part of a year, beginning in March 1948, as Creelman criss-crossed the country, she kept a field diary that formed the basis of her recom-mendations in the final report. Collectively, her diary entries paint a telling portrait of the inadequacies of the Canadian public health system and the chal-lenges experienced by public health nurses, especially in remote areas. Equally, they provide a snapshot capturing Creelman's own evolving outlook on public health nursing and the post-war transformation of public health policy. Overall, her observations reinforced long-held views on the greater preventative role and higher educational standards required for public health nurses. They also demonstrated her growing awareness of the diversity of factors that influenced the provision of public health nursing services within the provinces.

Creelman's sections of the report displayed an impressive knowledge of American and Canadian nursing leaders' research and writings. The report directly references the panel called "A Program for the Nursing Profession," convened by R. Louise McManus at Teachers College to review the quality and quantity of nursing services that would be required in the future.[19] Given Ethel Johns's close connections with both UBC and the Rockefeller Foundation, it was not unexpected that Creelman would have cited Johns's and Blanche Pfefferkorn's 1934 ground-breaking analysis of what nurses were actually doing on the job. Their definition of "good nursing" is repeated verbatim within the section of the report on the preparation of the public health nurse.[20] This defi-nition stressed the preventative function that all professional nurses should play, irrespective of their practice setting, and advocated more than a living wage and fair working conditions for nursing to be competitive as profession. The Johns-Pfefferkorn perspective served as a framework for evaluating the diversity of current public health nursing practice across the country. The goal was to formulate recommendations designed to improve public health nursing education and practice, to encourage recruitment and retention, and to ensconce nursing's presence within national and provincial policymaking bodies.

The Baillie-Creelman Report lamented that there had been no significant improvement in the ratio of public health nurses to the population served since the 1930 ratio reported in the Weir study. In short, over 1,500 more public health nurses would be needed to meet the desired ratio of 1:2,500.[21] Moreover, the lack of qualified nurses in official public health agencies, who carried the primary educational function, made that shortage even more acute.[22] Many of Creelman's recommendations dealing with public health supervision mirrored the model long advocated by the Rockefeller Foundation and aligned with her own administrative experience in British Columbia. Both predisposed her to promote modern supervision techniques to replace the old-fashioned view of the "snoopervisor" as the fundamental building blocks of a well-run public health nursing service. Not surprisingly, Creelman's section of the report stressed that "Canada lacks qualified public health nursing supervision"[23] and the necessary staff-education programs to sustain good supervision.[24] Accordingly, the lack of effective supervision was quickly identified as the major factor inhibiting the efficient delivery of public health nursing services throughout the country. That perspective triggered Creelman's stinging private criticism of the Hamilton supervisor whose failure to "talk the language of modern supervision" meant that "not a great deal would be left to the initiative of the nurses, more a case of telling her what to do rather than guiding her." She was especially critical of the supervisor's failure to make regular supervisory visits to pre-empt problems or to develop a staff-education program. As a consequence, the supervisor, overwhelmed with clerical duties, could not "see the larger picture."[25] Nor did she have the time to attend the committee meetings where health policy was set – which should have been, in Creelman's view, her key responsibility. Her field observations also substantiated Creelman's conviction that the use of well-qualified supervisors and administrators made public health nursing more attractive for new graduates[26] and led to better utilization of the public health nurses at current staff levels.[27]

While the family unit, not the individual, remained the focus of the modern health unit in Creelman's mind, she became increasingly critical of home visits where the public health nurse focused on the individual's physical condition but "did not touch on the social problems."[28] This view reflected her long-standing concern that public health nurses were simply handing off cases to social workers instead of using them as consultants.[29] In New Brunswick, as elsewhere, she found that too often public health nurses missed these opportunities because they had not kept abreast of the pertinent practices from relevant fields such as nutrition, mental hygiene, and social work: "There definitely needs to be more guidance from the provincial department nursing office. If only there could be someone appointed as Educational Director, to help the nurses keep up with the latest information in public health nursing and give them some inspiration ... As it is, more and more seems to be thrust upon them without any preparation for it, as an example, venereal disease. Now mental hygiene is being developed and they simply have not time to take on more and yet if they don't, other workers will be put into the field."[30] Her field observations across Canada reinforced a lesson she had learned in Vancouver and with UNRRA.

Proper supervision in tandem with ongoing staff education was vital to establishing clear operating parameters for nurses and other community health-care providers.

Not surprisingly, the report's recommendations, which championed the view that "the opportunities are unlimited in general public health work to help establish a healthy mental attitude in the people with whom we have contact," closely aligned with Creelman's own practice and earlier articles on mental hygiene: "There is a tendency to assume that unless an agency has a mental hygiene clinic it has no mental health program ... the public health worker in contact with the mother and child at the child health conference has an opportunity to do more for the mental health of the community than in any other way."[31] In Creelman's mind, the best clinical practice demanded that all public health nurses receive an extensive orientation in the work of the mental hospitals and, when a case was discharged, that the nurses handle the follow-up home visits. In short, she reiterated that the public health nurse should be used to the greatest possible extent as the fieldworker in the specific mental-health program.[32]

Creelman sought to identify the public health nurse's unique expertise and skills both as a route to personal satisfaction and as a tool to legitimize public health as a vital field of nursing. Despite her cool public persona, privately Creelman bristled when she observed well-qualified public health nurses engaged in routine tasks – such as weighing or measuring height – or consumed by clerical work that could have been assigned to nursing aides or, in some cases, volunteers. Even her stepbrother Prescott Creelman's tuberculosis clinic was not spared her biting criticism. The nurse in this clinic "is merely a clerical worker for the doctor in the office."[33] Over and over again, it seemed to her that, "when the nurse was assigned to a desk in out-patient departments or health clinics," she served "as an errand boy" and did "everything which nobody else seems to be responsible for."[34] After interviewing one of her former UNRRA nurses currently on the staff at the Hospital for Sick Children in Toronto, she despairingly noted, "This was a purely clerical job and not one which would be stimulating to a nurse with her degree and a great deal of experience."[35] Creelman's findings in this respect mirrored her earlier British Columbia study's conclusion that "public health workers were spending too much time on non-professional clerical work."[36] She believed that the failure to provide well-qualified public health nurses with interesting and diversified assignments went a long way to explain the low recruitment and retention levels. As important, she again linked the lack of adequate clerical assistance with nurses' inability to spend time with provincial officials, "the ones that direct policy."[37] These public health nurses, in Creelman's view, had an important responsibility to communicate the communities' changing health needs back to those responsible for setting public health policies and practices. Their failure to exercise this responsibility meant that doctors did not take nursing's assessment of public health needs and requirements into account when planning community-health services.[38]

Creelman envisioned the public health nurse's role as that "of health advisor teaching the prevention of disease" and providing a continuum of care within a community-based, generalized nursing service.[39] Time spent doing school service or home visits "in none of which any teaching was done" she considered "almost ... totally wasted."[40] Yet she was still quick to condemn public health nurses who, she believed, misdirected their teaching efforts: "What is the sense of trying to teach isolation for measles to a mother (low I.Q. often) with three children in three rooms?" At best, she contended, the effort should have been directed to preventing complications, and in this case she believed that the public health nurse's visit was redundant; the mother had already seen the family physician as well.[41] Lyle Creelman, like other public health workers of the era, was not immune to the class prejudice that related poverty to intelligence.

Her long-standing criticism of school nursing resonated throughout her diary and the report. With the exception of one rural area, she found that school services received most of the public health nurses' time,[42] thereby detracting from other maternal and child health-care programs. The former teacher believed that teachers were capable of doing much of the identification of cases, routine measuring and weighing, and health teaching. She envisaged the modern public health nurse as a consultant to the teacher, providing follow-up for cases referred to her and resources for the teaching of health classes.[43] On the basis of her experience in Vancouver, she knew that the nurses "will have a difficult time to get rid of some of these routines."[44] Indeed, her own discussions with Dr Murray during the course of the field studies shed considerable light on her past struggle to reorient Vancouver public health nursing services. "Dr Murray and Dr [Alexander] Willett, she recorded, "are very gullible. Dr Murray was more on the defensive than I have ever seen him. There was considerable discussion of the school program and routine physicals. Dr Murray thinks that these are important."[45] Creelman adamantly differed. The crux of the issue, she contended, was the failure to use teachers as partners in promoting healthy living within the schools because of the mistaken belief that they could not be trusted to weigh and measure the children or observe defects.[46] The final report therefore condemned the current practices within school services and made far-reaching recommendations that encourage a closer relationship between school health services and family physicians to eliminate many routine, time-consuming activities.[47] The voice of the young public health nurse in Revelstoke struggling to break the stereotype of school nurse was clearly discernible, even all these years later.

Creelman also challenged the prevailing medical practices in maternal and child health services. Here, as elsewhere in the report, her recommendations that implied a redistribution of nurses' functions were presented as steps to improving the efficacy of the existing health services. The idea that the easiest entry into the home was the school, in her opinion, "is no longer valid."[48] With few exceptions, she found, "health departments are unattractive places to which the average mother would hesitate to take her children or herself for health services."[49] She was appalled by the lack of privacy given mothers in many of the clinics she saw: "Must have been rather upsetting to the women to hear 'plus one', 'only fair', 'considerable discharge'" called out loudly by the doctor. She speculated that "the doctor would not use this approach with his private patients."[50] The lack of adequate maternal and child-care programs was an indication "of the 'poor relations' status of public health in the government's mind."[51] Hence, in the final report, she spared few words in noting that "in other areas where the facilities were poor with no privacy, and clinics not well organized, there seemed a tendency for such clinics to be considered charity services and were only attended in the main by low income families."[52] These visits convinced Creelman that appropriate space and clerical services be provided so that the nurse could arrange advance appointments for conferences with mothers and children.[53]

Creelman was equally critical of other outmoded policies that cast the public health nurse in the role of social police in the control and prevention of communicable diseases, especially venereal disease and tuberculosis. The final report concluded that "most of the control regulations now in existence are of no effect whatsoever in controlling an epidemic of the communicable diseases of childhood."[54] From the nursing perspective, the duplication of visits by public health officials and private practitioners to quarantined households meant that the public health nurses spent less time making other home visits that could have been of more educational value. She censored the use of public health nurses to make "defect visits" and "immunization visits," which focused on the individual patient instead of considering the family as the unit of community-health work.[55] She argued that public health nurses could not develop effective relationships if families viewed them as "social police." Their role, as she understood it, was to develop a treatment plan from the patient's point of view that simultaneously situated the patient's family within the wider community context.

True to form, Creelman did not hesitate to speak her mind during her nationwide interviews with public health officials and senior nursing administrators.[56]

In all aspects of public health practice reviewed in the report, she was quick to point out the inconsistency in public practice and lack of coordination among public health agencies that led to needless duplication of effort and consequent decrease in job satisfaction for the public health nurse.[57] The report left no doubt where Creelman stood: "The objectives of the post graduate public health training program are not to provide the community with a highly paid technician for administering immunizations."[58] She thought it a waste of time to have the nurse give these shots, especially when the physician was required to be present. Fortunately, Dr Baillie concurred with Creelman's view that the legal ambiguity on this issue should be cleared up.[59] Creelman's official stance that physicians should assume responsibility for community-wide immunization programs is understandable, given that the public health nurse's legal authority to give immunizations remained unclear. Privately, she wondered, "Why in the world can't [the public health nurse] do a simple intradermal test for scarlet fever and a little scratch for vaccination?"[60] As she knew, in rural Quebec public health nurses prescribed and sold drugs, and in other words "take the place of the doctor and are supported in this by the Ministry of Health." She cynically concluded, "Where the doctor wants the nurse to take responsibility for his own advantage, she is allowed to do it."[61] Over the course of the 1950s, these responsibilities and others would be delegated to nurses, as Creelman predicted, in response to the proliferation of new technologies, such as blood transfusion, that necessarily forced physicians to expand the scope of nursing practice.[62]

With respect to nursing education, Creelman, recognizing that university-based programs could not produce enough public health nurses to meet the acute shortage, advocated a gradualist approach stressing improvements in the public health training provided by the hospital-based nursing schools. She also favoured the expansion of clinical field placements to allow for increased enrolment within the public health nursing programs at universities. Even within the public health nursing field, Creelman never envisaged university-trained nurses replacing the hospital-trained nurse in the foreseeable future, but rather saw them as an elite cadre who would serve as teachers, administrators, and supervisors and whose expertise she never questioned would raise the overall quality of nursing.

Creelman consistently asserted that all nurses should be capable of taking part in the preventative as well as the curative aspect of nursing. Especially interested to observe how public health nurses created and handled teaching opportunities to promote healthy living, she found that, without public health training, nurses missed many such opportunities.[63] Time after time, the nurses interviewed by Creelman told her that the public health training provided within the basic three-year hospital-based program was inadequate. "Several instructors" said that they did "not have any idea of what we mean by incidental teaching. The nurses are not given this idea in the hospital and it is very difficult to pick it up."[64] Others commented that they lacked the necessary background on normal child development, nutrition, or public speaking essential to make them effective teachers.[65] Creelman urged that the basic nursing course be improved by integrating public health into the undergraduate curriculum and that opportunities for advanced public health education programs be expanded only when and if well-planned field placements were made available. Perhaps remembering her own experience at UBC, she warned, "No agency should accept responsibility for the student without a planned program (which should be in writing) and a staff capable of carrying it out."[66]

The Baillie-Creelman Report's recommendations on the preparation of public health nurses exposed the tip of the much broader debate then occurring throughout North America about the quantity and types of nurses required and where these nurses should be trained. Doubt that nursing was even a profession, combined with the lack of adequately trained nursing faculty, meant that, in the eyes of some, the inclusion of more women on campus threatened to disturb the traditional pattern of university life, without tangible return.[67] The issue would be debated for decades to come.

Common sense continued to sculpt Creelman's vision of public health nursing's future direction. She never abandoned her cardinal belief that "the ability to teach health is the foremost function of the public health nurse."[68] The report's recommendations, however, were tempered by her field observations indicating the continued need, especially in rural or remote northern areas, for public health nurses to serve as midwives and even to perform minor surgeries. While her field study revealed that "the shortage of public health nurses is both qualitative and quantitative," she always maintained that each province must undertake a survey to determine both its nursing needs and its capacity in order to plan effectively for the future.[69] Hers would not be a prescriptive approach. Creelman's extensive experience at home and abroad with UNRRA taught her that politics, economics, and culture coalesced to determine "the quality and quantity of nursing service" within a given country, province. or through an international agency in any given area.

For Creelman, the significance of her fieldwork went well beyond the written recommendations contained in the final report. In looking at current public health nursing practices, Creelman also paid careful attention to how the relevant agencies compiled and used statistics in planning nursing services for the community. Her interviews in the field more or less corroborated that "rarely is an analysis made of the collected information. A time study is useful but daily recording throughout the year should not be necessary."[70] Creelman's training

at Teachers College and her administrative experience deepened her appreciation of the political importance of gathering statistics to validate additional
funding requests and make programming changes.

Through the report, she sought to provide those responsible for the delivery of nursing services with the most current information to determine needs
and assess options. Nurses across the country participated in conducting the
activity-workload analysis included in the report. Creelman recognized that
"the value to individuals in being in on a piece of research is enormous and
a fine morale builder."[71] The activity analysis provided a national model of
how such research could be used to improve the delivery of the public health
nursing services on a cost-effective basis. More fundamentally, the technique
provided a scientific basis to reorient nursing away from those practices that
Creelman did not believe were part of the profession, such as driving patients to
the hospital or selling vitamins. Involvement in these studies, she believed, was
equally essential to develop nurses' political skills as advocates of progressive
health policy and social change.

Creelman also collaborated with the Council of University Schools and
Departments of Nursing (CUSDN) in preparing the survey sent to all universities offering a course in public health nursing. An early role model of the
nursing scholar, she doggedly pursued excellence in research at an early stage
in CUSDN's development as a vehicle to encourage nurses to think and speak
for themselves. She remained a firm believer that new approaches to nursing
practice and education should evolve from the grass-roots levels of nursing and
not just be imposed by the nursing leadership – an approach that became a
hallmark of her international leadership style. In this respect, her use of the
Baillie-Creelman Report anticipated the future direction of nursing scholarship. Although certainly not a straight-line trajectory, early nursing time-
motion studies that focused on the "practitioners, their education and specific
functionality of their work routines"[72] would evolve into a model that concentrated on patient-centred relationships. Creelman's long-standing support of
research-based nursing to improve the delivery of nursing services, and for a
collegiate system of nursing as the prerequisite for developing the skills necessary for scholarly inquiry, foreshadowed her later role as an international focal
point for the post-war evolution of what would be called evidence-based nursing care. In future years, she would look again to intra-country research initiatives within newly independent countries as a strategy to advance nursing's
voice in the development of sustainable and more effective nursing services
within those countries.

Overall Creelman's recommendations had sought to expose faulty assumptions, damaging stereotypes, and arrogant presumptions that had become
institutionalized as the way things are done to the detriment of public health

nursing. It drew attention not only to the need for better-educated nurses and better data about public health practices but also to the need to remove practice barriers. But at the same time, Creelman's recommendation illuminates the tensions undergirding the relationship of nursing and social welfare; nurses like Creelman promoted the ideal of social welfare programs but remained largely protective of their own identities. All proved enduring issues that would be hotly debated in the decades to come.

Some of Lyle Creelman's initiatives to clarify the status of public health nursing met resistance within nursing's ranks. In March 1948, at Creelman's request, the CNA had formed a subcommittee to outline the currently accepted functions of the public health nurse. Yet, even though she had cleared the way with public health officers when they had met in Vancouver in May, the CNA remained reluctant to undertake the task. At the meeting held on 18 June 1948, the issue of defining "accepted" by whom or on what authority proved such a roadblock that the subcommittee opted to use the Public Health Nursing Program and Function: the American standard recognized by the Committee on Nursing Administration of the National Organization for Public Health, the American Public Health Association, and the Canadian Public Health Association. The subcommittee thought it had fulfilled its mandate but Creelman requested that it continue to meet to provide advice after the fieldwork had been completed. At the meeting held in Montreal on 22 March 1949, the CNA's position remained unchanged: while it was "appreciative of Miss Creelman's efforts on behalf of Canadian nursing" and "very keen to assist in formulating functions for Canadian public health nursing across Canada," it believed that Creelman, "as the person with recent and personal contact with public health nursing across Canada," should formulate the tentative functions, which would then be submitted to the CNA for further study. At the April 1949 meeting, the members concluded that it would be inadvisable to attempt to formulate functions of the public health nurse until the CPHA survey with its interpretations of findings and recommendations was available for study.[73] Creelman's experience with this subcommittee illustrated the national nursing associations' limitations as an agent for change. Advancing public health nursing was not the sole item on the leadership's agenda at a time when nursing within hospitals was changing dramatically and striving to obtain an enclave within the federal bureaucracy.

At several levels, Lyle Creelman's odyssey across the country honed her art of political persuasion; excellent negotiating skills were crucial to navigating the political corridors within the multi-tiered Canadian health-care system. Moreover, Creelman's Canadian administrative career coincided with the lively discourse on social policy that accompanied the contemporaneous rise of the welfare state both provincially and federally. Two former UNNRA colleagues,

Harry Cassidy and Leonard Marsh, had influenced the creation of the Canadian welfare state. Marsh's 1943 landmark study, *Report on Social Security for Canada*, advocated federal government direction of an array of social programs dealing with housing, health, social security, and full employment. In 1943 Cassidy published *Social Security and Reconstruction in Canada*, and he would remain outspoken on the inadequacies of the Canadian social-security system throughout the 1940s. Cassidy and Marsh would remain important connections for the expatriate Canadian nurse on her visits home; both exercised considerable influence on the development of Canadian social work.[74] As important, Creelman's future employer and mentor, Dr Brock Chisholm, was appointed the first deputy minister of health in 1944, in which capacity he was expected to advise the government on health insurance; later, as the first director general of the World Health Organization, he would set an organizational tone that favoured a social approach to global health.

For many public health and social workers, it had become clear that health promotion and prevention required systems and policies directed at ameliorating the underlying determinants that undermined health. The entitlement to social services became associated with the rights of citizenship rather than charity. In Creelman's case, her elite educational public health background coupled with her public health experience within the nascent Canadian welfare state laid the groundwork for a rights-based view of global public health. In her view, public health was inextricably interwoven with human rights and economic security. Education, as always, would remain the connecting link. As we shall see, Creelman became a leading advocate for a "social approach to international nursing" that identified the socio-economic determinants of health. Her public health experience, gained within the Canadian liberal political tradition, would carry over to the next chapter of her career, when the stakes were considerably higher both for herself and for the advancement of nursing as a profession as the co-architect of global health.

The Baillie-Creelman Report epitomized Lyle Creelman's belief in the power of the written word to help the cause of nursing. According to the March 1951 issue of the *Canadian Nurse*, which every registered nurse in Canada received, the Baillie-Creelman Report awakened nurses from their complacency through its lucid portrayal of what it found and "alas! the things they did not find."[75] But how influential was the report beyond the nursing leadership? Every effort was made to publicize the report's findings. The CPHA discussed the report in Toronto from 12 to 14 June 1950. The CNA's Public Health Committee hoped that several of the nurses who had attended these panel discussions would assist with its discussions at its upcoming convention.[76] At its October 1950 meeting, the CNA's Public Health Committee discussed the possibility of provincial associations establishing study groups that would use the report as a benchmark to review current public health nursing practices.[77] It took until January 1951 to prepare and forward a study guide to all the provincial chairs, urging them to set up provincial study groups. Concerned about the limited circulation of the report, the CNA's Public Health Committee used the *Canadian Nurse* to publicize the report's findings among its membership. Eventually, several provincial associations reviewed the findings, and the statistical methodology used to compile the workload-activity analysis became the template for future studies of nursing practice.[78]

The Baillie-Creelman Report is purported to have established guidelines that would positively influence the provision of public health nursing across the country.[79] While the recommendations seem straightforward by today's standards, at the time they were considered controversial.[80] Tensions arose as public health officials attempted to reconcile the desire to improve the educational standards and standardize the practice of public health nursing with local prerogatives and traditions tied to community-based hospital schools. The influx of money required would have been significant at a time when the post-war shift to treating patients within hospitals decreased the perceived need for public health nurses and the value of community-health services. The Baillie-Creelman Report portended the medicalized conception of health, rooted in the seemingly unlimited achievements of medical progress, which caused developed countries, including Canada, to lose interest in public health systems in the decades following the Second World War. The WHO would afford a new leadership platform for Creelman to advance her views on public health – or, as it would come to be called, primary health care – but the task remained a challenging one.

Through the Baillie-Creelman Report, Creelman emerged as a powerful voice for a modern view of community-based public health nursing in Canada. Co-authoring the report raised her profile as a national nursing leader and, more significantly, established connections within the Canadian health-care community that would prove invaluable for her future WHO career. While the RF was not directly involved with the study of Canadian public health practices, Mary Elizabeth Tennant was kept well informed of the study's progress and reception. The private–public partnerships, with both the Kellogg and Rockefeller Foundations, that had characterized the development of Canadian health care at the provincial and national levels would be carefully cultivated by Creelman on the international scene. The Baillie-Creelman Report highlighted the capacity of "expert committees" to leverage scientific expertise to influence public policy. Both would become important strategies to advance nursing's international agenda. In the years to come, she would continue to use Expert Committee reports as vehicles to engage policymakers in the dialogue on nursing's future. Creelman's capacity to learn and adjust her ideas, coupled with her proven administrative prowess, earned the respect of medical colleagues at home and abroad. Her intellect, her dogged determinism, and her clear, simple, and direct language set the stage for her emergence as the voice of nursing around the world.

On a more personal level, advancing her career again took a toll. Long work weeks interspersed with a few stolen days shared with family or nursing friends foreshadowed her future solitude as an expatriate. The implicit distance from others inherent in leadership, combined with her natural social reserve and itinerant lifestyle, posed significant barriers to social intimacy during her working life. But she gradually developed a series of personal coping strategies to deal with the social isolation. She frequently spent the early mornings exploring and photographing the ruggedly beautiful Canadian countryside. Nature remained an important restorative refuge to balance her professional life. She developed a cordial professional and personal relationship with Dr Baillie and his wife. On several occasions she joined them on fishing trips before the workday began. Decisive, driven by logic and pragmatism rather than emotion, she had proven a reliable and industrious colleague. Professional and personal relationships blurred.

Her private records provide few details, but they do reveal that her return from UNRRA had been followed by a period of "frustrations & heartache" before she started work with the Canadian Public Health Association. With the fieldwork yet to be completed, she refused the first offer of employment from the World Health Organization in November 1948. But, when approached again the following April, she accepted the position as consultant in maternal and child health care. At that point, it seems that her relationship with Dick Pullen remained ambiguous; he was still dating another woman. All the same, joining the WHO, Creelman confided, had been "a very hard decision to make chiefly because of mother. Also on account of Dick. However, in respect to him, it is better that we be apart. He is very fond of me but something, I don't know what, holds him back."[81]

She left Vancouver for Geneva on 25 July 1949, at the end of a five-week summer vacation, with mixed emotions. The enjoyable time spent with Dick and her mother heightened the emotional turmoil surrounding her decision to leave. In the days to come, the physical distance from Dick made his emotional diffidence easier to accept but it did little to assuage her guilt about leaving her aging mother behind.

On her stopover in London, Lyle Creelman learned that Olive Baggallay had already left for Geneva as a nursing consultant. It would be interesting, she wrote, to see how everything worked out. Her excitement about her new position was tempered by her continued ambivalence about what the future held both personally and professionally. But her decision had been made. "Till Geneva and another new adventure!"[82]

Chapter Six

Joining the WHO, 1949–1951

On the last day of July 1949, as her plane made its final approach over the sunlit Alps, Lyle Creelman caught her first glimpse of the beautiful blue waters of Lac Léman surrounding Geneva – the city that would be her home for the next nineteen years. Recruited by fellow Canadian Dr Brock Chisholm, the first director general of the World Health Organization, Creelman was one of two nursing consultants appointed to the WHO Secretariat in 1949. Her work in this new specialized agency of the United Nations, envisaged as the permanent directing and coordinating agency for international health, would propel her career to new heights as the foremost international nursing leader in the early post-war era.

In August 1941 U.S. President Franklin D. Roosevelt and British Prime Minister Winston Churchill had issued the Atlantic Charter, a document that called for the creation of a better world – one that was free of hunger, disease, unemployment, and war. The creation of UNRRA had been the first step in honouring that pledge; the establishment of the WHO was the second. Creelman eagerly anticipated the new opportunities that awaited her as a maternal-health consultant with the WHO; to many at the time, the WHO seemed poised to usher in a new age of health blessed, in the absence of more wars, with the miracles of modern medicine. Yet she experienced an initial bout of nerves adjusting to her new life in Geneva – a city where the flower boxes reminded her of her native Vancouver but where the use of French made her profoundly uncomfortable. Her reservations about accepting the Geneva posting only deepened as she discovered more about her ill-defined role within the fledgling organization.

From 1946 until shortly after the ratification of the WHO's constitution on 7 April 1948, an interim commission had been responsible for targeting the most pressing global diseases and epidemics. The WHO had inherited the responsibilities of its predecessor: the International Office of Public Hygiene, the League of Nations Hygiene Section, and the UNRRA. The Pan American Sanitary Bureau was allowed to retain autonomous status as part of a region-alization scheme. The long-delayed, first World Health Assembly (WHA) was finally held June 1949 in Geneva, and by September the permanent organization was scrambling to find well-qualified staff to plan and carry out its work. The unexpectedly long existence of the interim commission had strengthened the candidacy of Brock Chisholm, the executive secretary since 1948, for the WHO's directorship. As for the WHO itself, its position was not as enviable. In the period leading up to its creation, other well-financed UN specialized agencies had initiated health programs interloping on what the WHO would consider its sole prerogative. There were also disturbing signs that the Cold War would have a particular salience for the work of the WHO, shaping both its policies and its personnel selection.[1]

In the year of Creelman's arrival in Geneva, the Red Scare reached new heights. The Berlin Blockade, the detonation of the first nuclear device by the Soviet Union, and the emergence of the People's Republic of China under Mao Zedong fanned the public's fears that the Soviet-backed spread of com-munism posed a clear and present danger to the democratic way of life. The Soviet Union's unexpected resignation from the WHO in February 1949[2] served notice that directing global health would not be easy as Cold War atti-tudes hardened and the nuclear arms race between the Soviet Union and the United States escalated.[3] The Soviet Union's resignation was quickly followed by the departure of other Soviet Bloc countries, which also expressed their extreme dissatisfaction with the organization's poor performance and demand for increased revenues.[4] Their withdrawal strengthened the possibility that the WHO would become entangled with the main objective of U.S. foreign policy: the containment of communism. The Cold War years signified the "promotion of a model of development aimed at repeating the evolutions of the capitalist countries" to counter the Soviet model of economic development.[5] This mod-ernization model assumed that all countries transitioned through similar stages of economic development and that injection of capital and technology, includ-ing health, could allow their economy to take off. Moreover, the Soviet Bloc's absence saddled the organization with a budgetary deficit that would constrain the breadth of its programming and left the WHO without a strong counter to the American view of Western medicine.[6]

Chisholm's ability to define a unified approach to global health was further complicated by the WHO's decentralized administrative structure. The WHO formally divided the world into a series of regions – the Americas (AMRO), Southeast Asia (SEARO), Europe (EURO), Eastern Mediterranean (EMRO), Western Pacific (WPRO), and Africa (AFRO) – but it did not fully implement this regional structure until the 1950s.[7] Politics figured as prominently as geography in determining what countries would be included in any particular region, and rivalry with the well-established Pan American Sanitary Organization (PASO) caused additional difficulties.[8] With permanent headquarters in Washington staffed by the members of the United States Public Health Service, PASO officially served as the WHO Regional Office for the Americas. In practice, however, it effectively operated as an autonomous administrative unit with considerable independent financial clout – increasingly being funded with monies well beyond those it received from the WHO.[9]

Given all this global conflict and bureaucratic politics, Creelman believed that the WHO was fortunate to have Chisholm at the helm. Others disagreed. A controversial and charismatic Canadian psychiatrist who lacked public-health experience, Chisholm was considered a surprising choice to lead the WHO in 1948.[10] The former director general of the Medical Services of the Canadian Army, Chisholm had been appointed deputy minister of health in the federal government in 1944. Since his eighteen-month tenure as the outspoken deputy minister had been contentious, both Ottawa and Chisholm were relieved by his appointment to the WHO's top position. His most recent biographer, John Farley, argues that despite the bad feelings Chisholm provoked as deputy minister of health – embarrassing and infuriating the Canadian government by public statements condemning family, school, and church that made him appear to be a godless iconoclast – he became more diplomatic once in Geneva.[11] Indeed, by the time of his appointment as director general, Chisholm had already deftly orchestrated the expansion of the health mandate contained in the preamble of the WHO's constitution. Incorporating a total concept of health as "a state of complete physical, mental and social well-being and not merely the absence of disease or infirmity," it "extended international collaboration in health well beyond previous more limited concepts"[12] to embody the belief that health, like peace and security, was indivisible. Chisholm, who exercised extensive powers as the chief technical and administrative officer of the WHO, looked to international cooperation in global health as the first prerequisite for world government.[13] Others regarded the WHO as a more restricted international instrument, designed to reduce the transaction costs of monitoring the worldwide threats of epidemics and to improve economic and social conditions to reduce the possibility of international conflict.[14]

By the time that Chisholm left the WHO in 1953, his personal philosophy and leadership style had left an imprint on the organization. Resolute, democratic, and ruthless, yet also patient, Chisholm favoured consensus over imposing decisions. Depicted by his first biographer, Allan Irving, as "Canada's first real guru,"[15] Chisholm thrived on making controversial and provocative statements designed to impel people "to think about modernity differently, to put aside past practices, superstitions, prejudices, intolerance and ignorance in order to avoid global destruction." Improving world health for him became the key to preventing world destruction. "It was nothing short of crusade for which he buckled on his armour."[16] His approach to international health reflected his bedrock conviction that economic progress and social development could not be achieved without improving the state of health worldwide – a world view to which Lyle Creelman also subscribed.

In most respects, but not all, Brock Chisholm was an ideal fit for the ambitious, independent, and equally internationally minded Canadian nurse. Both were a complex mixture of unassuming hospitality and approachability tempered by a discreet professional distance. Despite the controversies that his directorship would ignite, nursing leaders found in Chisholm a ready ally for advancing nursing's influence within the WHO.[17] Creelman in particular regarded him as a supportive colleague ready to listen and prepared to delegate leadership responsibility to his senior staff. Like others, she praised Chisholm's ability to maintain morale and lead through inspiration.[18] The two Canadians shared many common liberal humanistic beliefs and international goals that shaped their approach to promoting world health but diverged at times on the immediate steps required to achieve it.

Nursing's role within the WHO was defined within the overarching policy directives established by the World Health Assembly. In the early 1950s, as the first line of attack in combating infectious diseases, the WHO targeted malaria, tuberculosis, and syphilis, and it later expanded programming to include maternal and child health care, nutrition, and environmental sanitation programs. Underlying the public face of its programming efforts, however, was a fundamental schism within the WHO. Central to Farley's biography of "the man and the organization" is the argument that there was a deep division between those who, buoyed by the recent discovery of penicillin, DDT, and many new vaccines, "believed in the almost mythical potential of 'magic bullet medicine,'" and those who believed that, to improve health, "there was no substitute for the long hard slog of social and economic development."[19] Chisholm, a proponent of social medicine, stood squarely with the second group. He was convinced that "the causes of illness are not simply biological and physical; they need to be recognized as having economic and social causes." Social medicine, he maintained, "focuses on the entire individual and his or her milieu." Medicine must reach beyond the curative and preventative to encompass "social and industrial hygiene, mental health, rehabilitation, systems of social security and the enactment of workplace legislation."[20] In short, Chisholm and other proponents of social medicine, extrapolating from the successes of the burgeoning welfare states, underscored the need to move beyond the traditional focus on medical care and public-health interventions. For them, it was equally necessary for governments to address the added risk factors, such as poverty and economic insecurity, that contributed to poor health.

Lyle Creelman would have been aware of the competing approaches to global health and, indeed, would collaborate with several leading advocates of social medicine during her early years with the WHO. These ideas had been widely circulated and debated within UNRRA circles, and Creelman's own expansive definition of health had resonated throughout the Baillie-Creelman Report and set the stage for her subsequent endorsement of the fundamental tenets of social medicine. Proponents of this approach to global health believed first, that everyone was entitled to universal health care free of charge. Second, "disease campaigns had to be 'horizontal,' that is, directed at a broad swathe of diseases"; moreover, those campaigns required building public-health infrastructure and needed to be run by people who were knowledgeable about the society concerned. Third, "without social and economic development, efforts to eradicate communicable diseases were doomed to failure."[21] Fourth, by extension, the WHO should lead in the effort to codify the right to health through international agreements. To this end, the WHO would actively support inter-agency cooperation with the International Labour Organization (ILO), the Food and Agricultural Organization (FAO), the United Nations Educational, Scientific and Cultural Organization (UNESCO), and the United Nations International Children's Emergency Fund (UNICEF) during Chisholm's directorship.

Farley contends that, despite Chisholm's staunch support of social medicine, for a number of reasons the "magic bullet approach" prevailed. An almost unquestioning belief in the power of the new pharmaceuticals and DDT reinforced the ascendancy of the narrow technological and biomedical model of health within the WHO. At the same time, the Cold War mentality fostered a sense of urgency to demonstrate the concrete health benefits of capitalism: "In such a war, the 'hearts and minds' of people could more easily be won with rapid action 'impact projects' of DDT spraying, for example, than with projects to initiate genuine albeit necessarily slow social change."[22] In addition, Farley argues, the division of responsibilities within UN specialized agencies militated against a social approach. UNICEF, which received UNRRA's residual funds, had encroached on maternal and child health care and become a thorn in the WHO's side. Chisholm's attempt to reach out to the International Labour Organization to implement a broader social framework raised the highly charged issue of universal health care; it met with such hostility that U.S. funding to the WHO appeared threatened. "Chisholm had to play to the tune whistled to him by his political masters in the health assemblies and follow the concrete pronouncements of expert committees dealing with a series of individual diseases."[23] Thus, while Chisholm ably stewarded the WHO through successive political and financial crises, many of them created by a U.S. government that alternately demanded the organization's extinction or tried to make it an instrument of its own imperial designs, an overall public-health approach was put on the backburner. It remained to be seen whether the WHO under Chisholm's direction would "be able to weather the storms which are now brewing."[24]

Both Chisholm's biographer and, more significantly, the official histories of the WHO provide only cursory treatment of nursing's position in this struggle between the competing visions of global health and underplay its contribution to global health. That is a notable omission. Lyle Creelman spent much of her time navigating the political minefields in the WHO and receiving countries to define and advocate a social approach to international nursing.[25] Creelman's public speeches clearly enunciated her support for many of the constructs underpinning social medicine: "Without food, people cannot survive; without health they cannot win the food necessary for health; and without knowledge how to better both, they cannot improve either. Without the means of earning a decent living and without the sources for developing those means, they cannot ensure their material welfare and without material welfare they cannot achieve human dignity, or, indeed, their human rights."[26] In her opinion, " 'no man is an island.' His neighbour's sickness or his neighbour's health may mean sickness or health for him. Each of us has an inalienable right to health. But each and every one of us has an inalienable duty – our common responsibility for the welfare of our fellow men, not just in terms of our own community but the whole human race."[27] Public-health work was interconnected with the underlying determinants of health and human rights.

Just as Creelman understood the complications inherent in the efforts of competing jurisdictions of the modern Canadian welfare state to protect all of its citizens' rights to health and social security, she recognized the similar challenge that the WHO faced on the global level. She cautioned that the WHO was formed "as the servant of the people through the agencies of government. It is not a supra-national body. It cannot compel any nation to conform. Its only sanction is the respect it commands, and its authority is the value of the work it does." It demanded "the recognition of the principle, accepted and ratified by every government which joins the W.H.O., that 'unequal development in different countries in the promotion of health and control of disease is a common danger.' "[28]

An influential figure who helped shape Creelman's views on a social approach to nursing was the international statesman of public health, Dr C.E.A. Winslow, who acted as a consultant with the WHO in the 1950s. Creelman often incorporated Winslow's views on the economic and human value of preventative medicine from his 1951 WHO study, *The Cost of Sickness*, in her public addresses.[29] Well before health economics was born, Winslow pioneered an approach that recommended investing in health to roll back poverty. He argued that by preventing disease, the public health movement increased the potential efficiency of the population. He viewed disease as a cause and not just a consequence of underdevelopment. Emphasizing that most factors determining health resided outside the health sector, he articulated the need for an integrated approach to improving global health and insisted that public-health programs could not be planned but needed to be closely integrated with a broader program of social improvement. He also advocated that WHO health workers needed to collaborate closely with other United Nations agencies, particularly the ILO, the FAO, UNESCO, UNICEF, and non-governmental organizations.[30] All of these views would be clearly discernible determinants of Lyle Creelman's future course of action.

More immediately, Chisholm and Creelman differed on immediate tactics. Chisholm promoted the establishment of WHO health-demonstration areas and training centres, designed to demonstrate and develop, in relevant settings, methods of achieving a more complete realization of the WHO's mandate by working with national governments and other international aid agencies. Creelman fully supported these ideals but once in the field increasingly questioned whether free-standing demonstration centres created sustainable and efficient delivery systems for health care, especially given the limitations of the infrastructure within many of the countries receiving WHO assistance. For the moment, however, Creelman was the newcomer working in an untried organization. She needed the experience that only time in the field provided.

Olive Baggallay's and Lyle Creelman's appointments had been the first step towards implementing the 1948 WHA resolution calling for the appointment of nurses to the Secretariat. The driving force behind this resolution was a member of the United States delegation, Lucile Petry Leone, the first woman to serve as the chief nursing officer and assistant surgeon general in the United States.[31] A charismatic figure whose mantra was "Keep it simple, keep it friendly,"[32] Petry Leone would work closely on two of the five WHO expert committees on nursing with Creelman. Both adopted a practical, no-nonsense approach to nursing issues throughout their careers.

Ambitious and restless by nature, Creelman thrived in pioneering environments that offered important and challenging new work, and she was determined to secure a foothold within the new agency. Shortly after arriving, Creelman met with her chief, Dr Martha Eliot. A pioneer in children's health programs in the United States and an important architect of early post-war programs in Europe before becoming the assistant director general of the WHO, Eliot headed the Advisory Services from 1947 to 1951.[33] She had worked closely with Chisholm to have child health included within the WHO's scope of activity. The Advisory Services program, which received about two-thirds of the initial budgetary allocation,[34] oversaw the work of the expert committees and the fellowship program as part of a wider program of assistance for professional education. It provided assistance to build up national public-health services and for the tuberculosis, syphilis, malaria, and maternal and child health demonstration projects. The first meeting with Eliot did little to ease Creelman's mind: "Olive called for me and I was surprised to find that there were just to be the two of us. After tea, she [Eliot] proceeded to go over the new organizational chart that she was preparing for W.H.O. In it I could see myself set aside in the M.&C.H. [Maternal and Child Health] Section and almost completely away from nursing. I felt very discouraged. That was partly because of the strangeness, the fact that I was tired and homesick and fundamentally because I was not yet prepared to take the second position."[35] As important, although nurses were assigned to all of the WHO's projects, there was no indication that there would be a separate section with a significant administrative role in directing and supervising the nursing aspects of these programs.[36] Given her "unsettled state of mind," it is not surprising that Creelman briefly considered quitting. But within a few weeks her spirits rallied as she introduced herself to key WHO staff and came to the conclusion that she "knew more about the people and facilities than Olive did."[37] She was gaining confidence in her ability to do the job. Having ascertained that the administrative set-up was still being worked out on paper and knowing that her future prospects for advancement would be defined by those laying the groundwork, she was determined to be one of them.

Creelman had not been in Geneva very long before she came to understand that, although "the nurses have been made very welcome," they had "at some points been ignored";[38] the regional offices often negotiated directly with United Nations International Children's Fund (UNICEF) on maternal and child health-care projects without any input from headquarters. Both Creelman and Baggallay recognized that brokering nursing's interests within the nascent organization in an increasingly political, turbulent world would require the forging of strong alliances. They were up to the challenge. Once installed in their office, then housed in a little corner in the UN building, Creelman and Baggallay began re-establishing the connections among the nursing leadership that had been badly fractured during the war.[39] Creelman had strong professional and personal ties within the established North Atlantic nursing leadership that complemented Baggallay's broader ties within the international nursing network.[40] A well-respected and influential British nurse, Baggallay, who arrived in Geneva just two weeks before Creelman, had displayed great personal courage and commensurate political skill as the chief nurse with UNRRA during and after the Greek civil war.[41] She was a graduate of St Thomas Hospital, London, and had taken further courses in public health in Britain, Canada, and the United States. Both she and Creelman were Rockefeller fellows. While serving as a tutor at Bedford College, Baggallay had become the first secretary of the Florence Nightingale International Foundation, a position that she held at the time of her WHO appointment. She was especially well connected to the old guard of international nursing leaders in Europe and North America, known as the "old internationals," all of whom were graduates of the one-year advanced international course in nursing sponsored by the League of Red Cross Societies at Bedford College in London, and to American nursing leaders through her work with UNRRA in Greece and the Florence Nightingale International Foundation.[42] She and Olive compiled a list of nursing leaders whose expertise they could draw upon to strengthen nurses' voice within the WHO, either as members of its expert panel on nursing or as short-term consultants who could share their increasingly heavy administrative burden, especially in identifying well-qualified staff.[43] The selection of the forty-member expert panel members and WHO field staff was always circumscribed by the WHO's policy of equitable geographic distribution and sometimes by more overt political pressure from the member governments.[44]

An important part of Creelman's and Baggallay's efforts in these early years with the WHO involved organizing the work of the expert committees on nursing and attending international conferences. The expert committees provided the primary building blocks for attempts to advance nursing interests. Creelman would serve as the guiding spirit behind all five expert committees on nursing during the first two decades of the WHO's existence. In her capacity as the secretary to these expert committees, she was strategically placed to shape their agenda and membership.

Both Creelman and Bagallay understood that the significance of the expert committees on nursing went beyond the official reports issued. They viewed them as an important focal point in addressing the challenges presented by the new direction of medicalized care and the worldwide shortage of nurses. Outside the official sessions, Creelman solicited advice on these topics from some of the most outstanding and well-connected nursing leaders of the time and, eventually, from the new voices of nursing in the postcolonial era.[45] Moreover, since the reports of the committees were approved by the WHO's Executive Committee and reviewed by the World Health Assembly before their publication, they were instrumental in validating new approaches to nursing within the WHO's member countries and in strengthening nursing's voice, especially within the regional offices and in the allocation of scarce budgetary resources.[46] The first committee laid the pattern for its successors; it fashioned policy recommendations responsive to the new directions of health care in a manner that highlighted their advantages to both the WHO and its member governments, while simultaneously protecting nursing's rights to self-regulation and professional autonomy. Over time, the expert committees became an important transnational forum for re-envisioning nursing's international role.

When the first expert nursing committee met in Geneva on 20–26 February 1950, Creelman quickly surmised that considerable finesse would be required to broker the diverse agendas represented around the table. The committee's mandate, as stated in the *Report of the First Session* (1950), was limited to advising the WHO on measures "to ensure the recruitment of nurses in proportion to the needs of the country" and "to give nurses training in keeping with the numerous and complicated tasks which devolve on them."[47] Here and in subsequent reports, nursing leaders, however, had their own political campaigns back home in mind when they formulated their responses to those questions that mirrored nursing's uneven development worldwide.

Within developed countries, nursing leaders were under pressure to re-examine nursing education and practice from several sources. The dramatic transformation of the Canadian, American, and British health-care systems in the decades following the Second World War amplified the nursing shortage. The new drug therapies, medical technologies, and increased medical specialization raised post-war expectations for better medical care and shifted the focus to hospital-based care. The consequent dramatic expansion in government funding for hospital construction and health insurance schemes increased the demand for highly trained nurses, especially for the new intensive care and cardiac care units that were springing up within modern hospitals. These and other changes forced nursing to renegotiate the boundaries between medical and nursing knowledge and practice. As the number of hospitals and medical procedures grew more quickly than nursing schools, the shortage of nurses became more acute, leading to the training of auxiliary workers to share nursing duties in hospitals and health departments. The challenge nursing leaders and educators faced, here and on future expert committees, was to ensure an adequate labour supply to meet this growing demand without lowering the standards of the profession. At the same time, other groups – nutritionists, social workers, physiotherapists – also became involved in nursing care, further necessitating a clarification of roles. Taken together, these developments accentuated concern over the worldwide shortage of nurses and ignited a debate over the kind of education that nurses required.[48] Nursing leaders like Creelman feared that unless the nursing profession instituted changes, many "educated" young women would choose these new employment opportunities over nursing. Creelman was all too aware that other countries – either less developed or still recovering from the wartime devastation – lacked the health infrastructure or trained personnel to provide even minimal health care services. Their lack of resources complicated efforts to attract, educate, or retain nurses.[49]

To make the case for professional recognition and self-regulation of nursing, the committee's report highlighted both the worldwide shortage of nurses and the fact that "nursing is essential to the vitalization of the health programme": "When medicine is highly developed and nursing is not, the health status of the people does not reflect the advanced stage of medicine."[50] Nurses are required "in greater numbers than other categories of health workers because they have a direct, individualized and lasting contact with people, sick and well. In this sense, nurses are the final agents of health services."[51] The committee stressed nursing's curative functions and specialized knowledge rather than its "caring" function alone to validate its professional status. Having set the stage, the committee advocated the appointment of a chief nursing officer within each country to define the role of nursing within the national health-care system and to determine the types and numbers of nursing personal required. Coincidentally, strengthening the call for a CNO within national health ministries presented a tacit justification for a similar position within the WHO Secretariat.

The recommendations of the first expert committee on nursing bolstered the International Council of Nurses' (ICN) quest to establish paramount authority in setting educational standards[52] and also aimed at strengthening nursing's right to self-regulation. Founded in 1899 as a self-governing federation of national nurses, the ICN was one of the first NGOs in 1948 to be granted official status with the WHO, enabling it to speak for nurses at the UN General Assembly and to send observers to meetings of the WHO regional committees. The committee's request that the ICN continue to work on its guide for assistance to schools, establishing basic programs in professional nursing, reaffirmed the ICN's role in setting international nursing standards and as well as its authority as nursing's voice within the WHO.

The committee's discussions and recommendations closely aligned with Creelman's previously articulated core convictions. The first expert committee attributed the worldwide shortage of nurses to a number of factors, including women's limited access to education, inferior working conditions and pay, unsuitable learning and living conditions for nursing students, and lack of adequate financial resources for nursing education. Its recommendations to deal with the nursing shortage reflected the views and concerns prevalent among Western nursing leaders. In a letter to Margaret Kerr, then editor of the *Canadian Nurse*, Creelman reiterated that the real difficulty was to try to get young women "to become interested in nursing as a profession and not think that teaching, social work, law and medicine are much preferred."[53] The report echoed nursing leaders' conviction that "the elevation of standards for admission increased the number of qualified candidates for basic nursing programs."[54] Creelman's views on this score were reinforced by WHO nursing staff returning from the field.[55] The direction of nursing education was being hotly contested within many member countries. The expert committee's recommendations, however, were tailored to strengthening the Anglo-American nursing leaders' campaign to reform nursing education along the collegiate model rather than the old apprentice model, geared towards service. The move to university-based nursing education programs was designed to align the profession with new standards of nursing as experts capable of providing complex health advice. Reflecting their long-standing dissatisfaction with the nursing education offered by hospital-training schools, the report urged reorienting basic nursing education away from a "morphological and structural approach" towards a "physiological and functional approach."[56] This would, however, "require a change from the idea that nurses do *for* people to the idea that nurses do *with* people and that the nursing relationship is itself a therapeutic agent calling for insight by the nurse into her own personality." That belief, in turn, meant that a nursing student would have to be "taught by methods (active learner participation) she uses in her relationships with people."[57] Anglo-American nursing leaders believed that such a holistic patient-centred approach to nursing would carve out a meaningful role for nurses within gendered and highly specialized hospital-centred health-care systems.

Arguing for the need to expand nursing's role beyond curative services to encompass total health (both physical and mental), the committee's report similarly contended that, to be effective, health-education efforts could not function as "islands unto themselves." Instead, it championed teamwork with patients and other community-health professionals as the best way "of helping people to help themselves."[58] This was music to the ears of Creelman, who, as always, remained a strong advocate of broadening the scope of public-health nursing. The collaborative model for clinical practice mirrored that advocated to achieve global health on the international level.

Right from the beginning, Creelman struggled to reconcile the divergent nursing needs and educational requirements of the WHO's member governments. Like other North American nursing leaders,[59] Creelman had long advocated collegiate nursing education within Canada as crucial for both ensuring nursing's control over standards of practice and improving the quality of patient care. But, in keeping with her earlier observations of nursing services in Canada and abroad with UNRRA, Creelman supported the First Report's cautionary warning that "education efforts must be geared to the interest and problems of the people in local areas." Since "their traditions, culture, existing attitude and habits, ways of thinking, modes of living, education, available services and resources and related factors" all shaped nursing education's development, "no uniform international approach serve[d] the best interest of all." Rather, the real hope, the committee contended, lay "in dynamic 'local grass roots' efforts in which people are stimulated and guided to take a vital part in studying their health needs and to assume active responsibilities in solving their own problems. This process takes time, tact, patience and perseverance, and is considerably more difficult than 'doing things to people or for people.' "[60] Accordingly, the report emphasized that nurses engaging in international projects needed special preparation: "not only personal adaptation but also adapting their particular professional skills."[61] That viewpoint governed Creelman's direction of the nursing staff's work in the field. Yet, as she would learn, some nurses simply assumed that "guiding" would eventually lead to acceptance of Western nursing practices; the ideal of cultural adaptation proved difficult to achieve in the field. Indeed, there were still undercurrents of this approach in first expert committee on nursing's report.[62]

Despite the members' shared beliefs and educational background, disputes arose that required delicate handling. Privately, Creelman confided to Margaret Kerr on the difficulties they experienced in accommodating the clash of opinions over the role of midwives and licensure of auxiliary nursing personnel when the profession varied so greatly among countries.[63] The report's guarded language on this subject only thinly papered over the much deeper schism within the nursing community. The nursing leadership, preoccupied with safeguarding the public from unqualified nurses,[64] warned against relying upon auxiliaries too heavily in countries where the expansion of hospital facilities was imminent.[65] Explaining to Kerr why it was still premature to consider licensing auxiliary nursing personnel, Creelman wrote, "It is not so much the lack of teeth to grip with, to give adequate supervision, as the lack of any qualified nursing personnel whatever in so many countries."[66] She remained equally sceptical about the committee's ability to mandate that midwives receive nursing training.[67] Nurses, Creelman warned Kerr, "must face up to the fact that in countries of the world which have the greatest proportion of the world's total population, midwifery is recognized as a more desirable profession than nursing. For that reason I do not think that we would ever have midwives classified as auxiliary nursing personnel – or at least not for a long time to come."[68] Despite the fact that Canada did not recognize midwives, Creelman subsequently used the *Canadian Nurse* to urge her fellow nurses "to give some thought to encouraging more of our North American nurses to study midwifery."[69] Equally, however, she challenged midwives' assertion that public-health nurses were not qualified to supervise auxiliary midwives.[70] This would not be the last occasion when nursing leaders' attempted use of an expert committee to increase their political leverage at home exposed a rift over knowledge, skill, and identity between developing and developed countries.

It is, however, noteworthy that the WHO's Executive Committee and the WHA, in approving the report, chose to emphasize the importance of using auxiliary personnel to supplement the work of nurses, of fostering an understanding of the social and preventative aspects of modern health care, and of including preparations for public-health work in the training of all nurses.[71] Creelman and Baggallay were learning to navigate the political corridors at headquarters to reinforce specific recommendations by the expert committee within the WHO's policymaking circles. The ability to resort to common documents strengthened nursing's voice within member countries and at Geneva.

Domestic and international agendas became increasingly linked in other areas of the committee's report. For example, it gingerly approached the issue of gender imbalance within the nursing profession, making the qualified suggestion that "a larger number of men than are now engaged in nursing could be interested in nursing, particularly in certain cultures,"[72] where social convention precluded women from physical contact with males outside the family. But the committee did not miss the opportunity to highlight the "relationship of the status of women to world health and nursing in particular" or to stress that it viewed the improvement of nursing services and nursing education as a prerequisite to the improvement of the health of women worldwide. In this respect, it recommended closer cooperation with the UN Commission on the Status of Women so the WHO could "lend its support on a national and international scale to the improvement of the status of nurses."[73] As a result, when that commission met at Lake Success in May 1951, it had before it the report of the WHO's expert committee on nursing. It was the first time that nursing was an item on the agenda of the UN body.[74] Here, as throughout her career, Lyle Creelman would serve as the linchpin with other international bodies whose work influenced the delivery of nursing services throughout the world.

After the first expert meeting, Creelman could see the value of such committees for refining her ideas and, more broadly, for forging new global-health partnerships and providing opportunities to strengthen nursing within the WHO and beyond. In the process, of course, the committees justified the need for more such exercises – something that was not taken as a given at the time. Baggallay had written to Creelman expressing her frustrations with physicians' behaviour at an early nursing conference held in Uganda where they "suppressed all the working documents and all the translations before railroading the agenda, saying 'that they had nothing to consult them [nurses] about'"; the physicians also banned "any planning for group work. Result – no real conference – a lot of speeches & minutes and protocol." The one designated spokesperson for nursing was compelled to cut short her speech and then was ignored during the proceedings, except when Baggallay "forced the Chairman to call upon her." She became disillusioned and pulled "out of running the conference & I am doing that because it seems inevitable."[75] Expert committees on nursing were the first offensive in long battle for nurse-run conferences.

Creelman's attendance at the International Congress of Paediatricians, which met on 24–28 July 1950 in Zurich, only highlighted the inadequacies of nursing's voice within physician-dominated expert committees and professional organizations. Since this was the first time that nurses had been included in the congress, she was anxious that her paper on the role of the public-health nurse in the prevention of infant mortality be well received. Whatever her private reservations about the value of a conference where "we were limited to ten minutes [per speaker] and there was no translation so not all of our audience understood," her account of the congress – which was published in the *Canadian Nurse* – emphasized the positive aspects of nurses' inclusion.[76]

The first expert committee on nursing also recommended a joint WHO/ILO investigation of the working conditions of nursing, including salaries, hours, health conditions, and personnel policies. The study would consider, too, qualifications, adequacy of supervision, and problems of recruitment.[77] Some national associations contended that nursing, as a "reputable profession," should not have any connection with the ILO.[78] Finding it necessary to defend the decision to work with the ILO, even to Margaret Kerr, Creelman explained why there few other options: "I think ... the committee [members] were wise in their decision, since we do know that the ILO was planning to make this investigation anyway and it is probably better to be a joint investigation.[79] As a matter of fact, we have a very good relationship with their organization, and I really believe that, whatever is done will be in the best interest of the profession. At the same time I personally wish that nursing organizations would be more active in respect to the interest in the personnel policies of their members."[80] It should be kept in mind that the CNA had embraced collective bargaining as early as the 1940 but that very few provincial associations followed suit until the 1960s.

Creelman's definition of professionalism never precluded her from advocating better salaries and working conditions for nurses. Indeed, she would prove a fierce champion of higher salaries for WHO nurses and nurses around the world.[81] Moreover, Creelman clearly foresaw the value of strengthening nursing's voice beyond its own professional organizations so as to draw important nursing issues to the attention of the policymaking circles capable of effecting change.

Creelman's first opportunity to observe the ILO at work came at a meeting held in Geneva in mid-December 1951, which considered a broad range of topics pivotal to increasing employment opportunities for women. The delegates were provided with a detailed briefing on employment patterns and conditions for women within its member countries. Here, as in the UN's other specialized agencies, international meetings gave Creelman the chance to locate the professional development of nursing within the broader socio-economic landscape. She repeatedly impressed upon her fellow nurses that nursing's voice must be heard within international organizations to effect more fundamental change in nursing working conditions and access to education.[82] In 1957, after the ICN was included on the list of NGOs maintained by the ILO,[83] Margrethe Kruse, executive secretary of the Danish Nurses Association, was appointed to represent the ICN on the ILO committee tasked with studying the working conditions of nurses. At the time of Creelman's retirement, Kruse wrote to "thank you for many years of inspiration." She remembered "so well the help and assistance you gave me when I worked with the ILO in 1957/58."[84]

As a newcomer on the international stage, Lyle Creelman welcomed the opportunity to exchange ideas and views with leading public health officials from around the world.[85] The first year in Geneva had provided a useful orientation period during which Creelman strove to establish her own place within the nursing leadership network and to build support for an expanded role for nursing within the WHO. Given Creelman's and Baggallay's ongoing contact with the Rockefeller Foundation, and that organization's already well-entrenched nursing programs around the world, it is not surprising that, shortly after her arrival in Geneva, she and Baggallay met with its nursing officers, Mary Elizabeth Tennant and Elizabeth Brackett. Brackett, who had been the supervisor of student services at the East Harlem Nursing and Health Services when Lyle Creelman had been at Teachers College in 1939, had joined the Rockefeller staff in 1942 as the assistant director of nursing. Their friendships and common elite educational background further reinforced their shared initial view that the real challenge would be "how to develop and safeguard a professional group of nurses in those countries where the preoccupation of the day is the development of *numbers* to meet the emergency nursing needs."[86] Experience in the field would alter Creelman's initial evaluations.

While the Rockefeller Foundation supported the United Nations and its functional agencies from the beginning, it was not prepared to abandon its well-established reputation as a leader in international public health and nutrition and nursing education. Baggallay and Creelman and the RF's nursing officers quickly arranged to keep each other informed of their plans, to avoid duplication of effort. Just as important, the Rockefeller officers' extensive knowledge about the development of nursing in Ceylon, India, Iran, Pakistan, and Turkey was critical during 1950. After completing her first field assignment to Egypt, Creelman requested Tennant to change her itinerary to allow for a Geneva meeting: "She has many things she would like to talk about [the trip]."[87] As Tennant reported back, Creelman and Baggallay "appreciated MET's [Tennant's] coming to Geneva because they feel they are isolated in Geneva and have little opportunity of hearing what is developing in different parts of the world."[88] On the professional front, the Rockefeller connection proved a key intelligence corridor in other areas throughout Creelman's tenure. Rockefeller nursing officers regularly updated Creelman on the work of American nursing organizations, such as the National Nursing Accreditation Service, coordinated field trips to provide opportunities to discuss their organizations' future plans, and secretly shared confidential reports about countries where they had mutual interests. This crucial private-public partnership underwrote several joint educational and research nursing projects.[89]

In Creelman's social life, Elizabeth Brackett became a valued colleague and cherished travel companion; Lyle always looked forward to her visits to the RF's Paris office. A rare sentimental diary entry expressed her sadness on learning of Brackett's upcoming resignation in early 1951, recalling the thrill of sledding from the top of the ski lift at Zermatt and getting lost while seeking out Paris's finer restaurants.[90]

Despite the administrative hurdles, Creelman had enjoyed working on the plans for a joint research project with Elizabeth Brackett and the renowned Belgian physician René Sands, a leading proponent of social medicine and important international mediator, promoter, and coordinator of social work who revived the International Conference of Social Work after the Second World War. It would, however, take well over a year before she got the "the green light" on the study, to be conducted in cooperation with the Rockefeller Foundation and the United Nations Social Affairs Division.[91] Given Creelman's stand that public-health nurses needed to stake out their professional jurisdiction in relation to social workers in the provision of community-health-care services, it is understandable that she was intrigued by the study's mandate.[92] The two-year pilot study investigated the kind of workers required to meet family health and welfare needs in France and England. Specifically, it addressed the controversial issue of whether the community-health worker should be modelled on the *assistante sociale*, a combination nurse and social worker, or on two or more specialized health workers, as was the pattern in England and North America. Published in 1954, the study incorporated a social approach to determining the requirements of a national nursing service and, interestingly enough, presented an analysis similar to that in the 1950 Baillie-Creelman Report.[93]

By late 1950, Creelman was impatient to get out in the field. "Usual routine. Not really enough to do – probably I should get busy and make work."[94] Years later, she confided to a Canadian colleague that she had issued an ultimatum: "If I don't get out in the field, I am going home."[95] It worked. By December, she was busy getting ready to accompany Dr Dorothy Taylor, a maternal and child health consultant seconded to the WHO from the Ministry of Health in England, to undertake four weeks of intensive observation of Egypt's maternal and child health-care services.

Creelman's concern "to get out in the field" was well founded. When the World Health Organization opened its doors in 1948, most countries faced critical nursing shortages and there were a number of countries without a single qualified nurse.[96] As the WHO nurses entered the field, there were no theories of international nursing to guide their efforts to meet the overwhelming demand for nursing services in countries whose culture and rudimentary health-care systems were foreign to them. The challenge in the early days was especially daunting. Then, WHO nurses were requested as members of specialized teams concerned with malaria, venereal disease, or maternal and child health – often without Creelman's or Baggallay's input – and the appointment of regional nursing consultants within all the regional offices was still to come. Supporting these nurses in the field was critical to ensure their short-term job satisfaction and to create a cadre of "career" nurses who understood their role as WHO nurses. "Duty travel" helped Lyle Creelman to establish a key intelligence corridor with her field staff within the WHO's highly decentralized system that was critical for managing the nursing staff around the world and for acquiring an understanding of how local conditions shaped the WHO's regional nursing programs.

Taylor and Creelman's first stop would be Alexandria, the headquarters of the Eastern Mediterranean Regional Office. At the time of their visit, there were already indications of tensions within the regional committee. The following year, when Egypt barred Israel from regional committee meetings, the stalemate was resolved by a bizarre arrangement setting up two subcommittees: one for the Arab states and one for Israel. It soon became apparent that staff recruitment would have to balance these political schisms within the Middle East.

But at the time. Creelman was simply anxious to get started on their assignment. On the final leg of the journey to Alexandria, the brick-and-mud homes of the fellahin, or peasants, provided her with an instant reminder that "in spite of every facility being put at our disposal," it would be "not easy for us to obtain an adequate background of information on which we were expected to be so bold to make an evaluation of certain of the health services."[97] Nonetheless, that is precisely what she did.

There was little choice; the situation was dire. With fewer than 1,000 nurses in Egypt to meet the needs of 19 million people, it was impossible to reduce infant mortality rates that some said reached as high as 400 per 1,000 births. Creelman identified several factors that retarded the development of Egyptian nursing: the limited educational opportunities for women restricted enrolment, and cultural inhibitions against caring for the physical needs of patients meant that the status of nursing was not attractive to better-educated Egyptian women. Creelman was told of cases where nurses had their servants attend to the more menial duties of patient care, or where the *hakima*, nurse-midwife, sent out to assist in a home delivery would wait in the car until the servant ascertained the progress of the labour! She believed that, to overcome these cultural barriers, the educational experience needed to be changed. Only by ensuring proper ongoing supervision could Egyptian nurses and nurse-midwives be imbued with "the spirit of service which is an inherent part of nursing."[98] Cultural sensitivity was not always easily accommodated when it contravened what Creelman considered the core value of nursing practice.

Her recommendations attempted to reconcile the immediate demand for expanded nursing services and the longer-term development of the profession in Egypt. Here, as in most of the Middle East, midwifery was held in higher regard than nursing. Although dismayed to learn that under the current system it took five years to qualify as a nurse-midwife and that a public-health nurse required additional training on top of that, she identified the root of the problem as the "so-called schools of nursing." "If instead of trying to service the whole hospital the foreign personnel had been employed for training students using only the number of beds needed to supply the clinical practice," Creelman argued, "by now there would have been better qualified Egyptian nurses willing and able to accept responsibility on their own."[99] As a first step, Creelman recommended the establishment of a small demonstration hospital, staffed by well-qualified and experienced nurse-educators, that was financially independent and associated with hospitals only to provide the necessary clinical experience to train nurses in both curative and preventative aspects of nursing. She knew full well that "this would not relieve the shortage of nurses in a hurry, but it will do more than any other thing to attract a better educated girl and show that nursing is really a worthwhile and satisfying profession."[100] In planning future nursing education, Creelman believed that raising standards would make nursing more attractive to well-qualified young women; doing so was a challenge everywhere but especially so "in a country where the emancipation of women is really only now taking place."[101] At the same time, she recommended changes to improve the educational experience within hospital-training schools, as well as a postgraduate course in public health to nurses trained within the existing system and refresher courses for *hakimas* to bring them up to date in preventative nursing. Recognizing that raising the educational standards alone would not address Egypt's critical nursing shortage, Creelman stressed the importance of raising salaries for nurses to the level of those of other professional women in Egypt, the appointment of a chief nursing officer within the Ministry of Health, and appropriate nursing legislation to control registration, examination, and practice. All were aimed towards improving the status and self-regulation of nursing – strategies necessary to attract and retain nurses over the long term.

While the majority of her recommendations clearly bore the imprint of her own North American education and administrative experience, those supporting the continued training of auxiliaries contravened the mainstream opinion within the established Egyptian nursing service. The controversy foreshadowed what would be a continuing debate in the expert committees on the role and training of midwives and auxiliaries for many years to come. Creelman had begun to realize that both midwives and auxiliaries were needed permanently, not as short-term solutions to the worldwide shortage of nursing personnel. Recommendations typically combining long-term planning with more immediate measures to improve the quality of existing nursing services became the hallmark of her international work. Many of Creelman's recommendations on nursing services in Egypt would be reiterated in the report of the first expert committee on nursing. Perhaps it was her own uneasiness at being expected to set out a plan for the development of nursing in Egypt after a short visit that led to the inclusion of the section in that report dealing with the preparation of nurses serving overseas.

Laying the groundwork for the future development of nursing within the WHO presented exhilarating challenges, if one possessed the diplomacy, patience, and self-sacrifice needed along the way. Helping nurses communicate across borders to identify common grievances and, once these disagreements are identified, acting as an effective broker to clarify and integrate them not as zero-sum propositions but as achievable goals required more time on the job. The evolution of sustainable and culturally sensitive nursing programs developed only gradually; it could not happen without the development of a larger cadre of internationally experienced WHO nurses and, in many cases, the education of national counterparts with whom they could collaborate. It also required new initiatives that reached beyond the nursing leadership to encourage the lively exchange of resources, people, and ideas across borders at the local level. Baggallay and Creelman still had their work cut out to lay the foundations for a more transcultural approach to international nursing, within what Creelman like to call the "fast developing countries," during WHO's first development decade. But they were heading in the right direction.

Chapter Seven

Establishing the Nursing Section, 1951–1952

The year 1951 proved a turning point, both for Creelman and for international nursing. It was then that something she and Olive Baggallay had adamantly fought for – the creation of a Nursing Section within the WHO – came to fruition, with Baggallay as the section's chief nursing officer. Although officially her rank was public health nurse, Creelman functioned as Baggallay's deputy. The nature of her job did not change in its essentials, but the responsibility increased. Her promotion broadened her personal and professional horizons, setting the stage for her to assume the top position three years later.

The early 1950s were hectic as Baggallay and Creelman, working as a team, strove to put the Nursing Section on a sound organizational footing while endeavouring to meet the insatiable demands for assistance that crossed their desks daily. As the WHO settled into work, the budget rose from $5 million in 1948 to $8.5 million in 1954; the staff increased from 250 to 850.[1] Other challenges were emerging too. From 1950 to 1953, the Korean War drew greater attention to Cold War politics, heightening suspicion of further state intervention in medical or health services as "communist" and diverting funds towards increased defence spending. With all of this in mind, Baggallay and Creelman had to tread carefully as they went about their work, keeping the focus on nursing's role and responsibilities while remaining sensitive to the larger international context in which nursing operated.

The two nursing leaders carefully crafted both the agenda and the composition of the second expert committee, which met in Geneva on 15–20 October 1951. The committee was to consider "the contribution of nursing services in meeting health needs" and "the preparation of nursing personnel with special reference to those areas of the world where they are scarce or not immediately available."[2] It was also to examine the preparation of nurses for international service. Both Baggallay's and Creelman's first-hand experience in UNRRA reinforced their awareness that nurses did not shed their national identities upon joining the WHO.[3] Fostering a culturally sensitive and politically neutral viewpoint among the WHO's transient nursing staff would be one of their greatest leadership challenges.

Tehmina Adranvala, chief nursing superintendent, Directorate-General of Health Services in New Delhi from 1948 to 1966, and an "old international," was chosen as the committee's chair. Norena Mackenzie, Creelman's former deputy chief nurse in UNRRA and then the educational director at the Montreal General Hospital's School of Nursing, was its rapporteur. Given the committee's mandate, both were well suited to their roles. Meanwhile, although the selection of committee members from the expert panel on nursing had to be geographically balanced, there were no restrictions on the consultants chosen – and Creelman regularly took full advantage of that opportunity, to include nurses with the specific expertise required for the committees' work. These committees worked long hours, and at times tempers flared, whereupon considerable diplomacy was needed to prevent Lucile Petry Leone's "aggressive manner" from dissuading others to offer their opinions or from embarrassing Norena Mackenzie.[4]

While the second expert committee was more geographically diverse in composition than the first, eight of its members, including the chair, had ties with the Rockefeller Foundation.[5] Yet their presence brought first-hand knowledge of health problems in Brazil, Turkey, and other developing countries to the table. Moreover, the committee's mandate justified Creelman and Baggallay's request that the four existing regional nursing advisers attend the meeting in Geneva – and that, as it would turn out, happened infrequently during Creelman's era, since any travel authorization required the regional directors' approval. Early on, Creelman looked for ways to include regional nursing advisers in policy discussions at WHO headquarters, with the aim of providing uniform guidance for their supervision of the WHO nursing programs and of getting their feedback to improve them.

The committee's report heralded the gradual transition towards a more culturally diversified view of international nursing but still stressed professionalization through the raising of educational standards and state regulation of accreditation.[6] It built on the work of the first committee's report.[7] According to the committee, effective and efficient nursing services required that nurses be trained for specific functions they would be called on to perform, placed at appropriate levels of decision-making within the health-care system, and incorporated into health teams with a complete understanding of their roles in achieving the teams' overall health goals. It emphasized the need to collaborate with national nursing organizations so as to develop guidelines for state accreditation of both nurses and auxiliary personnel – a topic skirted in the earlier report. While the committee's public discourse stressed the need to protect the public's safety, the theme of regulation spoke to nursing's professional aspiration of distancing itself from auxiliary personnel.

The committee's findings reflected nursing leaders' desire to define more satisfactory professional and personal roles relevant to a modern health-care system. Its cautionary note that, above all, nurses must demonstrate "the human understanding, which is the essence of their contribution"[8] indicated nurses' ongoing struggle to preserve the notion of service and compassionate care within a modern health-care system in which new medical therapies and technologies centred in the hospital increasingly occupied centre stage. The new direction of post-war health care – away from private duty and public health nursing towards hospital-based medical care – also eroded nurses' individual social altruism and forced a reassessment of nurses' civic duty within their communities: "Her efforts should be directed towards stimulating community movements of a social, economic, or educational kind by working with lay leaders, clubs, and other social groups."[9] Defining an acceptable social stance for nursing in the Cold War era, epitomized by the anti-communism hysteria of McCarthyism, posed considerable risk. Viewed together, the committee recommendations melded the desire for social justice felt by nursing leaders with the professionalization of advanced nursing education with the hospital's needs for improved management of clinical practice, while preserving a veneer of social and professional respectability acceptable to both the public and the medical profession.

Many of the recommendations aligned with Creelman's own approach – one increasingly refined by her duty travel. The report stressed the importance of establishing a well-coordinated, community-based public health program that considered the local conditions in preference to ambitious building projects, as well as the need for long-term plans to develop a professional nursing workforce even while taking steps to provide immediate personnel. The regional nursing advisers were well positioned to validate the report's wisdom in this regard. Before the committee began its deliberations, the four regional advisers present, Agnes Chagnas, Elizabeth Hill (Western Pacific Regional Office – WPRO), Doris Pedersen (Southeast Asia Regional Office – SEARO), and Eli Magnusson (Eastern Mediterranean Regional Office – EMRO), reviewed the problems in their regions with their colleagues. The committee repeatedly heard of the success of public health nurses who reached out to the wider community and, conversely, their failures when local customs were ignored. In North Borneo, to avoid the gastrointestinal problems that often proved fatal, WHO nurses expanded their demonstration of the preparation of local food for babies to include local schools and indigenous midwives. In India, nurses in the malaria-demonstration teams had sought the assistance of the village headman, an initiative that "opened the door to a wide campaign of health teaching."[10] Village committees were created, the team helped build school latrines, and the health visitors worked with the local committees and schools in teaching rudimentary health rules along with treatments for simple ailments. The report viewed these as concrete examples of "helping people to help themselves." Creelman, as we shall see, supported using demonstration teams as bridgeheads to more broadly based community-health teaching along these lines. However, as Tennant noted, this approach avoided the real issue facing the committee: "the impossible task of trying to cover so much territory."[11]

The report addressed Creelman's growing concerns about the WHO's nursing education programs and its recruitment and orientation practices. Although nurses chosen by the WHO for international work were experts in their field of nursing, the report cautioned, "they have to be prepared for the impact of a different culture ... Nurses selected should have the capacity to appreciate cultures other than their own and an ability to adapt to local customs. They need a sensitive and imaginative approach to human relationships."[12] The committee recommended ongoing orientation, involving both the international organization and the recipient country, to ensure that nurses developed "a sympathetic understanding," allowing them to adapt their teaching and development of nursing services to the "sociological pattern of the country."[13] Yet, as Creelman repeatedly saw during her duty travels with the WHO, even the most carefully designed orientation could did not eliminate those whose motivation or personality precluded them from making a valuable contribution.

The report issued a strong warning that curriculum development in "areas where nursing is in the early stages of development" must at all costs avoid the "temptation to adopt a curriculum which has been prepared for other cultures ... it may be of little use and even a hindrance to acceptance of a more realistic programme."[14] The committee's recommendation of greater WHO support for educational institutions such as the All-India Institute of Hygiene and Public Health – as a training centre for both regional and international health workers – recognized the need for local control to ensure that regional needs and disease patterns were adequately addressed. The committee also looked to the ICN to update its 1949 booklet *The Basic Education of the Professional Nurse*, to ensure "that educational preparation shall keep pace with the changing needs of nursing services."[15] Once again, taken together these recommendations attempted to bridge the divergent requirements of developing countries and Western nations, where the nursing leadership placed greater emphasis on international standards and accreditation to advance nursing's professional agenda. Balancing the quantity and quality of nursing services remained a fundamental challenge during Creelman's career.

Reflecting on the work of the committee, Tennant questioned whether "this is the best way to prepare such important reports. A week is a short period to try to state essential problems and to set forth principles to resolve complex problems in all areas of the world. The order was far too large and too general."[16] While Creelman was certainly aware of the committees' limitations, she understood the opportunities they presented. Despite their limitations, the expert committees on nursing would continue to be an important venue to work out the conflicting perspectives over knowledge, skill, and identity that arose along the widening global north-south divide. They provided one of the few forums available to raise important nursing issues within decision-making circles in the physician-dominated WHO. Moreover, nursing leaders continued to look to recommendations from an "an authoritative body such as the expert Committee ... to strengthen their hands with their respective governments."[17] In addition, their social gatherings at the end of the workday served as platforms for building important relationships with representatives from the International Refugee Organization (IRO), the Food and Agricultural Organization, and the International Red Cross (IRC), while also providing the Nursing Section with networking opportunities among its geographically dispersed senior nursing staff.

Finally, the expert committees lobbied for more specialized committees or regional conferences, such as that on nursing education attended by Creelman in Geneva from 24 March to 5 April 1952.[18] During her home leave in late 1951, Creelman had recruited Kathleen Leahy, professor of public health nursing at the University of Washington and president of the Board of Directors of the American Journal of Nursing Company,[19] for assistance with the preparations for this conference. Although the two worked closely together, the conference's emphasis on a social approach to nursing and its format – designed to encourage broad participation – bore Creelman's imprint. Each nurse's summary of nursing education within her country was circulated before the conference. The agenda reflected the interests identified by the group, and each member took a turn presiding.

The talks focused on "the kind of nurse that is needed in all parts of the world." The conference participants' preferred educational strategy, known as the situation approach, combined the theory of nursing and previous experience to determine the best patient care. Moreover, since it incorporated the principles of psychology, sociology, and anthropology as well as nursing to gain a holistic understanding of the patients' background and needs, the situation approach was also well suited to adapting nursing principles to the cultural and socio-economic conditions within a specific country.[20] This was essential, in the participants' opinion: the "constant evolution of nursing services which results from general economic and social development, makes the organization of nursing services anything but static and abolishes all rigidity in the training of nurses."[21] Creelman would certainly have agreed with the fundamentals of an approach that stressed the underlying determinants of population health.

The discussions again mirrored ongoing concerns in Western countries over the scope of practice, professional responsibility, and consequent type of education required as nursing became more specialized and concentrated within hospitals. As nurse-historian Geertje Boschma notes, nursing leaders reacted to increased rationalization of hospital nursing care by redefining it "as a method, emphasizing the integrity or totality of the individual patient." A "pragmatic method of problem-solving was incorporated into this new definition of nursing as process, in which the needs of the patient were identified and the nurse was invited to assist." Increasingly, Western nursing leaders focused their attention on a holistic approach to hospital-based patient care to create professional space within the gendered medical hierarchy of hospitals rather than in the public health nursing community.[22] Creelman's brief journal entry noted, "Conference over. Very successful."[23] According to Ellen Broe, the Danish director of the Florence Nightingale International Foundation, there was wholehearted agreement among the nurses on most matters. The "principle of demonstration and of application in all teaching process in the school of nursing was very much stressed and patient-centred nursing care was felt to be essential."[24] Others were more critical, noting that the attendees may have been too uniform both in their composition and in their professional preparation and experiences to allow a wide-ranging discussion of problems with which they were unfamiliar: seven of the nine had done postgraduate work in countries with similar patterns of nursing education.

Planning and attending conferences continued to take up much of Creelman's time throughout the year. She was especially delighted by the invitation to attend the UN Casework Seminar held in Keurusselkä, Finland, on 21–27 August 1952; the seminar was to focus on in-service education and social casework. It provided a much-needed respite from the Geneva office while allowing Creelman to observe Finland's nursing services for the first time.[25] Her enthusiasm dissipated once the conference began.

Though quick to condemn her conference group leader as "washout," Creelman was in fact irritated by her own performance. Her first talk failed to convince the delegates that public health nurses were qualified to address mental-health issues and conduct family counselling. Public health nurses, they told her, were not trained to deal "with feelings ... [their task was] just weighing the children and discussing feeding." Typically, she left convinced that "it is the fault of nursing if sw [social workers] take these appointments from them."[26] Many public health nurses initially responded to this threat in a negative manner and clashed with social workers in the workplace. While never doubting that social workers potentially infringed upon the public health nurses' broader role and authority among clients and communities with whom they interacted, Lyle Creelman increasingly concluded that this non-collegial behaviour in the workplace was counterproductive.

Her second talk at the Finland seminar, on the common features worldwide of in-service training in public health nursing and social welfare, challenged the rivalry between the two professions: "Some of this is good but when this rivalry is based upon misunderstanding it is not healthy and it can easily be prevented."[27] After emphasizing the shared professional challenge to "help people help themselves," she pointed out that the public health nurse's responsibility, "of encouraging the patients to become more self reliant, to become more responsible for his own health," was not fully acknowledged by social workers. "It was recognized," Creelman told the audience, "that the preparation for any field of nursing must include the public health and social aspects."[28] Then she deftly extolled the benefits that public health nurses received by consulting with social workers: "The social histories had improved, there was a better understanding on the part of the nurses of the treatment recommended, and a better interpretation on their part to the parents. There were fewer cases that were not followed up ... The public health nurse has learned from the social worker how to improve her interview technique ... [and] more of the importance of human relationships," and "the patient and community are best served by an integrated generalized approach to health."[29] Citing a leading authority on in-service training within the social-work field, Catherine Manning, she added an effective twist in her closing remarks to illustrate the commonality of purpose behind in-service training for both professions. Quoting Manning, she told her audience, "I think that we might say that in-service training is an indispensable part of agency and staff development; that it should be broadly rather than narrowly defined; that it must be continuous; that leadership must be strong; that staff planning and execution is essential; that method and content must be fluid and geared to the movement of social work itself." Creelman suggested that her listeners simply substitute "public health" for "social work": since "the same principles apply, the same needs exist."[30] Delighted that her talk "had been clearly delivered and understood by the foreign group," she left encouraged by the overall future direction of European social workers: "They will not if they can help it fall into the error of too great a specialization in social work" – as had been the case in North America.[31]

As her talks to the UN seminar demonstrated, Creelman's speeches and writings frequently relied heavily on research drawn from broadly based social-science sources outside nursing to gain a hearing for nursing's viewpoint within the wider international health community. For her part, credibility and respect was exactly what she earned as, over time, she prepared to assume the mantle of the voice of international nursing as the WHO's CNO. In this regard, duty travel remained key to establishing her growing international reputation.

By early 1951, Brock Chisholm had informed his staff that they would have to "resign ourselves to more duty travel."[32] For Creelman, though, duty travel was not a burden but an essential part of her work, one that strengthened her reservations about some of the WHO's health initiatives.

Creelman had already cautioned that "as a World Health Organization, we cannot hope to do more than point the way which will, over a period of time, bring about improvement in infant mortality rates and in general health conditions. Above all the thing we must avoid in nursing is to try to force our western patterns on other countries as the pattern to be followed. It no doubt has many principles, which can be adapted, but each country must build on what they have now and develop to meet its own particular needs. If we can in some small way help them to do that we will have done much."[33] She questioned whether the WHO, by moving too fast and by imposing top-down technologically dependent programs, was building health infrastructures that would be too costly to sustain without permanent international aid. Instead, Creelman was more convinced that health programs should have started on a smaller scale and with the involvement of the local people.[34] She consistently warned against the error of over-specialization that many Western nations had made; instead, she preferred training local community health workers to do a range of services including tuberculosis or venereal disease case findings.[35] In her view, for example, the long-term nursing aspects of the malaria teams' work had not been thought through carefully. She acknowledged that the WHO nurses played a vital role in gaining the confidence of the local people to obtain the blood smears crucial for the malaria surveys; nonetheless, she argued less qualified auxiliaries might have been given the responsibility for taking the blood smears, thereby allowing the public health nurses to train additional local public health personnel. She questioned whether the WHO's malaria-prevention teaching would prove "very lasting" without any local community health personnel trained to carry on the work once the WHO team withdrew.[36]

Determined to help nurses within the developing countries in designing their own national nursing services, Elizabeth Brackett and Lyle Creelman had worked hard with a former UNRRAID and well-respected American nursing leader, Margaret Arnstein, to draft a practical guide that would help all seventy-three countries to survey their national nursing resources.[37] Recognizing the difficulty of preparing one guide to cover all these countries, Creelman insisted that the four existing regional nursing advisers try the draft guide out with their national counterparts and then provide Geneva with feedback on its usefulness.

During 1951, Creelman visited Greece, Yugoslavia, the United States, Central America, and Scotland to attend conferences and to view nursing's setup in these countries. With hardly enough time to catch up in the Geneva office after attending the International Council of Women's 1951 Athens Conference, Creelman left on 22 April 1951 for a twelve-day visit to Yugoslavia. Creelman's observation in the *Canadian Nurse* that "never have I enjoyed such hospitality or drunk such fine Turkish coffee ... one would never guess that it is very strictly rationed"[38] suggests how orchestrated her visit really was. After Tito openly broke with Stalin in 1948, Western nations took a more favourable view of his "communist" but "independent" regime. It is still striking, nonetheless, that Creelman publicly praised the virtue of a socialized system of health care amidst the Cold War. She came away from this trip with impressions of a people "filled with the spirit of enthusiasm to rebuild their country which suffered so much during the war years" and remained confident that the health ministry would work out a long-term plan to achieve its ambitious goals.[39]

In July 1951 Creelman embarked on the next leg of duty travel, this time to Central America, interspersed with some home leave late that year. Given that the Pan American Health Organization (PAHO) operated as a virtually separate administrative unit that seldom forwarded detailed reports on its nursing activities to Geneva, Creelman used the trip to Guatemala to strengthen her contacts with the WHO's and the Rockefeller's senior nursing staff. This opportunity was all the more imperative since Creelman could not use her Canadian nursing connections to garner information about the American Regional Office. The Canadian government, which viewed the PAHO as an instrument of American foreign policy, had refused to join the body; instead, Ottawa communicated with Geneva directly.[40]

On this trip, Creelman had a rare opportunity to assess directly the work of the nursing staff. In Guatemala City, she dropped in for part of a six-week workshop on administration, teaching, and supervision, sponsored by the PAHO and left convinced that the workshops were more valuable and cost-effective means of giving "more nurses the opportunity of learning how to solve their own problems" than could possibly done through fellowships.[41] This conviction would be embedded in the report of the second expert committee on nursing and dispels the view that the WHO nursing leadership unquestionably favoured international fellowships in the early years.[42] Later, while visiting

the School of Nursing of San Juan de Dios Hospital in San José, the capital of
Costa Rica, Creelman formed a favourable impression of the Portuguese WHO
nurse Fernanda Alves Diniz.[43] She later praised the former RF's teaching efforts
there in the *Canadian Nurse*. Undaunted by the overcrowded wards, where frequently recently delivered mothers shared beds, Alves Diniz had found a spot
in a corner to set up a makeshift teaching room – showing a level of initiative
that Canadian nursing schools should emulate.[44] The visit formed the basis for
an enduring personal and professional relationship that would ultimately lead
first to Alves Diniz's appointment as the regional adviser for Europe (1954–66)
and then to her return to Geneva to join the Nursing Section staff.

Typically, Creelman's schedule on this trip continued to be hectic, with work
often spilling over to the evenings. The evening that Tennant hosted a dinner on
the terrace of the Antigua hotel overlooking the Aguas Calientes volcano, however, passed too quickly. As the sounds of the marimba band filled the pleasant moonlit evening, Creelman delighted in the conversation with Dr Nevin
S. Scrimshaw, the founding director of the newly formed Institute of Nutrition
Central America and Panama (INCAP), whose groundbreaking work on nutrition and pregnancy in Panama had led to his appointment in 1949. At the time
of Creelman's visit, he was searching for solution to kwashiorkor – an almost
always fatal disease afflicting young children with a lack of protein in their
diets. His guiding principle – of building nutritional programs rooted in locally
produced lower-cost foods – left a lasting impression on Creelman. As she later
travelled throughout Africa and India, where disease caused by malnutrition
also ran rampant, her diary often recorded how these problems could have
been prevented by a shift to local produce. The efforts of the WHO's nurses
to address malnutrition by relying on local produce later were featured in the
technical reports of the expert committees on nursing.

In El Salvador, Creelman had her first opportunity to see the joint WHO/
UNICEF Bacillus Calmette-Guérin (BCG) team in operation. Certainly, by the
time of her visit, she would have been aware of the controversy swirling around
the WHO's decision to undertake mass immunization programs using the BCG
vaccine against tuberculosis.[45] The Americans were raising serious questions
about BCG's reliability and effectiveness in protecting against the disease. The
American medical community espoused a very different and more expensive
medical protocol "of watchful waiting," which was heavily weighted towards
treatment using the new antibiotics in American-style sanatoriums. But the
BCG program was particularly attractive to war-devastated European countries
that needed an immediate and affordable solution to an immense public health
issue. For the WHO, BCG seemed the only answer.[46] Creelman gave no indication that she questioned the effectiveness of the BCG program at the time, and
BCG has since been accepted as standard care for tuberculosis prevention.

For Creelman, "the visit in Central America came to an end all too quickly" but nonetheless created an indelible impression. Writing about her trip in the *Canadian Nurse*, she contrasted the uphill battle the organization confronted in overcrowded and economically deprived Central American countries with the wealth of her own native land. The vivid disparities in the standard of living led her to implore, as she had after her return from UNRRA, that "even at the risk of lowering our standard of living, which inevitably we must do if our population is increased to that which Canada can support, we must open our doors to the people from countries which are so overcrowded and over-populated."[47] At the time, however, few Canadians were prepared to liberalize Canadian immigration policy if there was any hint that newcomers would take away Canadian jobs or become a burden to the state.

Early in 1952, Creelman was off to Asia for a conference of the WHO's SEARO and duty travel in Burma, India, and Ceylon. As this visit approached, she grew uncharacteristically ambivalent about it. Work at the office had piled up as plans for the conference moved into full swing and staff wrestled with the knowledge that "many policies" would "have to be worked out before we have [a] smooth relationship"[48] with the regional director, Dr Chandra Mani, the Indian deputy director of health services. In 1952, India had been the first country to formulate a national family planning program, which was later expanded, to include maternal and child health. Her initial concerns about Dr Cicely Williams, then the maternal and child health consultant in India, weighed on her mind as well. Creelman feared that Williams would "continue to dictate re: nursing in S.E. Asia" and "make rash judgments and we will have difficulty."[49] Williams, the first woman physician to be appointed to the British Colonial Service, was a formidable figure. Imprisoned by the Japanese while serving in Singapore during the Second World War, she used her extensive knowledge of protein deficiency to save her fellow prisoners' lives. After the war, she helped develop a simple sweet drink that saved thousands of children's lives from "vomiting sickness" caused by ackee poisoning. But as Creelman correctly surmised, she was never happy at a desk planning an overall approach.[50] Deep down she knew there was no option but to go. As she admitted in the *Canadian Nurse*, travel gave her a perspective on the difficulties and complexity of fieldwork that was not possible from views acquired from her comfortable armchair in Geneva.[51]

The trip began in Burma, a country simultaneously grappling with the ravages of Japan's wartime occupation and the overwhelming political and economic challenges posed by its newly gained independence from Britain in 1948. Met at the airport by a lorry and five armed guards, she discovered that visiting the health-care facilities well outside Rangoon in the beautiful hill station at Taunggyi required special permission because of communist insurgent activity. Even once back in the riverside capital of Rangoon, when she found time to climb the gold-leaf staircase leading up to the famous Shwedagon Pagoda, work was always on her mind. She contrasted its opulence with the enormous health problems plaguing Burma's impoverished people, who, at Taunggyi as elsewhere, were housed primarily in bashas made of bamboo. She knew: "They need many trained personnel, doctors, nurses, midwives, sanitary engineers, and health educators, who will live in the villages and teach in the native language."[52] More immediately, the Burma team had pressing personnel and leadership issues that required her attention.

Creelman's frustration of being sidetracked by personnel problems instead of devoting her time to "policy matters and planning" resonated in her private correspondence to Olive Baggallay. She admitted that "probably many of the statements [in her report] should not have been made and some of them were modified later, but the writing of them did relieve my feelings at the time."[53] Her first impressions – "this is quite a situation ... the need for nursing leadership is obvious" – remained unchanged. After listening to all sides, the corrective action required gradually crystallized in her mind during the visit.[54] Creelman acknowledged that the team's problems derived in part from the government's political and financial struggles, but equal culpability, she soon discovered, lay with the WHO's nurses. Their demands for major renovations to their residence had created enough personal animosity with Daw Suu Aung-San, widow of the revered leader of Burma's fight for independence after the Second World War, that future WHO initiatives were at risk. Creelman admitted her own shock during a visit to Mandalay "when I saw how primitive the bathroom facilities [were]" but realized "that these people probably think us most unreasonable when we ask for these things that we consider as minimum for comfort."[55] Aung-San "certainly did not want any more nurses until the accommodation situation is corrected."[56]

By the end of the visit, Creelman had concluded that the WHO needed a more reliable selection process centred on in-depth interviews. The WHO VD nurse felt totally ostracized from the other public health nurses and complained "that she had never been in such a situation and was very worried by the lack of professionalism, the behavior and the continual gripping."[57] This team, she wrote, probably had "more than its share of problems but there are certainly three who are not really here for the purpose of the professional development of Burmese nurse[s] and are not pulling their weight."[58] After hosting a private dinner party for all the nurses, she was left with the clear impression that their "primary objectives in being in [the] WHO are based on female instincts and not related to professional nursing. They are out for a man."[59] The visit had also strengthened her conviction that cultural adaptability must become an essential selection criterion: "I am more than ever impressed with the need for our personnel fitting into the cultural pattern of the country, even at great personal sacrifice to themselves. Some of the team had not done that" on the job.[60] Creelman expressed concern that the WHO nurses socialized in expatriate circles to which few Burmese nurses had access: of the three clubs WHO nurses frequented, "only one has a color bar [but] few Burmese go to the others."[61] The racial tension had spilled over to the workplace. Aung-San had reprimanded the WHO nurses for their behaviour towards their Anglo-Burmese matron. Aung-San contended "that the reasons the WHO nurses do not pay as much respect and courtesy to [the matron] is because they probably consider her as only Anglo-Burmese."[62] Creelman concurred with the WHO nurses that Aung-San's reluctance to delegate authority over recruitment or programming equally undermined the matron's authority.[63] The matron's consequent "insecurity," both socially and professionally, led to Creelman's negative appraisal of her leadership: "She is not a very alert or intelligent appearing person."[64] Geneva's CNO's attitudes were not without contradictions: the individual professional performance, whether of the WHO nurses or their Burmese counterparts, remained the primary lens for Creelman's assessment of field operations.

Indeed, Creelman found other aspects of the WHO's nursing program in Burma equally disturbing. In evaluating the Burma program, she again distinguished between those WHO nurses "who [carried] on as at home" and those who "were doing some very practical teaching applied to the situation here."[65] She expressed "no doubt that this and all the other places are much improved since our people came." But the weakness, in her opinion, remained that "changes had not been made as a result of very much thinking on the part of the local group."[66] Before leaving, she encouraged the team to get together to discuss the public health nursing aspects of the WHO program and urged that their meetings include the European Advisory Commission (EAC) and BCG nurses in order to co-ordinate their agencies' work more effectively. They should, however, "not forget that what they decided in their meetings was not to be considered as the plan for Burma; the Burmese nurses must be brought in for this."[67] In the years to come, Creelman consistently repeated this message in conversations with the WHO's field staff.

Since many of these projects were designed as demonstration projects, she believed, building local competencies was crucial to their sustainability once the WHO team left. She could not help contrast the WHO's efforts to that of other aid agencies she visited. Her daily diary praised a Goodliffe mobile health project located in a community composed of six to eight hundred bashas housing up to two thousand people, many of them refugees from the insurgent areas: "The leader of voluntary group is a man who apparently has some private means and a genuine interest in the welfare of the people. They have regular meetings and they even have a MCH [maternal and child health] committee. They are planning to build a permanent clinic. This is a real 'grass roots' and I hazard will outlast the EAC project we saw the other day," that had no Burmese counterparts involved in their planned community project.[68] Creelman remained a strong proponent of "helping people to help themselves" on the terms set by the community involved. The Burma trip served as a case study for Creelman of the WHO's top-down implementation of health care and its failure to focus on sustainable practices or coordinate its efforts with other international aid agencies.

The Burma visit did little to improve Creelman's negative view of SEARO's regional nursing adviser, Doris Pedersen; the New Zealander's demeaning "scolding tactics" only compounded her tactical error of viewing the nurse-educators and public health nurses as separate groups. Creelman had failed to persuade her that public health should be integrated into all of the WHO's nursing programs or of the value of nurse-led team meetings. Pedersen's leadership deficiencies, in Creelman's view, reinforced the lack of coordination not only within the Burma WHO team but also with other international aid workers. In contrast, Creelman met with EAC aid workers to ensure that the timing of a request from the EAC health mission did not undermine the WHO's ability to secure a senior nursing adviser to the national government. In the end, she concluded that "if I had not been here this meeting to try to unify [the team] would not have taken place and there would have been no discussions about WHO activities in general."[69]

Other meetings with Burmese officials to encourage the inclusion of more public health training "fell on barren ground." Perhaps, she realized, "it was too much to expect an acceptance of this idea in these countries where every minute of the students' time is needed for service."[70] The visit confirmed her opinion that a country-based nursing adviser was required to bring about gradual change and curb doctors' tendencies to plan without consulting the nurses. But she was realistic enough to know that the timing was not right, especially after she learned that Aung-San had already told the minister that she did not want an adviser and would not reverse her decision. Instead, Creelman suggested sending Ruth Ingram, an experienced nursing educator and administrator who had been born into a missionary family in China and had later obtained her master's degree from Teachers College,[71] as the leader for the WHO team – but only after she had determined Ingram's acceptability to Aung-San. Typically, her upbeat account of the trip in the *Canadian Nurse* gave no hint of the difficulties that plagued the WHO's effort in Burma – perhaps because it, like all her articles, was screened by the WHO before publication and a negative account would have done little to aid her recruiting efforts in Canada.

The concerns raised during her Burma visit only intensified in Creelman's mind after she arrived in Delhi to begin an extended inspection of the WHO's nursing programs in India, another country of extremes. The opulent wealth of the Taj Mahal resided uneasily alongside poverty, dirt, unsanitary conditions, famine, and disease in a society "where nursing had not found its feet."[72] India had about 9,000 nurses to meet the needs of 380 million, as compared with 250,000 nurses in the United States serving a population less than half of India's.[73] Prime Minister Nehru used an effective strategy that interspersed Western fears of India as a source of contagious epidemic disease with India's entitlement as a new nation to modern medical science and technology.[74] The appeal was an effective Cold War strategy to gain aid from Western governments. Between 1948 and 1958, the WHO ran twenty-two nursing projects in India, representing 15 per cent of all its projects worldwide.[75]

Almost immediately after her arrival, Creelman was informed that the Delhi project was in jeopardy because of the government's failure to fulfil its obligations. She was given the impression "that Point 4 and the Colombo Plan[76] [other international aid programs] are hovering around like vultures waiting for WHO to step out so that they can step in."[77] Her staff's suspicions appeared justified as Creelman later discovered that the Indian government had requested two nurses under the Colombo Plan without any consultation with WHO representatives, even though the WHO was already installed in the hospital. Creelman simply "[could not] understand this lack of co-ordination."[78] Politics at all levels stifled progress. Matters were further complicated by the WHO's Regional Advisor Pedersen's willingness to request additional personnel that were not part of the overall nursing plan for the country. While nursing needed to be represented on the planning bodies, Creelman remained in "an uncertain mind whether to push it or not" because she thought it unlikely that "Doris [Pedersen] is going to be guided by any nursing policy other than her own."[79] In Creelman's estimation, being "very friendly and a good mixer in groups" did not compensate for Pedersen's inability to set long-term regional nursing plans.[80] More fundamentally, Pedersen simply did not share Creelman's line of attack. Whereas Creelman stressed slow, proper planning and laid emphasis on training local personnel for public health work, especially in villages, Pedersen favoured a more specialized approach: "As I anticipated when Dr G. Mettrop, the Public Health Officer, Regional Advisor, wrote up the meeting of the previous day with Dr Warner, he put down that two international nurses were required. No amount of persuasion on my part would make either he or Doris relent. It is a difference in concept, instead of going in and working with what is there, they want to push our standards on them as quickly as possible."[81]

For similar reasons, Creelman strongly disagreed with Pedersen over the WHO's current policy favouring international fellowships for study in more advanced health-care systems instead of regional fellowships for study within that country or a neighbouring one where the disease patterns and clinical experience would be more relevant.[82] Moreover, when she proposed holding a regional nursing conference because it would benefit a wider group of Indian nurses than sending a few nurses overseas to study, Pedersen remained unconvinced and argued, incorrectly, that Dr Mani would not support such a conference. Even when the regional nursing conference had been agreed upon, Creelman believed that "Doris will need a lot of help because I don't think she has the foggiest idea about it."[83] Creelman wanted the nurses from the countries involved to set the agenda – an approach clearly different from Pedersen's top-down style of leadership.

Creelman observed that Indian nurses worked and lived in dreadful conditions, often without support from the medical community, which regarded nursing students as cheap labour. Moreover, nursing challenged the prevailing social customs rooted in the carefully delineated hierarchy of the caste system, which relegated contact with bodily fluids to the untouchable caste and which disapproved of women providing intimate care to male strangers or working and travelling outside the home. The continued usage of the term "lady home visitor," designed to cloak the public health nurse's activities with the veneer of social respectability, reflected the prevailing social customs. The problem Creelman saw with "attracting the better class of girl is that she has never been taught to do anything in the home. And with the non-Christian at any rate it is beneath her dignity to do menial tasks. It will take time to overcome this."[84]

There were times during her visit when Creelman saw the advantages of local customs that appeared strange to Western eyes. While visiting Haldwani, an extremely wet area where malaria was all too prevalent and where thousands of refugees were being resettled,[85] she visited a young Hindu mother and her new-born, both of whom, according to local custom, had been removed from the family home and relocated in a hut in the garden for fourteen to forty days after the birth. In this instance, she saw that the local practice provided emotional support and protected the mothers' health: "It allows the woman, who normally works long hours and carries heavy loads on her head, to have a period of rest. It also keeps the baby from contact with many diseases and infections during these first weeks of its life."[86]

Creelman believed that maternal health practices must accommodate local traditions based upon indigenous knowledge that reflected local customs and values. However, she took the attitude, one still adhered to by the WHO today, that some maternal health-care practices, such as applying cow dung to the newborn's umbilical cord as was widely practised in India, should be discouraged because it increased the risk of neonatal tetanus. Other traditional practices were beneficial and should be promoted; others based upon local superstition could be ignored, if they did not endanger the mother's health.[87] In describing the local midwives, or "*dais*," Creelman told her Canadian readers that since they had "inherited" their profession from their mothers, aunts, or cousins, "their technique is questionable. They have little idea of asepsis."[88] In recounting WHO nurses' tales of maternal health work in countries in which women must veil the body from strangers (purdah), she explained that often the WHO nurses were often not allowed to assist in the delivery because it was the custom that the native dais cut the cord. Moreover, they knew that asepsis technique was followed only when they were present. She went on to explain that "these people will not allow the cord to be cut until the placenta is born as they have a weird belief that if it is, the placenta will choke the mother."[89] Even for Creelman there were limits to cultural adaptation; nursing's core ideal of caring sometimes required changing cultural attitudes over time that prevented a nurse from providing the best care possible under the circumstances or from choosing nursing as a profession.

In other areas, Creelman could initiate more immediate change. She determined that, in the future, headquarters should play a more direct role in senior nursing appointments within the regional headquarters. In their final meeting, Creelman let Dr Mani know that "I did not think he was getting as good nursing advice [from Pedersen] as he should be – that planning was not very good – that, after all, most of the planning had been spotty and it would not be fair to criticize unduly."[90] Here, as elsewhere, WHO projects involved a complex negotiation process to overcome powerful physicians' resistance. It would take several years to bring Mani around to her point of view.[91] Doris Pedersen's contract would not, however, be renewed at the end of her current term.

During her stay in India, Creelman endeavoured to strengthen India's chief nursing superintendent Tehmina Adranvala's voice within the WHO's policy-making circles. Creelman had worked closely with this outstanding British-trained Indian nurse and chief nursing officer during the second expert committee on nursing. While it seemed strange to Creelman to see Adranvala in a Western suit – perhaps Creelman underestimated the pressure Adranvala felt to gain acceptance as a modern woman within the medical community – the two quickly got down to business. Promptly identifying the need to involve Adranvala and other national counterparts more closely in the actual planning of projects, Creelman invited the Indian nurse to accompany her to Ludhiana, the largest city in Punjab. She insisted that Pedersen "bring Mrs Adranvala into the picture both in the initial planning and making the plan-ops."[92] Wanting to avoid a repeat of situation where a WHO nurse had been injected into a school without consulting the matron, Creelman suggested that a team leader be sent in first to work out the details of future projects with the local group – a suggestion Adranvala heartily supported. Creelman carefully listened to, and enthusiastically included in the operations plan, her Indian colleague's recommendation that greater emphasis be placed on refresher courses and staff training than on the introduction of more specialized nursing services. In exchange, she received Adranvala's support for her plan to focus the clinical experience on wards that were less overcrowded and better equipped. This would not be the last time that Creelman used an official WHO visit to strengthen the political and professional prestige of a CNO within her country.

On the trip to evaluate the Ludhiana project, Creelman quickly surmised that nursing in the local hospital associated with the Christian Medical College needed strengthening: "Miss Dennis [the matron] is a dear old lady and would be cooperative but has not much idea of nursing education, or of administration ... There is no staff education. The Sister Tutor is of the old school type ... She does not seem to have any plan for an educational level."[93] The hospital was understaffed because of the low salary levels.[94] Yet she concluded that a new nursing project was warranted for a number of reasons: the hospital facilities were to be enlarged, the medical community had a demonstrated interest in improving nursing education, including refresher courses, and the planned expansion into rural community work offered a real possibility of learning what the local needs really were. Equally, Creelman appreciated the need to build effective working relationships with local officials to enhance future nursing programs.

The Ceylon visit during the first week of March proved just as unsettling, since Pedersen again seemed prepared to exclude well-trained local counterparts. Creelman, in contrast, believed that "it would be fatal, of course, for a foreign person to be brought in when these Ceylonese girls have been prepared and are ready to take over."[95] When Creelman noticed that many Ceylonese nurses seemed insecure, she encouraged the WHO nurses "to work slowly and give the Ceylon nurses the security they needed" and "do everything they could to get the [Ceylonese] nurses to discuss their problems."[96] Over and over again, she had found it necessary to remind her staff that their primary function was to build local competencies and capacity.

Creelman met with Elizabeth Brackett of the Rockefeller Foundation twice during the trip. Towards the end of February, the two friends spent the evening in Delhi "swapping experiences and impressions." Just as important, Brackett gave Creelman advance warning of the requests for WHO assistance that she was likely to receive.[97] By the end of the trip, when they again met both nurses were at the same stage: "very confused about it all and finding it difficult to remember what one has seen and where."[98] Their field observations left little doubt of the·challenges their organizations faced in improving the quantity and quality of Indian nursing services.

As the time came to return to Geneva, Creelman was left dissatisfied with what she had observed. The SEARO trip illustrated the limits of her diplomacy. While she championed a more bottom-up approach to involve local nurses in the planning of nursing services on a horizontal basis, she encountered considerable opposition from doctors and some WHO nurses who wanted to impose a Western model. Unsettled issues within SEARO would demand her return to the region in mid-November 1953.

Creelman's expanded responsibilities opened the door to a career that was rewarding and empowering but, at the same time, emotionally, mentally, and physically challenging. She dealt with long hours in Geneva and on duty travel and contended with complex nursing problems without adequate resources. Her work demanded great empathy and, simultaneously, required maintaining enough professional distance to gain a level of insight beyond what could be provided by her own staff. Creelman had her own prescription for self-care, built upon a number of personal coping mechanisms – humour, physical recreation, hobbies, and travel. For her, relocating to Geneva meant making a new set of friendships in midlife. Over time, she forged enduring bonds with other single, well-educated, ambitious women whose professional aspirations for a more autonomous and rewarding career drew them to international work. Their friendship helped these expatriate women to define personal and professional space within the gendered community of global health workers, where physicians' influence dominated.

Shortly after Creelman's arrival in Geneva, Helen (Mardi) Martikainen[99] began her twenty-five-year career as the chief of health education of the Public Health Section. Sharing many common professional perspectives and challenges, the two women quickly became friends.[100] Both, in their different capacities, would be pioneer leaders in the effort to gain greater acceptance of health education as a vital part of the health-care system,[101] and both were devoted to identifying and developing indigenous leadership within the countries they visited "to help them help themselves." In her early days in Geneva, Creelman had needed somewhere to live in a city where accommodation was scarce and expensive. Martikainen provided the answer. Together, they rented a delightful apartment in Geneva's old town. Upon taking occupancy, however, they discovered that it needed a thorough cleaning and painting, which was a problem, since neither spoke French well enough to hire a painter. The two rolled up their sleeves and worked until well after 3 o' clock in the morning finishing the job themselves! Their friendship extended beyond the office; Helen proved an equally amiable travelling companion.

On a car trip in southern France to one of the charming but undiscovered Îles d'Or, Île de Porguarelle, Lyle and Helen enjoyed the fruits of the wine harvest and basked in the sunshine of its famous silver sandy beaches. One would have thought that, after all her duty travel, road trips would not have been Lyle Creelman's choice of a way to relax. But they were. She relished swinging her large Mercedes away from Geneva to explore the historic towns and enchanting villages within Switzerland and bordering countries. She delighted in trying new regional foods, such as crêpes and raclette, always carefully paired with fine local vintages. But sharing a rustic meal during an outdoor excursion was equally appealing to the native British Columbian.

Throughout her Geneva years, Creelman regularly escaped from the cares of the office by travelling to the surrounding mountain villages. Adventurous as always, she threw herself into new outdoor activities. Over the 1951 Christmas holiday, she joined Marjorie Bradford, a well-respected Canadian social worker and former UNRRA colleague who then worked with the International Refugee Organization, on a skiing holiday in Zermatt. As she recounted her alpine adventures to her stepbrother Prescott, "I used to do a bit of cross country skiing at home but thought that I would put that sort of life behind me when I came here. Apparently the outdoor life is still in my blood so I might as well give in."[102] Creelman frequently went hiking at the foot of the massive limestone mountain range of the Dents du Midi, or explored the trails from the village of Zermatt or around Champéry-Planachaux. But she particularly admired the beauty of the Engadine valley (St Moritz), known for its sun-filled landscapes dotted with lakes everywhere.[103] When time permitted, she and her friends made regular pilgrimages in June to see the bright pink alpenrose, edelweiss, and orchids at their peak. In late fall, the crystal-clear air beckoned her back to photograph the fabulous red and golden hues ablaze in the mountain meadows. Spurred by the physical challenge involved in completing difficult ascents, she often led the way for others and chided herself on the rare occasion when a noonday beer allowed Baggallay to capture the lead. On these outings, she could shed the formality of the office, sharing wine, fondue, and laughter with friends as they plunged into the cold mountain lakes even when they forgot swimsuits. These personal friendships, formed from a shared international purpose, provided a much-needed antidote to an ever-busy, ever-changing daily life. But Creelman needed longer periods away from the office, and from strenuous duty travel, to prevent burnout.

The WHO's home and study leaves were designed to permit staff members time for both professional and personal renewal. In most instances, Creelman's professional itinerary infringed on her private time with family and friends. During her 1952 study leave, she took up an offer to teach "Current Nursing Trends" at the University of British Columbia, believing that it "will be an excellent experience for me so think I should accept the challenge." Given her own appraisal – "would do it differently another time" – the course could at best be judged a moderate success. Yet, at the time, she contemplated teaching in a university after her work with the WHO was over.[104] Life within a university community gave her the time to read widely and engage in lively discussions with friends in the nursing faculty and leading social workers, such as Leonard Marsh from her UNRRA days. Her stay in Canada drew to a close all too soon.

Back in Geneva, it was time to reflect on the past and plan for the future. Creelman had used the expanded opportunities for duty travel and work related to the numerous expert committees to extend her sphere of influence within the worldwide nursing network, to form her own assessment of the WHO's current nursing program, and to envision the kinds of changes that would be needed in that program in the years to come. She had also sharpened her political skills and deepened her understanding of how to frame issues important to nursing in such a way as to gain a hearing within the WHO's decision-making circles. In the field, she had begun to understand the complexity of her leadership role as a social advocate connecting the highest policymaking levels to those who would advocate and implement new directions at the ground level. Field trips permitted her to identify and mentor international nurses, sometimes from outside WHO staff, for senior positions or to act as consultants.

The administrative challenges of running the Nursing Section were as all-consuming as ever. But no one was better acquainted with these challenges than Lyle Creelman, particularly when her stint as deputy chief of the Nursing Section culminated with her advancement another step higher in the WHO's organizational hierarchy. Her real work had just begun.

Chapter Eight

From Deputy to Chief, 1953–1960

In 1953 there was a changing of the guard at the top of the WHO, with Brock Chisholm being succeeded as director general by the Brazilian Marcolino Gomes Candau,[1] who would retain the post for twenty years. Whether pushed or simply disillusioned by the politics of the Cold War, and worn out by the years of struggle to achieve his ideal of global health, Chisholm had little interest in another term.[2] Creelman renewed her contract only after learning of Candau's appointment: "There could not have been a better choice," she wrote.[3] Creelman had become acquainted with Candau in 1950 after he joined the Secretariat. Within a year, he was appointed the assistant director general in charge of Advisory Services, a post he held until his appointment as assistant director of the WHO's Regional Office for the Americas in 1952.

Others agreed with Creelman that Candau was "ideally suited for the job." There was "no doubt that the United States was much happier with Candau in control than it had been with Chisholm"; his election initiated "a friendlier relationship between the [Pan American Sanitary Organization] and the WHO than would have been possible" with the former director general.[4] His appointment marked a shift towards an increasingly vertical approach to health and development along the lines advocated by the United States. In 1955, Candau was charged by the World Health Assembly with overseeing the ambitious malaria eradication campaign, conceived in the unbridled enthusiasm in the ability of widespread DDT spraying to kill mosquitoes. As American medical historian Randall Packard has argued, the United States and its allies believed that global malaria eradication would usher in economic growth and create overseas markets for U.S. technology and manufactured goods.[5] Designed to stabilize friendly democratic regimes, it would also win the "hearts and minds" of the local population in the war against communism. "This model of development assistance fit neatly into the US Cold War efforts to promote modernization with limited social reform."[6] At the time of his appointment, however, the Soviet Union and its satellites accepted Candau's neutrality and returned to the WHO fold. "The Soviet Union also wanted to make its mark on global health, and Candau, recognizing the shifting balance of power, was willing to accommodate."[7] In 1959, with considerable backing from the Soviet Union and Cuba, the WHA committed itself to another vertical program: a global smallpox-eradication program.

Candau's considerable diplomatic and administrative skills would be required to lead the WHO during the next two decades. During his tenure, 54 countries would gain their independence, which led to rapid growth in the WHO and its activities. In 1953 the organization had 81 members, a staff of 1,500, and a budget of US$9 million; by 1973, the WHO's membership had grown to 138 countries and it maintained a staff of 400 from 100 different countries and administered a budget of US$106 million.[8] The revolution in public health technologies and management techniques had to be adapted to the new postcolonial reality and the changed balance of power within the WHO.

Publicly, Creelman always maintained, "If we in the [Nursing] section fail [it] will not be for the lack of support and encouragement from our DG. Have been and are going to be very fortunate."[9] At first glance, the two had much in common. Both were Rockefeller fellows with extensive public health experience. Candau, an early advocate of the view that medicine is not only a biological science but also a social science, contended that social remedies might prove more effective than biological ones.[10] Creelman agreed; she and the Brazilian shared a deep appreciation of health as a vital factor in global strategies for development. At the same time, Candau and Creelman were both known for a keen intellect and a sharp, academic turn of mind, alongside a pragmatic approach to the WHO's work that constantly evolved to reflect new developments in science and technology. Both displayed a lifelong interest in education that underscored their common belief that "innovation is what we need in all countries. Innovation depends on knowledge. Knowledge is the bridge to achievement. But education is the bridge to knowledge."[11] While both recognized the importance of assisting developing countries to optimize their human resources and acquire the technology and knowledge they required, each forcefully articulated that "members of the health team must be trained specifically for the tasks they are intended to perform in light of their countries' needs and resources."[12]

There were, however, profound differences in their approaches to global health that became more apparent over time. Beginning in 1953, the WHO increasingly promoted a vertical, disease-specific approach to health. At the international level, it turned its attention to the prevention and control of malaria, tuberculosis, plague, cholera, yellow fever, and smallpox; at the country level, its programming focused on providing assistance through medical training and specific requests for medical technologies.[13] Mirroring the modernization development model of the time, it imposed technology without engaging the local community in either its development of implementation. Modernization theory assumed that nations transitioned through stages of economic development but that countries with the top-down infusion of technology and capital, the developing economies would "take off." It would take a decade, however, for the malaria warriors to realize that without a basic health service to back up and consolidate their gains, it was almost impossible to achieve their goal. As we have seen, Creelman had questioned the legacy of either the TB or malaria demonstration projects, if the establishment of permanent services for rural areas did not follow them up.[14] As time progressed, it became apparent that the two differed over what medical technologies should be prioritized. Equally disturbing from Creelman's viewpoint, modernization theory was underpinned by the assumption that cultural modernization would accompany and reinforce economic development. There were other similarly unsettling signs that the WHO was moving away from the "social approach" to global health that emphasized a rights-based approach to global health and long-term socio-economic growth rather than short-term technological intervention.

Under Candau's leadership, the WHO Secretariat would alter its health priorities and revisit its commitment to human rights. By 1966, the WHO was largely abandoning its "forceful" leadership role, forged under Brock Chisholm, in codifying the rights-based approach to global health contained in the WHO's mandate and its underlying emphasis on health determinants.[15] Candau also supported further decentralization of country programming to the six regional offices and shied away from engaging in collaborative health initiatives with other UN specialized agencies.[16] From Creelman's perspective, all this was alarming.

In March 1954 there was another change in the WHO Secretariat, this one involving Creelman herself. After two years as deputy chief nursing officer, Creelman learned that Olive Baggallay was stepping down and that she was now to assume the top post. She was not daunted by the prospect. On the eve of taking up her new appointment, she shared her excitement with her stepbrother, Prescott: "I look forward to the job as I like responsibility and I have been groomed quite well for it. Olive and I have worked very much as a team and I shall certainly miss her."[17] The CNO position gave her greater control over expert committees, recruitment, and senior staff appointments. It also afforded a more effective platform for cultivating relationships with other UN agencies,

NGOs, and international nursing bodies. A new chapter in her career had opened.

Even before becoming the WHO's CNO, Creelman had fostered close ties with the International Council of Nurses. She became a well-known figure at ICN gatherings. Members of the ICN contributed directly to the work of several of the expert committees on nursing and regularly attended WHO regional nursing seminars and conferences. In turn, the WHO's nursing leadership attended ICN executive meetings, while the WHO itself provided financial assistance to the ICN that enabled it to undertake four studies that contributed to the professional development of nursing within many countries.[18] At Creelman's suggestion, reciprocal arrangements were made to brief staff en route to new assignments. In short, the ICN and the WHO's Nursing Section shared a symbiotic partnership geared to extending their organizations' influence and strengthening nursing as a profession across the world.

In July 1953 Creelman attended the Tenth Quadrennial Congress of the ICN and afterwards participated in the WHO's Third Regional Nursing Conference, in Rio de Janeiro. While the focal point of the ICN Congress was the introduction of the first international code of ethics, Creelman understandably focused on her closing address. In a carefully crafted speech, she laid out her vision of an ICN-WHO partnership. She began by paying homage to the ICN's efforts to enhance nurses' professional status and improve the standards of nursing worldwide. Then, after lauding the ICN's role in fighting for a voice for nursing in the WHO, Creelman addressed the issue of WHO financial grants for the ICN's study of current post-basic nursing education. The tone now changed as Creelman questioned the prerogative of nursing leaders to set educational standards. The ICN guide *The Basic Education of the Professional Nurse* was a useful tool for curriculum planning within countries receiving WHO assistance. But, she warned, there "can be no set pattern" for nursing schools. "The national nurses and the international nurses must study together the needs of the country, the resources available and with this information develop the kind of the curriculum which will be most practical in its setting."[19]

In the midst of one of the oldest women's professional groups, Creelman also gently chided her fellow nurses for "our too frequent tendency to speak of nursing as though it was a profession whose membership is almost exclusively women. This may be so in many countries but is it not time to give more consideration to the recruitment and preparation of suitably qualified men for the nursing profession?"[20] Such a high-profile challenge to the gender barrier was directly related to the requests that came across her desk daily crying for more nurses and the difficulties she experienced in finding male tutors. What is remarkable is that more nursing leaders did not attempt to de-gender nursing to make it more difficult for governments and employers to discriminate against their profession. Creelman was not someone who believed that the old ways were necessarily the best.

Creelman also reminded nurses that the ICN, in essence, was an exclusionary force, for over one-third of the world's population lived in countries that either did not have a national nursing organization or were not yet a member of the ICN. Creelman assured her audience that the WHO was lobbying vigorously to further the ICN's goals of encouraging the formation of national nursing organizations and pressing governments to provide adequate resources for nursing education. Yet she reiterated that the real effort must come from within the countries themselves. This was strong language to use before an ICN meeting. Creelman served notice that it would be the WHO's responsibility to make certain that attention was paid to all nurses around the world, thus ensuring that the ICN's ideal of universalism admitted the necessity of creating a decidedly more culturally diversified definition in actual practice. Even before her appointment as CNO, the delegates left knowing that Lyle Creelman intended to be heard.

During the ICN conference, Creelman made a point of praising the increasing use of regional seminars and workshops, which encouraged ongoing discussions of common problems and sharing of practical solutions. As WHO nursing programs grew rapidly, she increasingly relied upon regional nursing conferences to provide direction, support, and resources to her staff and local nurses. These conferences not only widened the basis of local community involvement in decision-making but also identified and developed current and aspiring leaders. Her comments here and earlier on curriculum development, emphasizing the importance she attributed to devolving decision-making to the rank-and-file membership, trace their linage back to her work on the Baillie-Creelman Report and, indeed, to Stewart's earlier lectures at TC.

In Creelman's judgment, the international nursing conference held at Mount Pelerin, Switzerland, during the fall of 1953 turned out to be just such a gathering. Improving the coordination between hospital services and public health and strengthening the team approach to nursing and staff education provided the dual focus for the two-week meeting attended by nurses from twenty-one European countries. Creelman had looked forward to this conference, and, by her own account, she was not disappointed. "What a learning experience for everyone and me especially ... Ursula [?] and I carrying the load but probably Rosie thinks she did. First week has been most successful. A panel and role playing to finish on Friday. Quite an achievement for these people, most of whom know nothing of these techniques."[21] She derived particular satisfaction in seeing a nurse without any public speaking experience chair a plenary session and participate in a panel discussion. Creelman subscribed to the widely held belief that group work fostered democratic cooperation and built leadership skills that would have spill over into other areas of public life. Despite her initial scepticism about allowing each delegate one and a half minutes to explain how she would personally apply the knowledge gained at the conference, the closing sessions turned out to be one of the "snappiest" she had experienced. Creelman also applauded the conference organizers' decision to visit Dr André Répond, director of the psychiatric clinic in Malévoz, who was internationally renowned for his work with social workers. In her opinion, Répond was "doing outstanding work among the people of the remote and scattered mountain villages."[22] The conference concluded at the stunning thirteenth-century Chateau Chillon, on the shore of Lake Geneva. There, the lively conversation and refrains of local folk music filled the chateau's candlelit banquet hall late into the evening. As she drove home the next day, she "realized that no one could have gained more than myself from this rich experience."[23]

The invitation to preside over the Health Visitors Conference, which was part of the Congress of the Royal Sanitary Institute held at Bournemouth in the south of England in April 1955, attested to Creelman's growing reputation. Her address, entitled "Trends in Nursing and Public Health, Having Implications for Health Visitors," provides an important barometer of her own nursing agenda with the WHO. Creelman spotlighted the preparation of what she called the "comprehensive nurse" who worked in public health, the hospital, or midwifery. Like many of her contemporaries, she stressed that the "comprehensive nurse" made better economic sense, especially for the "fast developing countries," but admitted the challenges it presented in terms of curriculum and supervision. Creelman left no doubt where she stood on the new fashion in curriculum development: curriculum "should be dynamic, Socratic not didactic, teach principles rather than be overburdened with facts, and have adequate integration of theory and practice." To avoid imposing cultural norms, new methods of teaching placed greater emphasis on group discussion along with ongoing staff training to strengthen the nurse's ability to engage her clients in determining the course to recovery, rehabilitation, or healthy living. Changes in curriculum also needed to be based upon sound research and experimentation – what Creelman liked to call "action research, where a group may consider a specific day-to-day problem suggested by the persons involved and may investigate the various way of solving it."[24] She expressed her support, as well, for two other trends – greater collaboration with other community health workers and the generalization of nursing services – that had long been a mainstay of her approach to public health. Her summation succinctly embodied her definition of nursing ethics: "If we are to carry out in the best interests of the community the pledge we made on graduation, the theme of which is service, we must keep informed, be alert to the indications of the need for change and, above all, be willing to change."[25] Again, currents deeply rooted in past experience had matured on the world stage. The speech was classic Creelman.

In 1954 the WHO's third expert committee on nursing met in London under the capable chairmanship of Elizabeth Cockayne, the chief nursing officer in the British Ministry of Health since its inception in 1948. As it turned out, this was to be Olive Baggallay's last meeting. Even before the meeting opened in London on 29 March 1954, Creelman knew that she had been appointed as Baggallay's successor but she had little time to reflect on its significance. There was just too much to do before the conference opened.

Once again, Creelman's guiding hand was clearly discernible behind the scenes; she had carefully ensconced a Canadian, Ruth Morrison from UBC – whose views on nursing she knew and respected – within the committee. Officially tasked with advising on the principles of nursing administration to "assist in the world wide effort to improve the administration of nursing services," the third expert committee, like its predecessors, was framed to leverage nursing's agenda for greater authority and self-regulation from the hospital to the highest policymaking circles. Its recommendations buttressed the Nursing Section's requests to expand its programming through increased funding in the WHO's budgets for intra-regional conferences and workshops and championed nurses' participation in policy development. The manual on administrative nursing services prepared by the committee emphasized the importance of "good human relationships in administration," of an adequate in-service education program, and of the nursing director being given undisputed authority commensurate with the level of her responsibilities.[26] In the years to come, Elizabeth Cockayne would acknowledge Creelman's contribution to advancing nursing's interests through her work on the WHO's expert committees and during the 1956 WHA. In a private letter to Creelman in 1956, she wrote, "I realize fully that any success is largely due to yourself and your staff in the preparation and guidance to we mortals but it is a satisfaction that nursing was recognized on such a high level and I can only hope that the delegates will copy some of the attitudes demonstrated when they return home."[27]

The Ninth World Health Assembly, held in Geneva from 8 to 25 May 1956, was particularly demanding of Lyle Creelman's attention. "Nurses, their education and their role in health programs" had been designated by the WHA two years earlier as the subject of technical discussions at the ninth assembly, where nurses from twenty-one countries were to be part of the national delegations. In the two-year interval since, an immense amount of detailed planning in collaboration with the ICN, the International Committee of Catholic Nurses and

Medical Social Workers, and the League of Red Cross Societies had gone into preparing for the "big day." Pearl McIver, former president of the American Nurses Association and influential nurse director of the Office of Public Health Nursing of the U.S. Public Health Service,[28] worked closely with Creelman to finalize all the technical papers and also the questionnaire, intended to stimulate discussion on nursing's future direction, that was distributed to national nursing associations.[29]

The assembly allowed nursing leaders to showcase nursing's contribution to global health – at least for the moment. At the time it was heralded as "the first time, on an international basis, that outstanding doctors and health administrators have met with nurses to consider together the problems of nursing."[30] The discussions of the 1956 WHA echoed the concerns expressed in the previous expert committees, particularly over the lack of leadership and the nursing shortage, and, again like the committees, emphasized nurses' valuable contributions as leaders, administrators, and skilled clinicians with multiple roles, functions, and perspectives in the modern health-care system. Yet only eleven hours of the WHA's time were allotted to the technical discussions, with seven of the nine discussion groups being chaired by doctors.[31]

How effective were these presentations? Did they catalyse support for sufficient funding to establish nursing education on an independent basis equal to that of other professions and for a greater policymaking role nationally and globally? After the meeting, Dorothy Percy,[32] whose position as chief nursing advisor to the federal government had earned her a seat on the Canadian delegation, perhaps best captured the difficulty of assessing the long-term influences of any one conference. Admitting that there were times when she thought they were achieving little – "the same old problem we've been dealing with for years; the same old cliché we've being repeating for a long, long time, as we go round and round the mulberry bush looking for answers" – she nonetheless felt that "somewhere, sometime there may be something new because of Geneva 1956 … Geneva 1956 will be looked back upon in years to come as a signpost of no small significance."[33]

Perhaps, as Creelman suggested, its true significance lay outside the conference halls. National dialogues, she believed, probably formed the most useful part of the exercise, especially for those countries that included other members of the health team in their discussion groups. Tehmina Adranvala with the Indian delegation endorsed Creelman's position. She argued that preparing the national reports not only proved helpful in preparing for the SEARO nursing seminar but also fostered other valuable long-term outcomes: the "interest and the sense of responsibility aroused on being asked to prepare material for an international assembly, the occasion given for clarifying ideas on all aspects of nursing, the development of techniques of discussion and consultation which will carry over to other matters and the satisfaction of working together for a worthwhile objective – these are intangible gains but none the less far-reaching in their influence on the development of nursing."[34]

Geneva was a "signpost" in another respect. During Creelman's tenure with the WHO, the new international sisterhood of nursing leaders would increasingly function as a knowledge-based community; their expertise on how to deal with the worldwide nursing shortage became nurses' source of influence in leveraging their political agenda. Helping to cement this community at the WHA Assembly in 1956 were a number of social functions where Dame Elizabeth Cockayne, Lucile Petry Leone, Pearl McIver, Dorothy Percy, Creelman's fellow British Columbian Alice Wright,[35] Tehmina Adranvala, and Elizabeth Hill,[36] among others, networked and exchanged ideas.[37] These women formed an elite international sisterhood, forged in common experiences that began with their privileged educational backgrounds and professional status and was later nurtured in a series of professional associations, which transcended national boundaries and carried them onto the international stage. Their leadership, dedication, and shared professional values of service and caring helped to forge a common shared identity.

Long a proponent of researched-based nursing practice, Creelman eagerly anticipated the first international nursing research conference as an important step in that direction. Sponsored by the Florence Nightingale International Foundation and held in Sèvres, France, in October 1956, the conference centred on developing field studies and applied research to expand public health nurses' participation in the modernization of health care. Former UNRRAID Margaret Arnstein, head of the Division of Nursing Resources of the USPHS, directed the work.[38] Privately, Creelman depicted the conference as interesting but "poorly prepared" and lacking "flexibility."[39] Arnstein's private post-conference correspondence to Creelman lends credence to her complaint: "I appreciated so much your taking the time to be with us for the whole Conference at Sèvres. Your knowledge and experience gave me a feeling of security and your advice and counsel steered us into the best decisions a number of times. In addition, as usual, you were wonderful at seeing things that needed to be done, and without fuss or feathers you manned the boats each time we were in difficulties."[40]

In retrospect, the benefits of the international contacts – described by one participant "as a unique opportunity for nurses of widely different nationalities to meet on common grounds" – proved as useful as the knowledge of nursing research the participants absorbed.[41] Given that nursing research was still in its embryonic stage, even within industrialized nations, the Sèvres conference was a landmark in the uphill battle to gain recognition of its importance within the medical community. It was also an early indicator of the significance that Creelman attached to research as a key component of the modern nurse-scholar.

In October 1958 the fourth expert committee on nursing met in Geneva. Creelman's deliberate choice of public health nursing as the focus for the committee speaks to the ongoing resistance she encountered within WHO headquarters and some developing countries to "the concept that public health is one view of total nursing."[42] As she told the *Toronto Star* reporter in June 1958, "There are still many countries that lack any public health program ... We haven't quite got the idea across to the public that nursing means more than curative care in hospitals."[43] In the years following the Second World War, the WHO and its member governments lost interest in global issues and the development of public health systems attuned to the root determinants of health. Whereas Creelman advocated working with states to develop comprehensive public health systems, the new director general viewed WHO personnel simply as a catalysts who "would pass on to their counterparts the skill and knowledge needed to attack a specific health problem."[44] "Ignoring previously-recognized societal determinants of health," international aid agencies, "driven by the larger 'medical-industrial complex' that had sprung from the Second World War, imposed this biomedical vision of health on developing nations, emphasizing antibiotics, medical technologies, and private urban hospitals."[45] The primary goal was to achieve economic growth, not better health. The prescribed antidote of Western foreign-policy experts to communism – in line with what became known as the "domino theory" – was to strengthen economic growth within developing countries. Creelman had consistently advocated community-based public health programs as part of the larger strategy for long-term socio-economic growth rather than short-term medical interventions. The report of the fourth expert committee was Creelman's rebuttal.

In a curt journal entry after this committee concluded its work, Creelman noted that the proceedings had gone well, thanks in part to the able assistance of Liz Hilborn, formerly chief nursing adviser with the United States Operations Mission to Jordan. The committee's report provided a roadmap for the future development of public health nursing. While it mirrored the progressive perspectives on this subject that Creelman held in common with other nursing leaders, it bore her clear imprint. Its recommendations supported an approach to public health that focused less on "measures of control and environmental management" and more on "the broader social and educational approach."[46] The 1958 expert committee defined public health nursing as combining "the skills of nursing, public health and some phases of social assistance" and functioning as "part of the total public health programme for the promotion of health, the improvement of conditions in the social and physical environment, rehabilitation, the prevention of illness and disability." Moreover, in a familiar refrain echoing Creelman's earlier public statements, it emphasized the unique contribution of the public health nurse "as the channel by which many other public health and community services are brought to the public."[47]

Many of the recommendations of the *Report of the Fourth Session* reiterated the advice that Creelman had already given during her duty travel. The expansion of auxiliary nursing personnel should dovetail with the preparation of an adequate number of nurses to supervise their work. The development of generalized community nursing services was essential to avoid the costly mistake of over-specialization that Creelman believed Western countries had made.[48] The committee supported nurse-run and independently financed nursing-education programs in which curriculums were customized to the countries' requirements and resources.[49] It strongly recommended inclusion of public health education into the basic nursing curriculum. Once again, this committee triggered new research initiatives and an expert committee on auxiliary workers. It particularly stressed the need to expand the WHO's research activities at the regional or inter-country level, especially designed to identify and mentor potential nursing leadership below the upper echelons of nursing. The report moved the organization's nursing program towards primary health care aligned with local requirements.[50] In short, the report endorsed the direction long supported by its CNO.

In reviewing the report, Dorothy Percy praised it for its "recognition of the vast differences in the level of development of public health in various countries" and contended that the "emphasis on basic principles" would make it an invaluable "blueprint for countries engaged in setting up new health services and for countries with well established programs."[51] The report's clear language, in her opinion, provided guidance for the foreseeable future and did not lose sight of the individual nurse's therapeutic benefit for the patient's recovery; it met Percy's (and Creelman's) evolving vision of "the educated heart in the automated nurse."[52]

Extended periods of duty travel continued to complicate Lyle Creelman's increasingly heavy workload throughout the 1950s. By the time of her appointment as CNO, she had visited all six WHO regions. Duty travel remained critical to establish her authority as the WHO's CNO and exercise oversight over the growing number of nursing projects within more and more countries. Particularly important were private conversations in the field, which yielded a franker assessment of local conditions, especially within newly independent countries, than that gained during her carefully orchestrated itinerary set by the regional office. These conversations gave Creelman, renowned for corridor conversations with member-state delegates to the WHA or other expert committee meetings, valuable ammunition to influence the development of the WHO's nursing projects within their countries.

Visiting nurses in war zones and in remote villages where the notions of health or safe childbirth were unknown, while often profoundly disconcerting, remained essential for Creelman. Field visits refined her Western perspective on nursing, deepening her appreciation of the challenges her staff faced in tailoring the WHO nursing programs for non-European populations in resource-strapped countries. Often the WHO nurses functioned without the benefit of a common language or training or support from the medical community. On the 1953 trip to Thailand, Creelman seized the rare opportunity to combine a holiday with her scheduled duty travel. In Bangkok, "the Venice of the East,"[53] she took in the sights by canal boat while listening to fellow Canadian nurse Justine Delmotte's[54] moving stories of her adventures on a WHO/UNICEF yaws team in the backcountry. The use of a single dose of long-lasting penicillin made the widespread treatment of yaws, a crippling and disfiguring disease virtually unknown outside the tropics, economically feasible within these countries.[55] Afterwards, Creelman confessed she had no desire to exchange places with Delmotte, for whom home was a bedroll and whatever hut could be spared within the villages on her route. Lyle Creelman remained a visitor sharing their stories, where, for those in the field, adapting Western nursing principles to local conditions assumed a stark reality.

Creelman's professional growth continued as she travelled extensively in 1954 in preparation for becoming CNO. Her visits to the WHO nursing projects, in Manila, Borneo, Taiwan, Japan, and Tobago, wove a visual tapestry of the economic disparity, civil strife, and human cruelty that impeded the improvement of health services in these countries. While visiting Manila, Elizabeth Hill acted as her guide on a trip through the mountains of Luzon. She and Hill quickly found common ground; both were graduates of Teachers College and had served with UNRRA.[56] During the long drive, the two nurses reflected on the increased difficulty of providing rural health services in an economically depressed area where, "in spite of the fact that the mountain people toil from morning till night to grow their rice, they still do not produce enough for their own consumption."[57] But, just as important, Hill got an endorsement; she would shortly become Creelman's first deputy chief nurse.

During her subsequent stops within WPRO, Creelman contrasted the beauty of the blue-green, ring-shaped coral islands as her flight from Manila approached North Borneo with the political reality there. She found "the last stronghold of colonialism" to be "really sad. How can human beings treat each other so?"[58] There to visit the first school of nursing at Sandakar, Creelman left convinced that the island's health services, badly ravaged by war, needed many more midwives to improve the level of maternal and child care. Similarly, diary entries recording her visit to Taiwan noted the continued economic and political turmoil in which the WHO nurses lived and worked: "Political manoeuvres dominate everything ... Close watch for Communist[s] ... People shot every day."[59] Creelman's UNRRA experience seemed tame in comparison. After her experiences in Taiwan, a relieved Creelman "felt [she] was back to civilized living"[60] as her plane touched down in Tokyo. The visit to Japan sparked unexpected personal memories. Both surprised and touched by the Japanese nurses' thoughtful parting gifts, she was left feeling profoundly guilty as she confronted Canada's record on human rights during the Second World War for the first time. "It makes me feel very contrite about how we treated them in former years."[61] Realizations such as this eroded pretensions about the innate civility of Western society in Creelman's eyes.

On 4 February she caught an eighteen-hour flight from Tokyo to Vancouver for a brief visit. The impressions gained on her recent travels again triggered comparisons with the Canadian health-care system as she crossed the country renewing old contacts and looking for new recruits before returning to Geneva on 8 March 1954. Inevitably, as she compared these modern Canadian hospitals to those she had recently visited in less fortunate parts of the world, two things immediately caught her attention: "The children's wards seemed to be for children only. There are notices telling when parents might visit ... In my mind I saw other hospitals, sadly lacking in equipment and staff it is true, but the mother was there with the child providing the close link which we in the West are beginning to realize is such an important factor in recovery and which I suspect the people of the East have always instinctively known."[62] "Then I realized more than ever how much the countries of the East have to offer the West, if only the West will learn."[63]

After Creelman's appointment as CNO, duty travel brought new challenges, especially within newly independent countries. During these years, she further refined her own vision of international nursing and tested the limits of her authority. She was often called upon to arbitrate WHO relationships with local officials that had foundered on their government's failure to provide agreed-upon facilities, nursing students, or national counterparts. Frequently, her emphasis on long-term planning to create sustainable nursing services collided with the local government officials' agenda to construct showcase medical facilities to enhance the government's political prestige.

Her field visits and correspondence with Helena Reimer, first in Cambodia and later in Egypt, are illustrative of her emerging leadership strategies during the 1950s. Equally, they expose the limitations of personal diplomacy in addressing the problems that plagued the Nursing Section's efforts to improve nursing services within developing countries. In 1955 Creelman selected Reimer[64] to head a high-profile project: the first university-based nursing-education program in the Middle East, located at the Higher Institute of Nursing at the University of Alexandria. Creelman had become better acquainted with Helena Reimer in Geneva when Helena was en route to her first assignment in Phnom-Penh, Cambodia. During a weekend hike in the mountains, the two Canadians compared their very different experiences nursing with UNRRA. The challenges of Reimer's UNRRA assignment – nursing under canvas in the Egyptian desert – paled when compared to her subsequent harrowing experience of dodging bullets in remote parts of Formosa during the Chinese civil war. Throughout it all, Helena Reimer had demonstrated quiet courage, compassion, and resourcefulness. Creelman monitored Reimer's progress with considerable satisfaction and, at other times, with compassionate concern.

In a radio address, Creelman publicly featured the efforts of the three WHO nurses in Phnom-Penh – Reimer, Wilhelmina Visscher, and Alice Talbot[65] – to lay the foundations of the first "real" school of nursing there, one that met "the needs of Cambodia and not necessarily those of another country."[66] In keeping with her own past practice in the field, Creelman's radio address championed the dual-pronged strategy the WHO team had followed: establish a forward-looking plan, based on a survey of Cambodia's nursing needs and resources, that worked towards long-term goals by improving the nursing services already in place. Since the existing two-year program had a very limited curriculum with no opportunity for the teaching of nursing by nurses, Reimer accepted that it would take years to build a mature, multi-tiered nursing-education program. As a first step, here as elsewhere, the WHO nurses concentrated on helping existing nurses to improve their clinical skills and knowledge.[67]

Creelman had already showcased the work of the Cambodian WHO team as epitomizing the cross-cultural model for international nursing required in developing countries in *Nursing News*, the WHO newsletter,[68] and the *Canadian Nurse*. In the *Canadian Nurse* article, she cited Helena Reimer's reports to illustrate their shared belief that nursing and midwifery must be developed in conjunction with the communities and individuals they served. As Reimer described the Phnom-Penh team's cross-cultural education, "The Cambodian people are shy so it took some time to just get acquainted." But eventually Reimer's team placed itself "in a learning position and let them talk to us about their country, its people, its resources, and its needs ... they made me realize how important it was for us to learn something about the country if we are to develop a program to really serve the needs of the country." As they worked with two Cambodian nurses, Reimer recalled, they became fully convinced "that the only sound way of introducing a new program into a new country is by working step by step with some responsible person … even if it takes longer. Let it take root in their thinking as they help to develop it, so that it will be something that they have planted and watered."[69]

Creelman singled out Reimer's treatment of their national counterparts "as professional equals" who were consulted "about every plan we make and every step we take."[70] Her team carefully avoided embarrassing their Cambodian colleagues, who had only primary education, choosing instead to recognize that nursing leaders who themselves had not had the advantage of higher education could still be instrumental in raising the standards of nursing in their own countries. Reimer and Visscher made a point of introducing their Cambodian colleagues to the minister of health and including them in ministry-level discussions, even though the Cambodian nurses had "never sat down in these offices." The Canadian nurses took it for granted that "these, our colleagues, will be accepted wherever we are accepted, as the future nursing leaders of the country."[71] Reimer's approach to international nursing – which stressed cultural sensitivity and focused on building local competencies and creating a custom-designed and achievable level of nursing service – both reflected and reinforced Creelman's own thinking.

Creelman's laudatory *Canadian Nurse* article carefully avoided discussing the Phnom-Penh team's frustration in dealing with government officials and other WHO representatives who wanted health-care showpieces as soon as possible. Reimer's private letters speak to the enormous pressure many WHO nurses, including Creelman, faced for quick visible results:

> I was a fool … I should have started going into a hospital ward and sponging patients … and we could have reaped honour on our heads … But I do not care for honour nor a name for myself. Educating thousands of people in seven day courses will never establish nursing in a country. I am working against my conscience if I have to do something in a superficial manner just to have something to show … I cannot start building a house without knowing the ground it is to be built upon. Now we know the condition of the soil we are laying the foundation with good solid cement but the public will not see much structure until the building rises above the ground.[72]

Like so many other WHO nurses serving in virtual isolation in remote areas of the world, Reimer found that writing to Creelman for inspiration, encouragement, or advice when she was "feeling sad, angry and discouraged"[73] was invaluable. Creelman's visit in 1954 was her reply. Still, letters and field visits to nurses like Reimer could not adequately address the ethical dilemma many

WHO staff faced when their values failed to align with the harsh realities of fieldwork in poverty-stricken countries that often also lacked political stability.

Creelman's articles did not highlight how progress towards better health care often came at the cost of the WHO's nurses' own health.[74] After Creelman's visit, Reimer succumbed to a tropical disease and spent a year in Mathilda Hospital, Hong Kong, before overcoming the partial paralysis that accompanied the intense treatment. Creelman made a special effort to see that Reimer was well cared for during her recovery and included in the international nursing community during her subsequent study leave in France. There were other hazards too, ones again not conveyed by Creelman in her articles. For security reasons, the movements of the WHO nursing team in Cambodia were restricted, requiring them to travel by military plane when they visited other towns to conduct surveys.[75] Cambodia was embroiled in the struggle for independence from France and was to become fully independent in 1954 – the year of Creelman's tour. Not unmindful of the dangers in Cambodia and elsewhere, Creelman remained vigilant about the safety and well-being of her nursing staff. Many times, however, the distance left her feeling helpless to intercede in Geneva.

Creelman, an ardent traveller but dutiful daughter, abandoned plans to spend the 1954 Christmas with Helena Reimer in Egypt, in order to be with her ailing mother in Vancouver. Then it was not until the following March that she could break away from Geneva to handle the pressing problems brewing in Cyprus, Lebanon, Jordan, Egypt, and especially Syria and Iraq. Visiting this region had taken on a new priority since some of the WHO's nursing projects seemed to be closing down unexpectedly, and low morale among staff threatened further resignations.

In Syria, the WHO's future seemed especially uncertain: the WHO's regional office had been advised by the Syrian government that the Maternal Child Health (MCH) project started only three years earlier would be wound down at the end of April. Despite the Syrian minister of health's blunt warning that WHO nurses "were no longer needed in Syria," Creelman knew that this would be an item of further discussion with the Syrian delegate at the World Health Assembly's next meeting. She welcomed an opportunity to assess the situation on the spot,[76] but relations remained strained a year later. Without consulting the WHO team leader, the Syrian government had requested a former British WHO nurse to recruit a second hospital team.[77]

The Syrian project, Creelman discovered, was a case study in what could go wrong. Given that the nursing activities of the MCH centre and the responsibility for training the next group of auxiliaries would be left "in the hands of one competent nurse," Creelman could not help "feeling that WHO has failed in giving support of such quality and organization that the project can continue in a sound way after withdrawal of WHO personnel." She made it clear that she was not critical of the WHO nurses' performance but was merely issuing "a warning against the direction in which we have allowed our MCH projects, with their training activities, to develop."[78] This experience led Creelman to urge preparation of a senior Jordanian nurse to assume responsibility for the MCH program in that country, and that expansion of the MCH services in Iraq should proceed only after adequate supervision for auxiliary workers was available. That same North American emphasis on patient safety, as has been pointed out, made its way into the expert committees' reports and coloured the WHO's sometimes strained relationship with UNICEF.

Creelman's visits to these nursing projects were well timed to influence the direction of the WHO's nursing programs. In the end, the WHO would continue its MCH work in Syria. Creelman supported the recommendations of the WHO staff at the Syrian nursing school in Aleppo that clinical training should be improved, entrance standards raised, and salaries for locally trained nurses placed on a par with those for nurses educated in the United Kingdom. Similarly, she recommended the continuation of WHO support for the University School of Nursing, Damascus, at least until 1957 or until it could be self-sustaining.[79] Where she observed that a WHO project was providing good clinical experience for students, such as the tuberculosis program in Baghdad under the direction of a well-qualified Vancouver public health nurse, Queenie Donaldson,[80] Creelman not unexpectedly proposed including the prevention of tuberculosis in the basic nursing course for student nurses and graduates from other nursing schools.[81] The British Columbia public health department was a national and international leader in prevention of TB through public health measures and in ensuring that TB education was included in the basic nursing curriculum.[82] She also rallied support for Donaldson's request for a greater community-based public health nursing presence in the TB project itself.[83] By June 1955, Donaldson was writing to Creelman that "it has taken a long time to get nurses but they are seeing now that a public health nursing background is necessary," and that she would get her first group of graduate nurses in the fall.[84] This was only one of many cases where Creelman interceded to gain greater professional autonomy for a well-trained public health nurse on a TB team in order to extend the nursing component of community-based public health programs. She remained adamant that the nurse should retain control over the nursing aspects of the project, including the training of auxiliaries. Collectively, her recommendations in such cases followed the dual approach adopted on earlier trips: improve the level of current nursing services and lay the foundation for sustainable long-term development of nursing services countrywide.

Reimer's hope that Creelman's visit to Egypt in the spring of 1955 would "be of great inspiration to the team"[85] provided an early indicator of the difficulties encountered in gaining acceptance for the university-based nursing program at the Higher Institute of Nursing. Egypt, the first country Creelman had visited as a WHO maternal health consultant, held a special interest for her, as it did for Helena Reimer. The Egyptian government had insisted that either Canadian or American nurses who had university preparation – as opposed to WHO nurses from those countries that did not yet offer university-based programs – lead the program to establish the institute's international standing. To assist Reimer and complete the high-profile team at the institute, Creelman had selected two other Canadians: Lara Thordarson and Edith Green.

Reimer again insisted that a modern indigenous nursing curriculum and clinical service could be built in Egypt only from the ground up after a careful investigation of the cultural and economic forces that had shaped the prior development of nursing, and a careful survey of current nursing resources and needs.[86] Moreover, her curriculum design accented integrating public health into the basic curriculum. While her approach adhered to the recommendations of the expert committee on public health nursing, Reimer maintained that "the whole program is experimental and will be evaluated and adjusted as it progresses."[87] This was precisely the attitude that Creelman believed all WHO teams should embrace.

Yet, even when WHO teams attempted to tailor nursing-education programs to local needs, there was no assurance of success. Reimer was at loggerheads with the university over the question of modern facilities and with the government over its failure to appoint a national counterpart. Local opinion, she informed her chief, "bemoaned the fact that the Medical Institute building had sunk so low as to house a school for nurses" and others feared that each educated nurse would be a "half-baked doctor."[88] Moreover, there was opposition within local nursing's own ranks. Reimer cautioned that great care must be taken against giving the impression that "the new program will create a nursing aristocracy ... they will not be able to function alone"; success required the assistance and cooperation of the existing national nurses.[89]

At the end of the 1956 academic year at the Higher Institute of Nursing, Reimer resigned, citing her concern that she would "become a stranger to nursing in her own country." She had really never completely recovered from the tropical disease that had ravaged her health following her Cambodian assignment. Living from crisis to crisis had left her exhausted. The rest of Reimer's team resigned shortly afterwards when the Regional Office failed to uphold its recommendations against lowering entrance standards at the institute.[90]

The experience of Reimer's team provided an early warning of the road-blocks that would hamper the Nursing Section's efforts to promote and support nursing elsewhere. Cultural adeptness did not guarantee a WHO nurse's political astuteness, especially if the terms of the collaborative partnership were not clearly defined or regime change meant starting over again. Even qualified, experienced, and dedicated WHO nurses were worn down by their struggles to obtain the promised facilities and staff or to raise the stature of the nursing. Illness or loneliness led to others' resignations. Repeatedly, Creelman would learn that university-educated nurses on WHO assignments had encountered resistance and resentment within the autocratic health-care systems.[91] As CNO, she kept all these lessons in mind as she negotiated the terms of reference for future WHO nursing projects.

Reflecting back on her international nursing experiences with the WHO, Reimer acknowledged Creelman's "encouragement and support and her sane advice."[92] The rest of Reimer's team also preferred to sort out their futures with Creelman directly, rather than with the WHO's Eastern Mediterranean Regional Office regional adviser, Inge Götzsche, a Danish-trained nurse who held the post from 1952 to 1956. Letters from other WHO nurses indicated that dissatisfaction within EMRO was widespread; there were clearly leadership issues within the regional office that demanded Creelman's presence both in 1955 and a year later.

Developing effective working relationships with the regional nursing officers remained a vital function of duty travel, just as it was crucial to maintaining administrative cohesion in the field. The WHO nurses in Baghdad appeared as estranged from Götzsche as were the WHO team in Alexandria. Well before her visit, Creelman had received several confidential letters detailing the level of dissatisfaction that threatened the project's existence.[93] Creelman refused all transfer requests, however, and counselled that, despite the difficulties, progress was being made but would require more time. Several factors contributed to the unrest among the Baghdad team. Not only were the WHO nurses working and living amidst deplorable sanitary conditions, but supplies and teaching materials, though available, were tied up in red tape. The forced idleness frayed team members' nerves. One nurse wrote that, notwithstanding Creelman's "wise letter," "I am still thinking of resigning as it is a very unhappy situation, without any results in a country where things should be easier. Will you please stress that a nursing adviser to the Min[ister] of Health is a first essential who should be at the same time a philosopher and diplomat."[94] The nurses were still reeling from the dressing-down they had received from the ministry for "meddling" in domestic Iraqi affairs by making health-care recommendations and from their disappointment that "we cannot depend on even a little bit of support" from Götzsche.[95] The Iraqi government's obstreperous attitude only partially accounted for the team's dissatisfaction, however.

Creelman knew that EMRO was not listening to the nurses in the field: they "felt very discouraged and doing nothing does not improve the situation."[96] But she underestimated the challenges that pervaded the project right up to the regional adviser. "Certainly the nursing situation there is desperate but we must not accept it as hopeless and try to meet it [a plan for countrywide MCH services] only with auxiliaries and social workers."[97] Uncovering the real story proved difficult. All Creelman's correspondence to and from her nurses in Baghdad was either hand-delivered or mailed from outside the country[98] "because it had been difficult to get letters and material through Baghdad without censorship."[99] Consequently, Creelman requested that another member of headquarters staff who was visiting the region speak directly with members of the team. Creelman's leadership within a highly decentralized WHO field operation was predicated upon her ability to choose nurses who shared her transcultural approach to international nursing and who were politically adept at negotiating the political terrain to advance the level of local nursing services. In cases where she came to question a regional nursing officer's suitability, she frequently sought another perspective before taking action. Realizing the difficulties and complexities with which Götzsche dealt, Creelman reserved final judgment. Determined to extend her administrative reach as CNO, she would be a more active player in the future selection or reappointment of regional nursing advisers. This and other lessons gained from the WHO's past mistakes in the field provided useful guideposts for Creelman's discussions with local officials about future nursing projects, especially where the WHO was just beginning its work.

As 1956 opened, Creelman eagerly anticipated her first trip to Africa, where she would visit Tanganyika, Kenya, Mauritius, La Réunion, British Somaliland, Uganda, Zanzibar, Congo, and Bechuanaland. It would prove an interesting trip to compare the very different nursing education programs developed within those countries still under British or French colonial rule with those of the newly independent countries. On 16 January 1958 she again travelled to Africa for one-week visits to Gambia, Sierra Leone, and Ghana, in addition to three weeks in Nigeria. Since the first regional nursing officer for the African Regional Office would not be appointed until 1958, Creelman's trips served as a preliminary survey of future nursing needs and staffing requirements within AFRO. Despite her very full agenda of official visits and social engagements on both African tours, including some weekends, Creelman found "it was all so interesting" that she "had no complaints."[100] At some points, just acquiring the required visas and finding accommodations proved to be an adventure.

But, as she reassured her mother, "at the beginning of my WHO experience this sort of thing would have bothered me and now it does not worry me at all – things usually turn out."[101] Lyle Creelman had become a seasoned world traveller.

Routinely, she met and socialized with high officials and diplomats on her African travels – this is why a new evening gown was purchased and packed before leaving on the first trip. Intent on avoiding past mistakes, she took full advantage of these meetings to push for long-term planning of nursing services rather than "showcase" projects. Her approach during both African duty tours remained consistent with past practice: identify what could be built upon immediately as a foundation on which to improve both the quality and the quantity of nursing services. As always, she remained a fierce advocate of coordinating general educational plans with a community-based public health program. Meetings with WHO or local officials figured prominently on Creelman's hectic African itineraries. Throughout her visits, however, Creelman visited as many facilities as possible to draw her own conclusions on how the economy, demographic distribution, climate, and social and educational opportunities for women influenced the provision of community-centred nursing and nursing education. During her first trip, she concluded that Tanganyika, then part of German East Africa, was "the most developed from the health services point of view of any of the countries I have yet visited. They at least have the beginnings of public health – the rest are all curative services."[102] She continued to believe that hospital-based care was far too expensive and ineffective to meet the overwhelming health-care needs within developing countries.

Given Creelman's public health perspective, she made every effort to encourage public health teaching within the educational and health facilities visited. It was equally typical of her that, during her 1958 visit to the Yundum teacher-training institute in Gambia, she pointed out opportunities to extend public health teaching for the teachers-in-training: "Here baskets and cribs could be woven to put the babies in when they are not on the mothers' backs, thus helping them to avoid hookworm. Much practical health teaching could be given thus preparing the teacher to take part in health activities of the villages."[103]

After visiting Yundum, Creelman concluded that full-time tutors, residential facilities, and extra educational opportunities for nursing students, similar to those provided at Yundum for teachers-in-training, were necessary. Once again, their absence contributed to the reluctance of young women and parents to consider nursing as an alternative profession to teaching. Her views on this matter, however, clashed with the low budgetary priority given to health care and nursing education in a country geared to rapid economic development. Instead, she was told, the government's limited resources were aimed at raising the general educational level.[104] She left Gambia in 1958 believing that "we can do a lot if they will let us."[105]

Negotiating the terms of WHO's nursing projects without acceding to demands for "quick fix" solutions continued to be Creelman's major diplomatic challenge within these African countries. That campaign began almost immediately on her first visit to La Réunion, an island in the Indian Ocean, east of Madagascar and southwest of Mauritius. Creelman arrived on 7 July 1956 to discuss the government's request for assistance in nursing education. While recognizing "the need for some assistance to La Réunion in relation to the training of nursing and midwifery personnel," Creelman knew that there was "no hope that this assistance will be given in time to supply the needed personnel for the new hospital and, in any case, this should not be the specific objective." She adamantly resisted the pressure of the acting director of the department of health, Dr Gouère, to provide nurses for immediate service. Instead, she recommended assigning "the first WHO educator on a six months contract to study the situation and with the Government draw up plans for a long-term program of assistance."[106]

The same message had to be repeated on her next island stop, 125 miles southeast in Mauritius – a British protectorate until 1968. From 11 to 18 July, Creelman was the houseguest of the British chief matron, "an open hearted Welsh woman, as broad as she is tall and really quite mad." Instead of doing "a real nursing job" as Creelman understood it, the chief matron "runs around all day to clinics, [and] hospital dispensaries." Accompanied by the matron and the wife of the governor, Lady Scott, Creelman noted that "everything was laid on" for her official visit to three hospitals.[107] By the end of the week, "a rather tired" Creelman had decided to forgo the daily rounds with the matron and instead visit the WHO nurses in the tuberculosis program. When she was again pressured to provide additional WHO personnel, Creelman made it clear to government officials that a survey of nursing needs must be the basis for the WHO's plan of operations; that it be adapted to the needs of the country; and that considerable emphasis be placed upon public health, midwifery services, and the extension of domiciliary services.[108] The visit once more spoke to the overwhelming pressure WHO nursing staff faced in resisting local officials' demands for more hands and showcase facilities.

Advancing nursing interests in a way that Creelman believed would have some hope of permanence required more active intervention during the June 1956 visit to Zanzibar Protectorate. She was firm in handling the director of medical services' request for assistance in training health visitors. The director, who "tried his hand at being a missionary once ... knows nothing about nursing and he therefore tries to run nursing himself. He thinks that the W.H.O.

nurse who comes should have what he calls 'the missionary spirit' and be happy to live in a rather inferior housing in the natural area. That is because there happened to be a flat that [the WHO nurse] could have on top of the maternity hospital. It won't do at all and I have told him so!"[109] Creelman's earlier contention that WHO nurses should have the "dedication" of missionaries and be prepared to live and work under difficult conditions did not mean that she was prepared to acquiesce when nurses' work was undervalued.

Creelman worked late into the night making the revisions necessary to the "draft plan of operations" that had been "dreamed up." Again, she "strongly recommended" that the first group to be trained with WHO assistance be the local midwives, who then could assist in the training and supervision of less-qualified home visitors. But steps needed to be taken to train a national counterpart to supervise the less-qualified health visitors and midwives. Moreover, she urged that the chief matron's responsibilities extend beyond the Zanzibar hospital to allow her to act as the nursing adviser to the director of medical services in all matters related to nursing.[110] On a more general note, Creelman found the lack of public health nursing to be a glaring deficit: "The Colonial Service certainly need to get some nurses with an appreciation of public health."[111] As it turned out, the colonial era would soon draw to an end; on 10 December 1963 the Zanzibar Protectorate acquired independence from Britain and became known as the Sultanate of Zanzibar, but the regime was short-lived. On 12 January 1964 a violent coup following a disputed election resulted in the deaths or expulsion of an estimated one in five of the Arab population. A month later, Zanzibar was incorporated into the new state of the United Republic of Tanzania. This changing of the guard would bring new recruiting challenges for the WHO's chief nurse in the years to come.

In other cases, a clash of professional perspectives within the international nursing community on nursing education and services created a cultural gulf that Creelman was unable or unwilling to bridge. During a five-day visit to Uganda, still under British colonial rule, on her first African trip, Creelman noted the difficulties in providing health services in a country where people did not live in villages but were scattered throughout the rural regions. The purpose of the visit was ostensibly to explore the possibility of future assistance to improve the nursing situation but also to buttress the prestige of the matron-in-chief, Margaret Oswald Clark Bonthron, of the Queen Elizabeth Colonial Nursing Service, stationed at Medical Headquarters, Entebbe. Bonthron had served on the second expert committee on nursing. During their discussions, Creelman pointed out the advantage of seeking WHO fellowships for African nurses that would be held not in Canada, Britain, or the United States but in countries where "the conditions might be somewhat more similar to

Uganda."[112] In her mind, if the WHO was to give assistance in the future, the first step would be to help with the clinical teaching and the integration of public health into the nursing curriculum – a recommendation that was eventually followed.[113] Creelman, however, had more immediate issues to resolve. Several British matrons opposed the appointment of WHO nurses, fearing that they would be saddled with high-powered Americans and that the WHO's high salaries would ignite dissatisfaction among local staff. Privately, Creelman chaffed at their parochial attitudes: "They can't see beyond their own noses. They have done some good work in nursing but with assistance it could be so much better."[114]

Creelman questioned both the leadership and direction of nursing on her next stop. Arriving in Gambia on 19 January 1958, Creelman clashed with another British-trained matron, Miss Gray. She simply did not warm up to Gray, "a north country English woman who has to have time to get to be really friendly," and found little in common with her – "not even in nursing."[115] Privately, Creelman confided to her mother that "WHO can help but I do not really think the authorities understand when I am talking about an educational program for nurses. It's hard to find a common basis."[116] Creelman's observation of the health visitors only confirmed her belief that public health officials "miss so many opportunities to do good work because they have no notion of teaching."[117] Given the repeated stories she heard of infant deaths, she was disappointed that the recent staff appointments were "not being used to their best advantage"; they should be used to train more auxiliary workers for the health centres, home visiting, and domiciliary midwifery.[118] The root of the problem was clear: "There are no medical specialists in Gambia. This means that there is not even a paediatrician nor anyone prepared or interested in MCH. There is no training for midwifery outside the hospital nor is there training of indigenous midwives. I was not told of any active plan for the development of this MCH work in the future."[119]

There were instances when all the factors cited above came into play but, in the end, it was the government's trump card that terminated negotiations on Creelman's 1958 visit to Sierra Leone. On the professional front, her visit to Sierra Leone, under British colonial rule until 1961, was unsatisfactory on several grounds. She initially took a dim view of the principal matron's failure to meet her upon arrival – until learning that she was, in fact, hospitalized. And her accommodations, shared with another WHO nurse, were the worst she had ever experienced in a British colony. She fully expected that local medical authorities would present "a cut & dried program which I shall have to make them change."[120] In fact, shortly after her arrival, the WHO's CNO was informed that the government had withdrawn its request for a WHO tutor and had instead approached Chief Nurse Florence Udell, in the British Colonial Office, to engage a sister tutor.[121] Nonetheless, Creelman carried on with the planned itinerary. Her diary recorded her visit to Bo, about 175 miles into the protectorate: "The roads were terrible – rough and dusty and [I] … was a very dirty looking specimen when [I] arrived." Here, she stayed with the British matron, who ran "the so called school of nursing,"[122] which, as far as Creelman could figure out, "is pretty much a lecture program with memorization and giving back at examination."[123] In Creelman's view, the matron at Bo had far too many duties – housekeeping, ordering supplies, and managing diets – that had nothing to do with nursing. While her report to Geneva highlighted the deficiencies in the nursing services, it took a more positive view of the efforts being made in the rural health centres she visited elsewhere.[124]

Both of Creelman's African duty tours highlighted unique nursing challenges. Independence raised expectations of a better life, including improved health care. Yet, as Creelman witnessed, the vestiges of colonial rule left many countries ill-equipped to meet these expectations; most notably, they lacked the indigenous trained medical personnel to guide the work of the postcolonial bureaucracies. Her visit in the first week of June to British Somaliland, where there were no trained nurses whatsoever and, in several centres, no hospitals, epitomized the challenges that lay ahead.[125] Since about 90 per cent of the population followed a nomadic life and "virtually all women [were] illiterate in English and Arabic," Creelman concluded that WHO assistance would require at least a six-year commitment – especially because any assistance the WHO could provide would have to await the completion of English-language instruction for the students selected for nursing training.[126] She candidly admitted in a telling letter home, "I should not want to be the nurse recruited for the job."[127]

In other instances, political decisions spurred by a rising sense of nationalism compounded the challenges of addressing the shortage of health workers within African countries. Such was the case in Ghana. After 100 years of British colonial rule, the Gold Coast achieved independence in 1957, becoming the new state of Ghana. Creelman's visit the following year provided an opportunity to appraise current facilities and future needs. All British nurses were to leave in 1959.[128] Following independence, the government implemented a policy of Africanization to encourage the replacement of expatriate white workers with Africans. Given this mandate, Creelman was interested in observing the state of nursing in the first former colonial country of Africa that had obtained reciprocity in training with the United Kingdom.

While Creelman considered nursing in Ghana more advanced than in Gambia or Sierra Leone, she thought the country had made a fundamental error in attempting to have reciprocal standards with Great Britain, which lengthened the training period required.[129] She also criticized both the colonial authorities and the new regime for their lack of cultural insight in designing new facilities or nursing-education programs. The government's decision to train doctors locally at the University of Ghana necessitated the enlargement and modernization of Korle-Bu hospital in Accra to turn it into a teaching hospital. In such an institution, nurses with more specialized clinical skills were deemed necessary to complement the medical program. At the time of independence, the two government-run training schools in Accra and Kumasi prepared nurses to qualify as state-registered nurses (SRN). Even though the majority of nurses were men at the time the SRN program was established, the decision had been made to admit only women to these schools. The gender shift in nursing preparation in part may have reflected the continued influence of outsiders on Ghanaian nursing education.[130] Moreover, the facilities at the Kumasi Central Hospital were not well planned for the country. Mothers, living a significant distance away, would not bring their sick children to this hospital because there was no place for them to stay.[131] Believing, however, that consideration of the total training program was "rather urgent" and that the Ghanaian nurses as well as the UK staff should be involved in the planning, Creelman fully supported the request of the chief medical officer, Dr Eustace Akwei, for a WHO nursing adviser to assist in the overall planning of nursing administration, education, midwifery, health visiting, and legislation.[132] Creelman's evaluations would influence how WHO assistance would be offered in the 1960 budget.

Before leaving Africa in 1958, Creelman spent several days in northern Nigeria, whose nursing shortage, she already foresaw, would continue to be acerbated by the Muslim population's strong aspirations for political and cultural autonomy: "They are Muslem [sic] and education for women has been very backward. They are wanting self government and in addition they want to employ only people from this region. Many of the 500 nurses [for a population of 18 million] are what they call 'Southerners' – that is they are from the tribes of the Eastern and Western Regions. So politically they talk of both 'Northernization' and 'Nigerianization.' They have a long way to go."[133] Indeed, after Nigeria gained independence, violent ethno-religious conflicts between Muslims and Christians would endanger the country's nascent democracy and complicate the WHO's efforts to establish nursing-education programs there. Ethnic clashes that reached across the artificial national boundaries created by the colonial powers would render the politics of global health in Africa volatile throughout the rest of Creelman's tenure as CNO.

Political turmoil, corruption, poverty, and underdevelopment within many of these newly independent countries, coupled with the repercussions of apartheid in South Africa, all circumscribed the WHO's efforts. Long before theories of economic development had matured, Creelman observed first-hand the widening economic gap not only with the developed countries but also within the developing countries themselves. Uganda, in Creelman's mind, was a perfect illustration of the dilemma faced by many developing countries: "the trouble," she thought, was that economic development "will come too fast" and its benefits, as she saw elsewhere in Africa, were unevenly distributed among the population.[134] Civil unrest compounded economic disparity in Nairobi, Kenya, another country on her 1956 trip, threatening to retard nursing's progress. After completing a carefully orchestrated tour of flagship hospitals, the WHO's CNO drew her own conclusions as she drove through the countryside with the chief matron. Images of splendid homes on the tea and coffee plantations stood in stark juxtaposition to villages where members of the Kikuyu ethnic group, the core of the Mau Mau resistance against the British colonial administration, had been rounded up and where a nightly curfew was still in effect.[135] In a letter home, Creelman described her visit to one of these villages, where the recent installation of a pump meant that the villagers would no longer have to walk miles to obtain water. While she admitted that the village system might make it easier to administer health services and provide safe water, to her it was not at all clear whether people would "continue in these villages or go back to homes on their own plots of land."[136]

These trips to Africa provide a window on Creelman's observations about racism. Her back-to-back visits to La Réunion, under absentee French administration, and Mauritius, under British administration, gave rise to private comparisons in this respect that were not without contradiction. In her diary, in referring to Mauritius, Creelman confided that she "thought that the difference in discipline and standards was probably preferable to a complete absence of color bar. It is the French who are more color conscious."[137] Nevertheless, her letters home depicting La Réunion's great beauty but abject poverty noted one good thing: "There is no color bar. In a British territory one is always conscious of the differences made between the European and the African."[138] But none of this detracted from her enjoyment of the African people she met in Uganda. Her letters home made it clear that she "like[d] the Africans very much. They are very kind and friendly and also very clean. The little villages are very tidy and clean in comparison to those which I have seen in Eastern Mediterranean and Asian countries." Similarly, she found that the "nursing is also a higher standard, although they are not so highly qualified. They are very good at practical work."[139] Nursing sometimes provided a narrow perspective from which Creelman could understand and evaluate African society.

On both trips, she made her last stop Brazzaville, in Congo, to catch up on her report writing and discuss what she had seen with AFRO's regional director, who was the key player in securing budget approval and implementing the nursing programs. As she prepared to head back to Geneva after the first trip, Creelman knew that even when the reports were all done, her real work had just started. She thought that five countries would want WHO nurses. "After I go back it will be a job trying to find suitable candidates. As all but one are British countries, it will be British nurses who will fit in best."[140] On her second visit, she welcomed the air-conditioned office and quieter social life in Brazzaville as a welcome sanctuary where she could complete her duty reports on the African countries and prepare her speech for the upcoming meeting of the Canadian Nurses Association. She caught the ferry to Leopoldville several times to see what nursing was like in Congo. From her observations, she perceived "a little contrast between the development of the African in a Belgian country from the British countries. There is no doubt that the latter have done much more."[141] From a nursing point of view, however, she contended that the total absence of female African nurses in Congo, despite the educational limitations, should have been addressed more aggressively. These private reservations were communicated to her mother with a strict warning: "If you read my letters to anyone, don't let the wrong people have my statement on the differences between the Belgian Congo and the British countries."[142] Her letters written during this Brazzaville interlude were illustrative of the public circumspection and diplomatic acumen that characterized Creelman's conduct as the WHO's chief nursing officer.

As the WHO continued to expand its nursing programs worldwide, well-chosen lieutenants became more critical for keeping in contact with staff scattered around the globe. In 1958 she lingered in Brazzaville, awaiting the return of the regional director to discuss the appointment of a new regional nursing adviser. "He agreed to the person I wanted so [I] supposed it was worth waiting."[143] Louise May Bell would serve as regional nursing officer in Africa from 1958 to 1964. Bell, who had been trained at the Nightingale School, St Thomas's Hospital, in London, had held a variety of positions in Tanganyika. She had served as a sister tutor with the Colonial Nursing Service before returning to St Thomas's as a sister tutor. She attracted Creelman's attention for her current work in launching the University College Hospital, School of Nursing, in Ibadan, Nigeria. Although Creelman had handpicked Bell, theirs would be a tumultuous relationship.

In 1960 the bilingual New Zealander Edna Valerie (Ted) Metcalfe was appointed as the nursing officer for Congo and subsequently joined the Brazzaville staff in 1962 as the regional nursing officer responsible for WHO nursing programs in the French-speaking countries in AFRO. Creelman's close personal and professional relationships with the New Zealander endured well past the WHO years.

By the end of her African duty tours, Lyle Creelman had glimpsed the difficulties that the WHO nurses encountered daily in designing and implementing WHO's programs within newly independent nations. The tours apprised her of shifts on the political horizons; she witnessed the rising tide of nationalism within African nations that would dramatically affect future WHO programming. There was no doubt in her mind that Nigeria "will have its independence before too long. Many people believe that Africa (including South Africa) for the white man is lost. Eventually they will all have to get out."[144] It was equally clear that the battle to promote community-based public health programs was still ahead.

For Creelman, first-hand observations were vital to setting realistic expectations for and refining the WHO's nursing programs. Through the WHO's first development decade, her vision of international nursing continued to mature. Face-to-face visits personalized the danger, lack of infrastructure or back-up, language difficulties, illness, or yearning for home that were part of WHO nurses' daily lives. Creelman strove to inspire and support both WHO nurses' efforts in the field and their professional growth to ameliorate the hardships of life in the field. While she became more adept at persuading others to adopt a longer-range vision of building nursing services within developing countries, often hers was a lone voice competing for scarce resources. Geneva's CNO and her regional advisers could actively advocate the development of long-term nursing plans with a significant public health component, but they could not achieve their goals alone. Ted Metcalfe, like many WHO nurses, recalled, "Our goals were to have strong healthy families. I was a jack of all trades and did the best I could with what there was." But front-line WHO nurses also confessed that it was difficult "to make progress unless the governments take an active role in improving general education and the socioeconomic conditions … The nurse doesn't work alone; there are the team, the counterparts, and the government which must have an ideology and commitment to healthcare."[145] Gradually, Creelman came to understand the limitations of leading from Geneva and attempted to foster new avenues to strengthen nurses' voices within their own countries.

Viewed as a composite snapshot, Creelman's and these WHO nurses' stories from the field discredit the view that the WHO's nursing programs represented a top-down donor-driven process that uniformly imposed Western biomedical models. Instead their diverse cross-cultural field experiences suggest that the WHO's nursing programs were more experimental and deeply imbricated in the tangled personal and professional relationships that defined power within the contested local terrain. Some WHO nurses never developed the feeling of belonging; others worked collaboratively with their counterparts to improve local health services. Constructing the WHO's nursing programs remained a highly negotiated process, not only between the WHO's field staff and local the populations but between Creelman and the region's medical officers and politicians. The WHO's nursing programs were necessarily adapted to the host countries' practices, political priorities, and institutional infrastructure as well as to the institutional prerogatives of the WHO's Nursing Section, whose authority would remain disputed during Creelman's tenure.

Creelman always maintained that the selection and retention of an international nursing staff was her most important and challenging responsibility – but one over which she never exercised complete control. Duty travel was an important, but limited, vehicle for extending her administrative reach within the WHO's sprawling field operations. Personal contact during these visits permitted Creelman to support the WHO's nurses, even while assessing their suitability and leadership potential. As the WHO's nursing contingent continued to expand numerically and geographically, she would continue to devise other means not only to sustain and evaluate her far-flung staff but also to extend its authority worldwide.

Chapter Nine

Lyle's Secret Service, 1954–1968

Creating an internationally minded cadre of well-qualified nurses, at a time when there was a global nursing shortage, remained a critical challenge throughout Creelman's tenure with the WHO. As CNO, her responsibility to forge a sense of shared identity and provide effective oversight for her staff – recruited from different countries and, often, with different training backgrounds – presented administrative challenges well beyond her previous international experience in UNRRA. Despite repeated requests for additional staff to meet its expansive administrative responsibilities within the WHO's increasingly far-flung operations,[1] the Nursing Section at headquarters remained incredibly small. In these circumstances, the selection of senior nursing staff within the regional offices and the retention of experienced field staff were crucial components of Creelman's job, which required new management techniques and a different style of leadership.

Over time, Lyle Creelman would fashion several strategies to circumvent the organizational complexities of recruiting and retaining well-qualified nurses from around the world. Her established connections with nursing leaders proved useful in this regard. But Creelman also networked outside formal channels to orientate, support, and evaluate her nursing staff in the field. This vertical administrative network functioned as a vital underground intelligence and communication corridor within the WHO's sprawling field operations.

Lyle Creelman had the added complication of navigating a highly decentralized administrative structure that, under Candau's leadership, increasingly accorded extensive regional autonomy to both selection and program development.[2] Until the establishment of the Nursing Section, regional offices recruited nurses. Even afterwards, the WHO nurses worked within all other functional divisions of the organization under the control of a male-dominated medical profession that influenced staff appointments and daily life in the field.[3]

Appointments to "career" positions, for which staff were eligible after five years of service, and of nursing staff in non-nursing projects did not require the CNO's concurrence. Moreover, politics influenced nursing appointments at every level. A nurse's national background had to be acceptable to the host government; many former colonial countries did not want American nurses, but at other times nurses could not be sent to their countries' former colonies. Sometimes, as in the appointment of the nursing adviser for the Western Pacific Regional Office in 1955, Creelman's preferred candidate fell prey to the political necessity of preserving "geographic distribution."[4] The New Zealander Alice Reid, who lacked any previous experience with the WHO, was selected over the Canadian Lillian Turnbull, who had responsibility for coordinating all WHO nursing programs within Malaya.[5] In this case, other factors may have been at play. Elizabeth Hill, then the WPRO regional nursing adviser, speculated that the resistance to Turnbull's selection also reflected "the fear often expressed towards better education for the nurse." Turnbull had butted heads over this issue with the physicians who blocked her appointment within the Selection Committee.[6] Two years later, when Reid resigned to marry, Turnbull received the nod and served as the WPRO nursing adviser until her appointment as chief nursing officer upon Creelman's retirement in 1968.

Carefully ensconced regional nursing officers served as vital intelligence sources for Creelman within the WHO nursing network. To avoid the development of politically embarrassing situations, she corresponded privately with the regional nursing advisers and the regional directors to vet a particular nurse before either received the "official" memorandum recommending the appointment.[7] Even when an experienced applicant had been identified, obtaining all the clearances within the regional offices and country missions involved considerable persuasion and backstage political manoeuvring by Creelman and the regional nursing officers.[8] Also, inter-regional transfers had to be negotiated with the regional directors, who were frequently reluctant to approve the release of staff to other regions. When Turnbull heard that Creelman was considering appointing her to EMRO in 1966, she wrote to let her chief know that the regional director "strongly protest[ed] such move" and indicated he "would not take the decision lying down."[9] It was not uncommon to have the Nursing Section's prospective recruit overturned at the country level, as was the case in 1952 when Vietnam informed Geneva that appointing a public health nurse "would not be desirable." Vietnam "produces ... doctors who in the field of public health know their jobs better than nurses."[10] Doctors not understanding the nurses' preventative role, either in the hospitals or in the community, remained a major obstacle for the Nursing Section's efforts to call attention to primary health care within many countries. For Creelman, building a nursing presence across the WHO's functional divisions and throughout the regional offices remained a formidable undertaking.

Privately, Creelman vented her ongoing annoyance with what she termed the "administrative muddle" surrounding recruitment.[11] As early as 1951, she complained that her heavy workload at the time was attributable to the task of recruitment, which remained "a frustration more than anything else."[12] Earlier, Creelman would have gladly delegated the "routine responsibility" of recruitment to others, or at least distributed the workload more evenly. In 1955 she raised this possibility with her newly appointed deputy chief nurse, Elizabeth Hill: "If Headquarters' Nursing Section became less interested in finding bodies and paid more attention to so called leadership activities would the regional offices take more responsibility?"[13] While Hill shared her new boss's concern that "we should be giving leadership, and the first requirement is that the technical staff should be relieved from donkey work as highly paid clerks," she told Creelman that "finding bodies may be routine, but this office [Western Pacific Regional Office] would be totally unprepared to cope with it. Gosh, we bog down in getting the bodies placed that are found."[14] Hill would be frequently dispatched on recruiting missions to Canada, Europe, and the United States. But often it would be Creelman who followed up the initial contacts to close the deal. The continued need for the "personal touch" in recruiting senior nurses or consultants meant in practice that most home leaves became recruiting missions.[15]

More irritatingly, often the "mad rush" to find people was followed by budgetary cutbacks, when the director general failed to get sufficient approval. Other times, a project was suddenly cancelled because of a change of government after a nurse had been appointed. Eventually, Creelman "learned to take a calm attitude towards it all."[16] A 1949 diary entry exposed the crux of the problem: "They don't know what to request."[17] Many of the newly independent countries lacked the experience to determine what assistance was required to improve nursing services nationwide. Creelman always made a point to be in Geneva during the World Health Assemblies and became extremely adept in explaining to country representatives the benefits of using the WHO's assistance to develop a long-range plan for national nursing services before undertaking specific projects.[18] But it remained a struggle to avoid showcasing projects that served short-term political needs. Sometimes, she knew that governments recruited WHO nurses to undertake assignments in parts of the country where their own nurses refused to go. In other instances, the WHO stepped in after other international organizations had refused. And, as Creelman candidly admitted after her retirement, it was sometimes necessary to meet these requests so that more effective long-term planning could be undertaken.

In time, Creelman fine-tuned the screening and orientation procedures to improve the utilization of the WHO's nursing field personnel, but she never succeeded in drawing up official selection criteria beyond the stated professional qualifications.[19] In practice, nursing leaders worldwide acted as scouting and screening agents. Early on, however, she acknowledged that the interviewing done within the candidates' home countries was flawed: "It is a very difficult thing to make a selection and then employ people without personal interviews. We cannot expect all our interviewers to know as much about the characteristics required for international work as we do now from our experience and there are bound to be mistakes."[20] Creelman compensated by relying heavily on her Canadian contacts;[21] the Canadian nurses, she always maintained, were better screened than those in other countries because she handpicked nursing directors whose judgment and approach to nursing she could trust.[22]

In her own mind at least, Creelman had a very clear picture of, and was outspoken about, the professional credentials and personal characteristics required to be a WHO nurse. On a visit to Canada in May 1958, she told a Vancouver reporter that "the brisk type" should be "avoided like the plague." As a WHO nurse, she told the reporter, "you have to let someone else do a job that you know you can do better. The authoritarian aggressive person is absolutely wrong for the work. Most Asian and African people are too polite to contradict her but they will resent her attitude." Creelman believed that the "quiet person achieves the most"; a WHO nurse "must drop her own sense of superior knowledge" and learn to adjust "to living conditions – physically difficult, isolated, perhaps both." She must possess "inner resources." She is not "a missionary but she must have the same quality of dedication."[23]

During the 1958 visit, Creelman spent a week in Ottawa catching up with nursing friends and left with the hope that "time has not been harder on me than most of them [but] ... [I] feared it has."[24] She was there to address the Fiftieth Anniversary Biennial Meeting of the CNA being held that week – the first she had attended since joining the WHO. Knowing that "normally it is not possible for HQ staff to attend national meetings," Creelman had obtained permission by portraying the gathering as "an opportunity to do some recruiting which is sorely needed."[25] Her address again singled out cultural adaptability as a prime prerequisite for successful international nursing: "Westernizing was not necessarily the answer ... Today the culture of the country must be considered to make the new approach to health appeal to the people."[26] Creelman constantly reminded Westerners "that our customs are queer to them. Always look for a reason before you criticize."[27]

Recruitment of nurses, she knew, was only the preliminary step; their appointment to appropriate postings and their ongoing support and evaluation were essential to maintain staff morale. Geneva's CNO understood the need for a direct line to her nurses in the field. At best, field reports provided a preliminary assessment of a WHO nurse's adjustment and agency.[28] Official reports were scrutinized to eliminate politically sensitive material before being distributed to the member governments and headquarters.[29] Commenting on the value of nursing reports, Ted Metcalfe said, "Oh we wrote monthly reports but they are probably lying in the regional offices."[30] Another former WHO consultant commented that the practice of creating "positive" quarterly reports made it extremely difficult to evaluate an individual's performance or the progress of any project.[31] Moreover, all official correspondence between headquarters and the region had to be routed through and reviewed by the regional office, which constrained Creelman's ability to provide advice on sensitive issues that involved other regional staff members. On top of it all, shortly after Creelman established a quarterly newsletter as a lifeline for nurses in remote areas – an innovation that unabashedly promoted her own approach, stressing cultural adaptability and the preventative aspect of the WHO's nursing role – it was discontinued. The other divisions, it seems, were not pleased that the Nursing Section was setting up a separate enclave.[32]

Career WHO nurse Mary Abbott aptly described Creelman's strategies to compensate for the administrative restrictions encountered in managing her staff: "We became Lyle's secret service – in a good way."[33] This intelligence network outside formal channels allowed Creelman to circumvent the administrative roadblocks and political intrigue enmeshing the WHO's selection process at every level, and to ensure better utilization of staff once appointed. By providing a franker strategic assessment of nursing programs and personnel, it also served to refine her ideas about the delivery of nursing services around the world.

Creelman took full advantage of the policy that nurses – except those serving in the Region of the Americas – going to and from the field must pass through Geneva. She used the opportunity of every face-to-face meeting with her nurses to acquaint them with the complexities of working within a developing country or with their future team. Like many other WHO staff, Verna Huffman Splane, a well-qualified public health nurse with previous WHO experience in the Caribbean,[34] vividly remembered and commented upon the sound professional and practical personal advice she received from Creelman. She had left her "official" briefing sessions increasingly anxious about the possible difficulties of being the only woman on an all-male team in Libya, an Islamic country where women still wore the veil, and working with a team leader who was not convinced that "a nurse was necessary or qualified to be a member of a national health planning team,"[35] Splane also commented that her discussions with Creelman upon the completion of her assignment "relieved my concern and added to Dr Creelman's file for future use."[36] Splane had made sure that Creelman received a copy of her "unedited" report on Libya's nursing conditions. Addressing returning staff's concerns and conveying a sense that their work was valued and was important, especially when, as in this case, Creelman wanted to draw upon their expertise in the future. The Geneva briefings laid the groundwork for future professional and personal relationships.

While other headquarters staff took care of the administrative aspects of the Geneva briefing, Creelman made a point of meeting and socializing with as many of the nurses as possible during their stopovers. As she confided to her stepbrother, Prescott, a good deal of her leisure activities involved entertaining WHO nurses passing through Geneva: "I have been all day in the fresh air and am soon going to have to take to my bed. There is a Vancouver nurse here en route to India so that I thought I should show her a little of this beautiful country before she goes to the heat and the dirt of India."[37]

Eva Williamson, or "Billie" as she was called, who had been a member of Lyle Creelman's staff at the Metropolitan Health Committee in Vancouver, wrote a letter home that typified the warm welcome awaiting WHO nurses whenever their chief was in Geneva: "Miss Creelman met me at the airport on Sunday and brought me here to deposit my bags before taking me to see the big parade of the Fête de Genève. What a sight it was – gorgeous floral floats, numerous bands and contingents of citizens from the cantons of Switzerland and joining French provinces all in native costume ... After the parade we drove along to Lausanne, a short distance, for tea." Later that evening, they witnessed the confetti parade: "Confetti was everywhere – it seems to be part of any celebration here to throw confetti at anyone you meet, especially if you have your mouth open. The noise continued most of the night so my sleep was nil." Williamson, assigned as a sister tutor in public health nursing in Colombo, Ceylon, appreciated Creelman's personal support during a time of anxious transition within "the imposing headquarters of the Organization," as she struggled to stay on top of the "mountainous piles of [pre-posting briefing] reports" and find out what she was supposed to be doing.[38] But seemingly casual social interactions served other purposes as well.

The chief nurse increasingly viewed these meetings as a final safeguard to determine a prospective candidate's suitability for a proposed assignment. Some did not recognize that Creelman's subtle testing – socializing in several languages or vigorous hikes – was vital for their future career. Often diners at her Geneva apartment were really in-service training in a social setting. In 1954 Eva Williamson joined nine other nurses in transit for an evening at Lyle's apartment, where they enjoyed an evening of slides taken while on duty travel.

Right from the start, Creelman emphasized to each nurse that the goal was to develop the expertise of her national counterpart and not to promote her own career – or, to put it another way, they were to "work themselves out a job as soon as possible."[39] She listened carefully and quickly assessed a new appointment's character and suitability for her prospective assignment or future leadership role.[40] There were cases where Creelman would have preferred to give a new recruit three months' notice in lieu of sending her into the field to fail, but given the demand for WHO nurses, that did not always happen.

While the initial orientation was essential for setting out institutional and professional expectations, most staff still required time in the field to work through their individual personal and professional adjustment to unfamiliar conditions. They had to learn to cope with civil unrest, non-Western standards of public hygiene and health care, and profound cultural differences. One WHO tuberculosis nurse captured the dangers that WHO nurses in many Asian countries experienced: "At the time it was not acceptable [in northeastern Thailand] for women to travel up country as it was considered to be dangerous. I was offered a revolver, which I did not accept."[41] Others told similar stories. Elizabeth Barton recalled, "It was an on the job learning experience. Nothing can prepare one for that first assignment."[42] After her initial briefing in 1962 by Creelman, Dorothy Hall remembered that she left Geneva for India "with a sense of being part of a larger humanitarian initiative capable of bringing change; the idealism of the early post-war years had not totally dissipated yet." These expectations made the cultural shock of navigating a very different health-care system all the greater. India's relentless poverty and cultural milieu, where physicians, who were drawn primarily from the Brahmin caste, were reluctant to touch the children of a lower caste under their care, shaped the delivery of nursing services. Nor had the Geneva briefing prepared Hall for the delicate task of being dispatched by her male WHO colleagues to chastise local physicians who thought that student nurses were there to serve them tea or provide "other pleasures" in the afternoon. Hall later complained that SEARO physicians, "the last great colonial empire who treated the nurses as natives," were prepared to accept her as their social equal at cocktail parties but not in the professional world. It would be Hall's national counterparts who helped her understand the nurse–patient relationship within countries of the Far East.[43]

Once in the field, nurses of all nations and ranks looked to Creelman to alleviate their sense of professional isolation.[44] From Gambia, one WHO nurse wrote, "Sometimes I feel rather like the man who takes a watch to pieces and is surrounded by the bits wondering how to put them back together. Of course there is great interest in what I am doing but no understanding of it and a total inertia in contributing."[45] Recognizing the limitations of "armchair" briefings remote from the field, and admitting that it became increasingly difficult to keep track of her nurses once they moved to their station,[46] Creelman always encouraged the departing nurse to write her about work and life in a foreign country. They told their friend and chief things that they would not discuss with others.[47] As one WHO nurse confided to her, it was a relief to be able to share her feeling of being overwhelmed, "like Alice when she found the 'Grow Tall' tablets in her hand and swallowed one."[48] Their chief nurse was the knowledgeable and empathetic confidant to whom many wrote, whether to vent their frustrations, to gain perspective on arduous working conditions, or to gather up the courage to continue against what seemed overwhelming obstacles.

Both male and female WHO nurses wrote to the chief describing how gender barriers and conflicts with physicians, who failed to understand the importance of public health, deterred their projects' progress. One WHO male community nurse posted in Addis Ababa wrote "without dictionary" to "pour out his feelings" to Creelman in Geneva, though not without cautioning that his revelations of "difficulties, frustration and disappointments ... is one not for the files." His physician team leader, he stated, had declared that a sanitary engineer "in our team was not necessary. When clean water supply is ... essential. This after he wrote ... the *male* community nurses could do a better job. Well, some village people threatened to kill me and one of the community nurses, if we look at the female genitals during delivery. And they would have except that the delivery was carried out successfully, and the clergy protected us." Yet, despite all this, he could report, "I love my work here," and although "it is *not* written in the plan ops ... today I have started to plan a program for public health orientation for nurses ... they need this knowledge so very much."[49] Such letters from the field serve as a reminder of the importance of individual WHO nurses' agency outside the parameters of official operation plans approved in Geneva.

Graham, like other WHO nurses, sent letters to Creelman to discuss sensitive problems – such as her strained relationship with her fellow regional nursing adviser, Doris Pedersen, and the lacking of planning – that could not have gone through regular channels. Others sent sensitive messages via nurses going through Geneva en route home or to other assignments.[50] Creelman, in a move to strengthen nursing's voice within SEARO, had had Graham, a well-educated and experienced hospital administrator, appointed as regional nursing adviser alongside Pedersen. She counted on her close friend and former classmate at the University of British Columbia to send frank private briefings on nursing programs within SEARO. But, just as important, Graham's appointment ensured that views closer to Creelman's would have a role in determining the future direction of the WHO's nursing programs within Southeast Asia. Graham had been involved in a nurse-run, financially independent demonstrator-nursing school in Canada that was designed to educate academically superior nurses in two years. Creelman believed it should be considered as one option for some nursing schools within the developing countries. Whatever the intention behind Graham's appointment, however, the experiment could hardly be deemed a success. Graham encountered considerable resistance from Pedersen to sharing the job for which she had previously had sole responsibility.[51] Moreover, Graham conceded that it would have been better if she had had field experience before being appointed to the regional office.

Although she had decided by January 1955 to "stick it out here," with the implicit understanding that she would succeed Pedersen after March 1956, Graham's correspondence with Creelman was a lifeline throughout this difficult time. As she wrote in one letter, "Lyle, I hope that you understand that it isn't that I have minded being second in command. That would have been fine if only I could have known what was going on … I can't help thinking that too many projects are started without sufficient planning, especially the MCH ones, and so often they have no nursing education aspects. Doris and I must be more insistent in getting in on the early planning stages … thanks so much for your ready response when I air my troubles … I think I will be able to handle matters from now on."[52]

For Creelman's part, Graham's remarks on Pedersen and the ill-advised MCH projects merely confirmed her negative impressions gleaned during earlier field visits. Creelman took steps to ensure that Graham would replace Pedersen in SEARO. Nor would Pedersen receive Creelman's support to be reappointed elsewhere.[53] As Creelman confided to Elizabeth Hill, "It was a hard thing for me to do but I just could not reverse previous impressions. Mike [Sacks], Chief, Programme Co-ordination, would like us to agree that Doris could be transferred to the Western Pacific or that her contract could be extended beyond 1956. I could not do so."[54] Creelman was not given to snap judgments, and her action regarding Pedersen was fully supported by others.[55] Yet, at the same time, she orchestrated a dignified exit for Pedersen and even sent a parting gift. On the eve of her departure, Pedersen wrote Creelman expressing her thanks for "your many kindnesses, your wise guidance and your friendship during my assignment."[56] The iron fist had a velvet glove.

Private letters to the chief nursing officer indicated who needed simple encouragement and who required more dramatic intervention: either reassignment or non-renewal. Requests to Creelman for transfers were not uncommon. The exchange of letters acted as a safety valve for the staff to air their concerns between field visits and provided Creelman in turn with the opportunity to ward off unwanted resignations. They also alerted Creelman to trouble brewing before her visits and provided follow-up monitoring and support afterwards.

Such was the case when Creelman exchanged a series of letters with Elizabeth Barton, a British midwife/public health nurse, and the Canadian nurses Dorothy Potts and Nan Kennedy before and after her three-day visit to Pakistan in March 1954.

Potts was in charge of establishing a basic school of nursing at the Medical College Hospital in a predominantly Muslim country facing seemly insurmountable problems and plagued by continued political turmoil since the partition of India and Pakistan in 1947.[57] The WHO nurses and their Pakistani counterparts shared cabins behind the hospital in a compound enclosed with barbed-wire fences and with guards at every corner. The tall, statuesque Potts, an independently minded and resilient former Canadian army nurse, thought nothing of living there despite the fact that the cabins – small cement cells with tin roofs and interior ceilings made of straw and bamboo – lacked any modern conveniences. She believed that "unless you know what makes a nation laugh or cry then you don't know how to deal with them."[58] Creelman soon learned that primitive living and arduous working conditions were not Potts's greatest professional hurdles. The need to work effectively with professionals from other countries was clear to Creelman and her staff, but it was easier said than done.

Potts, the former director of nursing at Belleville Hospital in Ontario, was respected as a skilled administrator with a forward-looking approach to clinical practice. Yet her British colleagues on the MCH team remained aloof because Potts was not a "sister tutor" with training in midwifery.[59] Eventually, Potts reported to Creelman that she had secured the MCH team's agreement to add a public health component to the curriculum. But Creelman knew from their subsequent correspondence that this assignment continued to test Potts's resourcefulness, resilience, and, indeed, physical and emotional resolve.

Writing afterwards to Creelman on "one of those rare days when one feels one is riding the crest of the waves," Potts good-humouredly recalled, "If you knew how many proposals of one sort or another that I have sent to the Director for apparent consignment to the waste paper basket, without a word of acknowledgement, you would appreciate my feelings of jubilation." She then recounted for her chief how she had finally succeeded in getting her curriculum proposals accepted. Fed up with his complaints that the WHO had little to show after three years, she confronted the medical director. With "fire in the eye," she entered his office "to remind him that we could do nothing without the bodies to train and there would be no increase in the number of bodies to train unless they took action to make the training facilities passable and acceptable to the people." Potts's earlier letters also exposed her initially strained relations with the East Bengal Nursing Council, an "august body" that, Potts complained, "has only recently appreciated the fact that the WHO nurses could be of some assistance to them." Nonetheless, she eventually obtained the council's support to train ward aides and auxiliaries to alleviate the students' heavy workload and to reduce students' obligatory service conditions from six to four years following training, both of which discouraged candidates from entering nursing, But, as she confided to Creelman, the real issues had yet to be addressed: "I did a tour last week and was heart-sick at what I saw. The hospitals are bad and no mistake about it. But what really depressed me was the attitude of senior officials … towards nurses and nursing … sheer indifference and even disrespect. I suppose it is the result of man's age old concept of the 'place of women.'"[60] While Potts had developed effective professional and personal relationships with Pakistani counterparts with whom she lived and worked, the battle to improve nursing services and conditions took its toll, as manifested by her condescending attitude towards the Pakistani nursing leadership. Her letters to her chief underline the immense difficulties even well-trained and well-meaning nurses experienced in negotiating culturally sensitive and sustainable nursing services.

Looking back on her time in Pakistan years later, Potts admitted, "I don't think that a foreign group can enter a country without creating some problems … It is important for consultants to realize that people must be helped to do things the way they think it should be done and not coerced into doing it 'our way.'"[61] For many WHO nurses, the personal and professional adjustment experienced in undertaking their first WHO assignment was enormous and usually a clear indicator of who was up to the challenge. While Potts regretted leaving Pakistan, she realized that she needed more public health training if she were to continue working for the WHO. Creelman supported Potts's request for a study leave to obtain her master's degree at Teachers College and afterwards endorsed her appointment as the regional nursing officer for EMRO (1959–66). Creelman, like her nurses, had to learn from experience that cultural sensitivity was achieved on the job and that professional leaves were required to provide perspective on conditions in the field, to set realistic professional boundaries, and to rekindle the desire to undertake another international assignment.

Elizabeth Barton's letter requesting a transfer had alerted Creelman to the tensions brewing within the team in advance of her arrival. Creelman wrote a letter to Barton in which she apologized that Barton had received the notice of another WHO posting too late to apply. Empathizing with Barton, she encouraged her to hold on until the arrival of an experienced public health nurse with whom she was sure Barton would enjoy working.[62] Creelman identified Barton as a midwife with great skill and dedication. She would guide her professional advancement, successfully encouraging her to renew her contract and later arranging a WHO fellowship for further study in Canada that led to a life-long career of valuable service with the organization.

Following the Pakistan trip, Creelman, as promised, strengthened the WHO team in Dacca with the appointment of a lively, independent, and widely experienced British Columbian public health nurse, Nan Kennedy.[63] Kennedy had become unexpectedly available for this assignment when her earlier hopes for a Burma post were shattered by the outbreak of civil war in that country. In Pakistan, she told Creelman, she quickly realized that the program in the maternal and child health centre was unrealistic; it was impossible to send young nurses out from the very protected environment of the MCH centre to do rural midwifery, often without the assistance of a doctor, in a country where women played no role in public life. Kennedy discovered the difficulties of negotiating, as a woman and a nurse, with medical officials to obtain a small rural MCH centre outside Dacca, where the students could do the final months of training. During the next two years, she frequently accompanied her students on visits to villages where she met with village officials to ensure that her nurses had physical protection if they were called out to do home deliveries in the middle of the night. Wading through the floods to help her students on their hut visits built a strong bond of mutual respect and friendship but did not remove the frustrations involved in gaining a voice for nursing within a male-dominated society.

The Dacca team's correspondence illustrates the wide spectrum of WHO nurses' experiences in sharing knowledge and learning from their counterparts while serving in the same geographic and socio-economic location. It also underscores the achievement of Creelman's vision of working with local nurses to improve nursing services, which depended on the locale, length of international experience, temperament, and agency of her field staff. Not all were up to the challenge. Some requested transfers; others resigned or were not renewed.

While most nurses drew comfort from writing to their chief, this was not the case for the British Columbian public health nurse Margaret Murray Campbell Jackson. Assigned to Iran, an Islamic country where religious restrictions, lack of educational opportunities, and low cultural status impeded nursing's development,[64] Campbell Jackson, the former assistant director of public health nursing,[65] experienced a profound personal and professional cultural shock in poverty-stricken Tehran. The Nursing Division within the Ministry of Health had been established only two years earlier.[66] WHO nurses assigned to Iran had been carefully briefed not to expect the democratic environment of their home countries. The country was still reeling from the 1953 coup that had ushered in the military government under Mohammad-Rezā Shāh Pahlavi.[67] As the nurse on the WHO team, she was expected to launch a public-health nursing-education program and to train a counterpart to take over an MCH centre without the requisite authority to implement the changes required.[68] She became increasingly discouraged by the venality of government officials – "who were only interested in lining their own pockets and obtaining service from WHO's staff" – and by their failure to provide the promised facilities and students. As an experienced public health nurse "who had come to Iran prepared to teach," Campbell Jackson chafed at the professional constraints of working in a clinical setting where the Swedish physician expected her to be content with seeing "babies day after day"[69] and where her administrative contribution went unrecognized.[70] These workplace-related disappointments fostered a pejorative attitude towards her first national counterpart, whom she characterized as "pretty useless and beside not too clean." Her lack of training, aggressive nature, and inadequate command of English, in Campbell Jackson's view, "made her an unfortunate choice."[71] Even after she negotiated the appointment of a more acceptable British-trained counterpart, Campbell Jackson continued to compartmentalize her professional and personal relationships.

Contact with Creelman was one of few avenues open, outside the immediate circle of WHO nurses assigned elsewhere in the city, to overcome her sense of professional isolation and frustration in a place where "we get absolutely no magazines … on nursing – or any professional stuff at all except a tiny bulletin put out by the WHO."[72] Campbell was determined to set Creelman straight about what was really happening: "It's a cinch she knows nothing of Iran."[73] Sometimes she "wonder[ed] what Miss Creelman is doing in that office. She surely takes on her share of duds, I am learning."[74] In fact, Creelman already shared Campbell's reservations about the suitability of another WHO nurse whom Campbell censored for regarding her work as a year-long vacation and for the lack of discretion she displayed in her personal life. In July 1955, "terribly fed up,"[75] Campbell wrote Creelman in the frankest terms possible, explaining why the whole project was a mistake and requesting a transfer. Creelman's reply did little to alleviate Campbell Jackson's unhappiness: "I was quite disappointed in it. I don't know what help I expected but certainly more than what she said – they can't do anything about the project but certainly they are concerned. And she knows that often an international team find that they can't contribute anything. And that a conscientious person would feel the way I did. They would be glad to offer me a position, if and when a position was available, but she hopes the situation will resolve itself. That would be a miracle."[76]

The exchange exposes the limits of the Nursing Section authority and Creelman's personal diplomacy, practised as it was from her distant office in Geneva. Creelman letters could not rectify Campbell Jackson's Western sense of superiority. Equally important, it exposed the highly contested political terrain in which the WHO's nursing programs at all levels were negotiated. The Nursing Section often had little say about a specific country program. The Creelman-Campbell Jackson correspondence reveals one of the chief nurse's retention strategies – an empathetic response to prevent immediate resignation until a more suitable position became available. In Campbell Jackson's case, she ultimately turned down a transfer. Instead, after being appointed team leader, she deftly manoeuvred, sometimes outside official channels, to obtain her proposed freestanding MCH clinic that would be the cornerstone of her field-training program.[77] Still dissatisfied, she chose not to remain beyond this assignment.

Letters between Creelman and Lillian Turnbull were particularly illustrative of the formative influence that Geneva's chief nurse had in shaping the direction of nursing leadership within the senior ranks of the WHO's Nursing Section. After her appointment in 1957 as the regional nursing adviser in the WPRO, Turnbull struggled to express her appreciation to Creelman for her kindness and advice during her Geneva briefing: "My feelings are really too deep to express in words on paper. I cannot tell you how much it has meant to me to have this chance to know you, to learn your strength of purpose, your faith in the Organization, and your faith in us who have been working with you in the field, we have made many mistakes, have been weak when we should have been strong and many time let self become before service but it is a comfort to know that these weaknesses have been viewed with tolerance and most of us can have another chance to do better."[78] While Turnbull believed that "the advice and counsel you have given me will be a real resource to remember and use in difficult times," she knew "that you will be there for advice and help when I need it ... I know that there will be times when I wish you were in the next office and not half way around the world but I will try to give it my best and hope to learn and grow on the job and that I will be able to keep up the good reputation that has been established by our Nursing Section."[79]

In Turnbull's case, she had grown "tired of cold formal memorandums which have a tendency to make you feel like [an] essential item on an inventory and make it seem that the distance between Geneva and Manila [is] so great that it cannot be spanned." She relied upon personal correspondence with Creelman both to humanize the bureaucratic channels and to convey the details of the "battle of the Budget" within the regional office where "some of the assaults and offensives have been a success while in other cases a graceful retreat has been necessary." In one of these letters she confided, "I don't know how I like this job. Some days it's fine and then come days when I am sure that I will end up with a gastric ulcer and, perhaps, a warrant for frustrated murder."[80] Her often humorous exchanges with Creelman provided a much-needed emotional release for insecurities that could not easily be shared with her own staff. She once anxiously wrote about her role in the upcoming regional nursing conference: "I have lot of hurdles to clear and a lot of pit-falls to fall into and try to crawl out of gracefully ... I'll feel your presence with us in Tokyo. Carnations and Roses are my favourite flowers in case of any personal disasters."[81] Turnbull's respect for Creelman never wavered. As she prepared herself "for the horrible fate" of replacing Creelman as CNO in 1968, she lamented that "it will be a sad day when our Chief decides to leave us. Many people will remember ... with respect and admiration your support and judgement and the place you held so admirably in the World Constellation of International Health Workers."[82]

None of Creelman's relationships were more important than those with regional nursing advisers. Only rarely could Creelman meet with them as a group: their meeting in 1964 was the first since 1951. Moreover, their cooperation was vital because Creelman's infrequent visits to any region were possible on the basis of regional requests. These women then mounted the first line of defence against any encroachment on the nursing aspects of the WHO's health programs in the field, and, consequently, Creelman paid particular attention to their selection and ongoing development. She identified those who shared her transcultural approach, such as Elizabeth Hill, Lillian Turnbull, Dorothy Potts, Dorothy Hall, Evelyn Matheson, Ted Metcalfe, Louise Bell, and Mary Abbott. Geneva's CNO then took steps to ensure that they acquired a breadth of field experience or upgraded the educational qualifications required for future career advancement that reinforced that approach. Creelman discerned their views from interviews, letters, and reports and often incorporated excerpts from their field reports into her speeches.[83] These women understood that WHO nurses needed to plan educational programs "based upon local situations to such an extent that all the driftwood in the conventional school of nursing curriculums will be left behind." They looked for nurses "with confidence, courage and vision to be original."[84] Prior to Hall's appointment as SEARO's regional adviser, for example, Creelman arranged a study leave for her so she could obtain her master's in nursing at the University of Washington on one of the Rockefeller fellowships reserved for WHO personnel. Creelman knew that Hall's time there would be valuable for her work as an adviser to India's Ministry of Health, where her responsibilities included teaching her national counterpart the principles of curriculum building. In this Hall followed the University of Washington model, which stressed the necessity for nursing educators to determine what their students needed to know to meet the health-care needs within their country.[85]

Creelman's relationships with these nurses, while obviously crucial, varied immensely among the regions and the personalities involved. Some regional advisers respected her while holding firm to their own views; others were somewhat intimidated by her extensive knowledge of nursing conditions worldwide. Dorothy Hall, who had joined an American nurse, Lucile Holsinger (1957–62), as the second regional nursing adviser in the SEARO office in 1962, was independent and self-reliant in temperament. A former Northern Ontario Outpost nurse, Hall would earn a reputation among her WHO colleagues as "a power in the land" during her twenty-six years of service with the WHO.[86] She had met Creelman only after joining the WHO, but the two of them spent many weekends relaxing at Lyle's chalet whenever Hall came through Geneva. During the 1960s their chalet visits provided the occasion for long and animated discussions about changes to the nursing curriculum in SEARO. Both women could be blunt at times and neither tolerated fools well. Yet, despite their friendship and cordial working relations, Hall always contended that it was impossible for Creelman to grasp fully the gruelling conditions that many of the WHO nurses experienced or prepare them for what lay ahead.

Creelman understood the limitations of staged visits for furnishing anything more than a snapshot of the health landscape within any country, and so she relied on letters from regional advisers to provide an invaluable corrective to sanitized field reports. Often letters from nurses on the spot, especially staff she already knew personally, gave a more frank assessment of relationships within a team or how individual nurses were adjusting than could be put in official reports.[87] They often provided candid accounts of WHO nurses' difficulties with physicians or the dangers posed by war, such as in Vietnam, where the nurses had to be rescued from jail. Alice Reid, after visiting Saigon with Elizabeth Hill in 1957, compared the WHO difficulties there to those of UNRRA, "with the nurses on the whole doing a good job, and too many doctors riding on their coat tails."[88] Sometimes, private assessments also led to the difficult but necessary decision not to renew contracts of Canadian nurses whom Creelman knew or had recruited.[89] If Creelman determined that a regional adviser, such as Doris Pedersen, was not suitable, she secured her removal as soon as possible. Occasionally, however, the termination process was complicated by the incumbent's attempt to withdraw her resignation, as in the case of the regional adviser for the Eastern Mediterranean Regional Office, Inge Götzsche. Having admitted that "ambition, drive for appreciation, approval and success has in many cases prevented me from being of help to people around me," Götzsche appealed to Creelman in 1956 for permission to remain in the WHO to engage in "the ideological fight which is becoming more intensive for [sic] every day."[90] Her departure, not surprisingly, was not delayed.

Whenever the budget allowed and approval from each of the regional directors could be obtained, Lyle Creelman brought her regional advisers on an individual basis to Geneva to assess staffing issues or thrash out the future direction of programs.[91] Fellow British Columbian Margaret Cammaert[92] recalled making such a visit to Lyle's chalet over the Christmas holidays while serving as the regional nursing adviser for the Americas. Afterwards, Cammaert always felt a bond with Creelman, whom she regarded as "having a kind heart under the austere outer veneer" required of Geneva's chief nurse. Lyle, she recalled, "was a brisk no nonsense kind of woman on the outside. She was straight talker and [you] never left with the idea that she would manipulate you for her own advantage." In her opinion, Creelman's strength was her ability to lead her regional directors "indirectly." She provided direction in a way that was not confrontational. Cammaert contended that the sense of collegiality that characterized the WHO's nursing leadership derived from their common challenge of advancing nursing in politically fragile and economically strapped developing countries and from a shared international perspective that "you needed to see things through their [locals'] eyes and not ... western eyes that valued efficiency and time management."[93]

WHO nurse Maura Leavy's recollections of her early days in the field suggest that, by 1961, the presence of carefully selected regional nursing officers had led to greater continuity between the Geneva briefing sessions and the ongoing orientation in the field: "On joining I was impressed by the idealism & calibre of the staff ... and it seemed that everyone's contribution counted & was under constant scrutiny in a constructive manner to ensure that progress was being made ... A maternal/paternal eye was kept on new recruits to ensure their safety and suitability. Monthly reports were required and were read and commented upon and all field staff on their first assignment had a visit from their Nursing Advisor within the first 6 [months] ... This was great."[94] Creelman had taken steps towards correcting the troublesome staffing issues identified on her early field trips.

Even at times when the writer professed not to have any business writing personal letters to their chief, the letters allowed nurses to express their frustration at the lack of professional respect shown for them in countries where the authoritarian atmosphere reflected the "great white father attitude" rampant among international workers. The letters exchanged with Eleanor Kunderman, a well-educated and broadly experienced Vancouver public health nurse,[95] spanning the twenty years of Creelman's tenure, illustrate both the personal and professional dimension that linked staff nurses within the WHO's nursing network. In 1959 Kunderman arrived in Geneva for a general orientation from Lyle Creelman and Elizabeth Hill before going on to EMRO for a more detailed briefing about her first assignment just outside Tehran, at the Red Lion Sun School of Nursing. Over the next eighteen years, she worked in India, Sri Lanka, Nepal, and Burma until her retirement in 1977.

Notwithstanding warnings from Creelman and Elizabeth Hill during her Geneva briefing "not to try to set the world on fire" and that she "would not find things as democratic as I was used to" in Iran, Kunderman grew impatient with the lack of progress. Expecting "that people in international work would naturally be superior types," it came as a great "shock to find out that they could even be inferior." She frequently wrote to Creelman to "validate my feelings that I was proceeding in the right direction ... I can be honest with you and it helps me in my perspective. These are things that one does not tell to people at home, because as far as they know I am having a real ball – and I am too but it is appropriate for me to tell you my real feelings because you understand and I have always been able to talk with you easily."[96]

As Kunderman candidly admitted, "I am the type that has to be 'belted in the mouth' with this kind of advice before I learn."[97] Her letters, indicative of the professional difficulties many WHO nurses encountered, describe the Geneva briefing's influence on her own journey of cross-cultural adaptation:

> Your words lit up like neon signs at the first team and counterpart meeting ... It seems that a group of students had refused to write an examination and it was announced at the team meeting that their caps had been taken away for two weeks, nobody had asked the students why ... [Subsequently] it was decided that the students be withdrawn from the wards and two weeks added on to their training ...I sat in shocked silence that this was accepted as the right thing to do – I felt it was a bit soon in my international experience to question this ... Then the pattern of the whole project began to become clear and one meeting after another was taken up with discipline and punishments to the exclusion of anything constructive.[98]

Then a more experienced Canadian WHO nurse, Evelyn Matheson, arrived and Kunderman found "she had a soul mate." Working together with their national counterpart, Sirkka Leva, the three nurses succeeded in changing the tone of the team meetings: "One would never recognize these nationals as the same frightened, intimidated girls as I first saw them; the way they speak up at meetings is wonderful." Kunderman confided to Creelman, "I am still awaiting the 'cultural shock' but nothing has happened." But she assured her chief,

> I have had the professional shock and this will require compromise and adjustment but I think that I can handle myself in the situation. Evelyn [Matheson] is like an oasis in the desert and we have planned all kinds of activity for the next two years ... I am enjoying my work in planning a nursing arts course with my counterpart and we are also trying to produce a procedure book before fall class ... My counterparts are beginning to accept the idea that they are actually teaching the

course and not just interpreting my words. Please tell Miss Hill that her advice about this being "their program" still echoes in my ears and I am so grateful for the careful briefing I got from her – her message came through loud and clear & I will remember it.[99]

Once in the field, Kunderman grasped the core message of the Geneva briefing and gradually developed a more realistic view of what could be expected in a project. Her definition of international nursing echoed Creelman's and Hill's philosophy: "The most important thing to realize in international work is to realize that you don't go in and say this is the way we do it in Canada and it has to be like that … there is no way that a paediatric ward in Canada can be like a paediatric ward in Madras. You can't compare them. So you can not super-impose your western ideas, or your culture or your western beliefs on to these people. You start where they are at and you work with what you have and you must be satisfied with the smallest return, with small satisfactions but in reality tremendous satisfaction."[100]

Kunderman's letters, expressing her gratitude to Creelman for her personal friendship and professional support, echo comments by other nursing colleagues from around the world about a chief "who sustained us wonderfully."[101] Equally, Kunderman's letters capture the extent to which the private and professional spheres of Creelman's life were intimately connected, her nursing colleagues being part of an extended family network. In 1966 Kunderman wrote about their shared time: "Real cheese, good bread, friendly cups of coffee and glasses of wine. Open windows, blankets, sleep and 'bed-coffee' provided warmth for body and soul. Long walks, wild flowers, painting benches in the cold air and warm sun. Good talk and comfortable silences in quiet communion. Friendship and affection. The sharp mind of a friend … How lovely it was – and is – and how grateful I am for the time."[102]

Knowing that her staff lacked the "comforts" of home, Creelman routinely addressed her nurses' personal needs by sending small personal gifts or favourite food items. Her actions set the tone within the administration for other regional nursing advisers and consultants. Katharine Lyman, a distinguished American nursing public health educator, expressed the sentiment of many former WHO nurses when she wrote in 1961, "Really the thing that makes WHO tick in my mind is the myriad of personal things that you and Elizabeth [Hill], Alice [Reid], and Lily [Turnbull] over the years did – letters in your own handwriting, cards at the holidays."[103] Creelman always believed that the WHO doctors were envious of the close rapport she and her nurses had, despite the intermittent nature of their get-togethers.[104]

Most WHO nurses were single career women who chose international careers to gain greater professional autonomy than they could have aspired to in either military or civilian nursing. Letter writing was one expression of the female friendships that fostered a sense of kinship among expatriate nurses. Exchanging letters helped them to create a shared sense of personal and professional space within the gendered global-health medical hierarchy that few back home would have understood. Often, correspondence also provided valuable insights into local political conditions that inhibited WHO health programs within a country. As one WHO nurse explained to Creelman, "It is always a pleasure to write to you, but you probably noted that I write more frequently when I am out of the organization than when I am in – always afraid of offending the 'proper channels.'"[105] In the early 1960s, letters from her staff continued to provide Creelman with a frank assessment of the WHO's position in many countries. One of these was Cameroon, where the WHO had a strained relationship with government officials. A WHO nurse there, Olive Manning, wrote to Creelman in 1962, "I fear the chances of job-satisfaction are extremely remote. To begin with it is pretty obvious that the present administration does not want (though it badly needs) any assistance from nurses in planning or running its services and in particular the French medical advisors in the ministry want nothing of W.H.O. I could give lots of examples of what I have seen of the waste and misery which could have been avoided if the advice of a nurse had been sought, but you asked me for the lighter side of life."[106]

But even personal letters had to be used cautiously. In a letter written to Eleanor Graham upon her resignation from SEARO, Creelman candidly acknowledged, "I have to be very careful in some of my statements as I could send only personal letters to the regional office. I was not sure if all personal letters reached the addresses unopened. There were often times when I would like to write you and give you more explanations."[107] The fear of prying eyes explains why Creelman habitually sent private correspondence, as in this case, with WHO nurses going through the regional offices en route to their posts.[108] Her actions speak to the political sensitivity with which regional autonomy was guarded in setting and implementing the WHO's programs, and underline as well the expectation that its representatives remain strictly neutral.

Götzsche and Pedersen notwithstanding, Creelman displayed considerable ability to work with a wide range of colleagues. While some of her field staff sometimes viewed her as set in her thinking, she generally listened and considered all the factors shaping the advancement of nursing before taking a position. Certainly, her serious nature, drive, and determination made her a difficult colleague at times. Yet she was an able administrator who allowed, indeed expected, her senior staff to have the freedom to experiment in order to customize the nursing program within their regions.[109] Creelman recognized that, as one person in a huge organization, she had only a limited ability to effect change; accordingly, she found people with the skills and capacity to act independently and told them to get on with the job. She counted on her deputy chief nurse, regional advisers, and consultants to act as her agents; she imbued them with the principles of cultural adaptability and expected them to convey back new ideas to refine her own transcultural approach. She never adopted a monolithic view of international nursing; she believed that both the local community and the nation were important, especially in countries where large segments of the population had been displaced.[110] Over time, she developed a deeper appreciation for the work and human experience of the ordinary nurse in the field but could never entirely stand in her shoes.

Some WHO nurses felt that Canadians got the choice placements under Creelman,[111] and there was some truth to that view. Creelman, as she had in UNRRA, relied upon Canadian nurses whom she knew to be supervisors or team leaders able to act as troubleshooters or to keep an operation afloat in difficult and physically demanding settings.[112] In 1965 Canadian nurses held at least one of the two regional nursing adviser positions in all but the European Regional Office. Even there, Alves Diniz had a very close personal friendship with Creelman and was the holder of a Rockefeller Foundation fellowship at the University of Toronto. In addition, over a hundred Canadian nurses received field appointments, second only after the United States, during Creelman's tenure. Their selection had sound administrative grounds; many former colonies did not want American nurses, and bilingual Canadians with university degrees were actively recruited for French-speaking countries in Africa during the 1960s. In fact, finding more French-speaking nurses had become such a priority that Creelman dispatched Elizabeth Hill on a trip to Canada from 25 January to 8 February 1961 to enlist the aid of Canadian government officials and nurses in key positions in recruiting French-speaking staff and to explore the interest of selected schools of nursing in forming a cooperative liaison with schools in Africa.[113] On a subsequent trip of her own to Canada, Creelman made inquiries along the same lines. From her earlier field observations, she knew the importance of having nurses who could live and work together without a language barrier.

While Creelman may not have deliberately given Canadians preference, there is no doubt that she viewed Canadian nurses as well qualified and more likely to be culturally sensitive than their American counterparts. Like many Canadians of her generation, Creelman naively assumed that her country's lack of colonial possessions made it well suited to play a constructive and politically neutral role in the developing world.[114] But the reality was that newly developing countries demanded nurses with degrees to launch their university-based programs, which further limited the countries from which nurse-educators could be chosen.[115] Many European and Commonwealth countries launched university-based nursing education programs only in the decades after the Second World War.

Creelman's highly personalized administrative style relied on personal loyalty and a shared sense of corporate purpose with her staff, as well as her personal and professional contacts within the established leadership circles worldwide. Its success attested to her growing international reputation and administrative acumen. There was no guarantee that a less adept or well-connected CNO could replicate it successfully. But, for the moment, as the WHO's nursing staff swelled in size, Creelman concentrated on gathering intelligence and forging a spirit of corporate identity among her field personnel; her approach represented a shift in values from an elitist or faith-based concept of duty to one of advocacy and collegiality in the effort to achieve the right to health for all. Her correspondence with WHO nurses illustrates her ongoing battle to establish a more culturally sensitive approach to designing national nursing services within the WHO and its member countries. Even those who "made [themselves] invisible and pushed the national nurses forward,"[116] and who "had a feeling of belonging"[117] still remembered the enormous difficulties they faced: "the lack of water, the materials and immunization that didn't arrive, the teaching that seemed to make no sense, the routines of feeding and hygiene that were Western and seemed strange to the population."[118] There was always an inherent tension in relying upon Western-trained nurses to implement a more transnational approach to nursing within the WHO. Cognizant of the structural dependency, Lyle Creelman sought new opportunities to engage nurses from the developing world in the regional or intergovernmental policy dialogue that would shape the future direction of nursing services and education within their own countries.

Work remained Lyle Creelman's central focus, leaving never enough time for family and friends outside nursing circles. In her personal life, a significant relationship remained ambiguous throughout much of Creelman's time in Geneva. Her sporadic contact with Dick Pullen during trips to Vancouver left many questions unanswered. During a 1952 visit, Lyle recorded that she "had some wonderful times with Dick, but wished she 'could really read his mind.' He seemed interested in how long I planned on staying with [the] WHO. He is really in a spot with his Mother ill ... We became closer than ever."[119] By 1954, however, her diary suggests that she realized the limitations of the relationship: Dick was "the same as ever. Guess he will always be there but that seems hardly enough."[120] Creelman reconciled herself to accepting "pleasant evenings" and "pleasant memories." A letter she wrote to him in 1958 recalled the "pleasant memories of the three weeks ago this evening, and also of other times. Too bad one has to live on memories, but they are nice to have," ending with simply "Cherrie."[121] Dick would continue to pick her up at the airport on most visits and take her out for dinner as time allowed. Whatever the hopes of her youth, she had little expectation that her return would change their relationship after all these years. As she said so long ago, she simply had no luck with men.

But in reality Lyle Creelman had chosen an international nursing career over marriage. Her heavy workload and prolonged absences from both Canada and Geneva offered few opportunities for courtship or even for female relationships beyond nursing's ranks. As a single expatriate career woman, often living out of a suitcase for months at time, her social network within the nursing community became increasingly important both for professional validation and for personal rejuvenation.

Chapter Ten

The Voice of International Nursing, 1960–1968

During the 1960s, a period of particular global turbulence, Lyle Creelman became the unparalleled voice of international nursing. Respected by colleagues, she directed the WHO's Nursing Section with skill and confidence, and nurses around the world routinely turned to her for support and advice. In turn, friendships formed within the international nursing community, sustaining both her social and professional networks, were especially important to Creelman as she navigated these hectic years. She continued to rely upon the leadership network for direct help, political intelligence, and reassurance. Recognizing, however, that WHO nurses could not effect sustainable change alone, Creelman also encouraged the development of more advocacy and communication networks within countries at the grass roots, where the WHO ran nursing programs. Functioning as a cross-cultural broker between these social and professional networks, Creelman acted as a catalyst to change the face of international nursing. She reached the peak of her influence in this period, but her achievements came at considerable cost in her private life.

In the WHO's second development decade, the politics of the Cold War had a special salience for the organization's policies and personnel. The year 1964 alone brought heightened international tensions: China exploded an atomic bomb, and Vietnamese communists successfully waged the guerrilla warfare against the American-backed regime of South Vietnam. The year also witnessed widespread unrest and discontent in Africa. The Federation of Rhodesia and Nyasaland dissolved. There were revolutions and riots in Zanzibar, Tanganyika, Uganda, and Kenya. In Congo, the last UN troops withdrew, leaving in power Moise Tshombe, who defied international opinion by using white mercenaries against local rebels. South Africa was barred from the Olympic Games in Tokyo because of its apartheid policies. The next year, Rhodesia unilaterally declared independence from the United Kingdom. All these events demonstrated the complex social and political conditions that Creelman would encounter at the height of the Cold War, which diverted funds from health issues to the arms race and yet at the same time made global health an important instrument for forming new anti-communist alliances in the post-colonial world.

During the WHO's second decade, the Nursing Section expanded both the scope and the reach of its programs. From 1958 to 1968, WHO nurses took part in 160 country projects and conducted sixty regional workshops and conferences.[1] In 1958 Creelman had responsibility for 155 WHO nurses serving in forty-four countries – approximately one-fifth of the total WHO field personnel.[2] By 1963, the WHO had 183 nurses, with 163 engaged in fieldwork in seventy-three countries,[3] and by 1968 there were over 200 WHO nurses. Budgetary restrictions forced the WHO to concentrate on improving or initiating educational opportunities to complement the growing role of the WHO nursing consultants in advising national governments.[4] Nonetheless, the Nursing Section expanded its mandate to include the promotion of research relevant to nursing issues throughout the world.

Moreover, by the end of the decade, the vertical approach used in malaria eradication by U.S. agencies and the WHO since the 1950s came under increasing criticism. Within the WHO there had always been tension between the social and economic approaches and the technology- or disease-focused approaches to population health. The emphasis between the one and other shifted, depending on the larger balance of power and their changing interests and the philosophies and personalities of the directors general. In 1968, the year of Creelman's retirement, Candau called for a comprehensive plan to integrate preventative and curative health-care services that ultimately led to the acceptance of a primary health-care perspective in the 1970s. A new director general, Halfdan T. Mahler (1973–88); new international actors; the re-entry of China into the WHO and the accompanying widespread interest in Chinese barefoot doctors; and the advent of new developmental theories during the 1960s and 1970s that drew on the grassroots experiences of non-governmental organizations and medical missionaries all shaped the future direction of WHO policies. During the 1960s, the Nursing Section would put forward its own proposal for health and development, as the future direction of the organization began to be re-thought.

All these factors increased the magnitude of Lyle Creelman's role as the international gatekeeper brokering nursing's advancement worldwide. As CNO, she continued to rely on the advice she received from her extensive contacts within the nursing leadership network while also taking steps to broaden the representation on the expert panel on nursing.[5] With many of these colleagues, Creelman had strong personal ties. One such figure was Sheila Quinn,[6] who served on the administrative staff of the ICN from 1961 to 1970. Quinn fondly remembers Creelman as a delightful companion and a valued colleague, "both a mentor, and a great point of reference."[7] To the ICN, Lyle Creelman was a familiar personality – "a quiet interested figure never pressing her opinion, but always ready with sound advice when called upon." Lyle was a "brisk voice at the end of the phone with a snap answer to whatever question was put to her."[8] The two had become friends when Quinn, a relative newcomer to the ICN, unexpectedly had to take over as executive director from Helen Nussbaum just as the ICN was preparing to move its office from London to Geneva in August 1966. Creelman was especially supportive of the newcomer during the transition to Geneva and continued to prove "a fount of useful information on global nursing matters" throughout her term.[9]

Quinn, however, "could not imagine Lyle not giving her considered opinion in a very forthright manner" at ICN meetings,[10] and Creelman herself freely admitted to being "a very active observer" at the ICN Congress in Melbourne in 1962. Ellen Broe, director of the Education Division, had proposed holding an international seminar based upon data collected solely from countries with specialized training. When it became "obvious that members of the [Education] Committee did not like this idea, but avoided making any other suggestions," she "finally suggested how we might approach a similar problem at WHO – hence consultants."[11] By hiring consultants, the background survey for the international seminar could be expanded to allow for extensive participation and feedback from the membership "to learn whether they want to move toward a more generalized education or not, and to define what they thought generalized education should be." In making this suggestion, Creelman "had in mind the very good response we had in 1956 from the nursing association in preparation for our technical discussions on nursing [at the WHA]. They are still talked about."[12] Creelman was not reticent in recommending to Broe two consultants, Katherine Lyman (American) and Helen Mussallem (Canadian), both of whom she knew personally and held in high regard professionally.[13]

As Quinn recalled, "Lyle was waging an awful battle to get nursing established within the new organization and perhaps hoped the ICN's closer proximity [after the ICN relocation to Geneva] would allow for greater coordination and more widespread influence."[14] Just such an opportunity occurred in 1967, when Quinn included Creelman in the initial discussions triggered by the ILO offer to develop an instrument of international law on the status of nursing personnel. Knowing that the ILO would take this action in any case, and believing that the legal change envisioned would be of "real value," Creelman used the ICN as a shield to overcome the WHO's reticence to become entangled with the ILO again or be placed in a position where it might be expected to ensure its member governments' compliance with other UN specialized agencies' conventions dealing with human rights or the social determinants of health.[15] Her proposal that the WHO collaborate through the aegis of the ICN in the preparatory work but without any financial commitment was finally accepted. While the ILO report of 1960 had failed to produce any immediate significant results, this time the ICN-ILO collaborative partnership eventually led in 1977 to the adoption of the ILO Nursing Personnel Convention (C149) and accompanying recommendation (R.157) as international labour instruments.[16] According to Creelman's successor, Lillian Turnbull, this caused "turmoil in the WHO Executive Board. There was some ambivalence regarding bargaining privileges for nurses."[17]

Quinn maintained that Lyle Creelman acted as a particularly effective ambassador for the ICN. Creelman constantly "stressed to WHO nurses that 'the ICN was the professional association in the country and WHO had the responsibility to interpret to the government the role of their own professional organization.'"[18] During her duty travels, she always informed the local CNOs of ICN work and the procedures for becoming a member. In fact, Creelman often dropped by the ICN office to suggest which national nursing officers had "gotten off track" or needed the ICN's assistance to gain admission to the organization. "Lyle's most striking characteristic," Quinn said, was her internationalism, which, coupled with her detailed knowledge of nursing around the world, meant that others often consulted her.[19]

Given the demands placed upon the small staff at Geneva headquarters, Creelman sought the ICN's help to shoulder some of the workload but never hesitated to make her own views known on the task at hand. While she remained adamant that the ICN should take the lead in fashioning the guiding principles and content of nursing legislation,[20] she opposed applying the legislation of one country to another. "We do not do this in relation to nursing curricula, the philosophy being that we help the country to develop its own. I think the same applies to legislation but we can, however, be somewhat more specific in this field ... It seems to me we need a document which outlines what should be included in an Act and what in By-laws and why."[21] In the end, her lobbying paid off: after the formation of its Nursing Service Division, the ICN undertook this responsibility.

Creelman's counterparts in other international organizations remained some of her most important sources of support; they offered an opportunity for frankness and comparison of experiences not always possible within the WHO, where discretion was advisable. One such figure was Lucile Petry Leone of the USPHS, who provided great personal support for Geneva's CNO and regularly tried to schedule the annual meetings with American agencies or organizations engaged in international nursing projects at times when Creelman could attend.[22] Key nursing leaders, including Creelman, often met over cocktails before working dinners at Petry Leone's home to prepare for these meetings. At one such meeting in 1964, Dr Leona Baumgartner, appointed the head of the U.S. agency for international development in 1962, was one of several influential guests invited to brief the nurse representatives from ten organizations with international health programs.[23] Creelman used such gatherings as sounding boards to air controversial professional issues and to strategize on how to advance nursing's interest in global health within international forums. At the time of Petry Leone's retirement, Creelman thanked her for her personal and professional support. Referring to the meetings in her home, Creelman said that "their informality has made them so valuable to all who participated and the most recent one, held earlier this month [January 1966] was indeed a highlight."[24] These meetings were especially important for Creelman, given that PAHO operated as a virtually independent fiefdom within the WHO and limited the official flow of information on nursing activities to Geneva. Her praise for the meetings, however, did not preclude Creelman from contending in 1961 that, unless minutes were kept and circulated, nothing would come of the discussions.[25]

As always, Creelman's off-the-record conversations and letters with the Rockefeller Foundation's nursing officers were designed to short-circuit potentially divisive staffing issues or determine the likelihood of RF financial backing for a joint project before these matters were raised in Geneva.[26] She developed strong personal and professional ties with the RF's Virginia Arnold. Arnold and Creelman had shared formative experiences while working with UNRRA.[27] Both were indefatigable advocates of preventative as well as curative public health services, both fought to establish a stronghold for nursing within their respective organizations,[28] and both consistently had to convince their medical colleagues that nursing made an essential contribution to international health programs. Arnold so respected Creelman that she considered spending the final years of her career working for her in Geneva.[29] Moreover, it was Arnold who asked Katherine MacLaggan to nominate Lyle Creelman for an honorary doctorate from the University of New Brunswick, which was granted in 1963.[30] On the occasion of Creelman's retirement, Arnold wrote a private letter to her friend to let her know that "I have always felt a closeness and kinship for you. I felt that you also knew what I was trying to do. At the same time I felt that you had a more difficult task in WHO than I had in the Rockefeller Foundation by the very nature of the WHO organization. May I say that you have done the job amazingly and with the greatest effectiveness?"[31] As director of the Rockefeller's Nursing Section, Arnold was responsible for liaison with the USPHS technical-assistance program, which ran nursing-education programs in Latin America, the Middle and Far East, and Southeast Asia. When their paths crossed in the field, Arnold and Creelman frequently exchanged intelligence on matters that had the potential to impede either's work in the area, just as Arnold's predecessors had done with Creelman in earlier years.[32] The two chief nursing officers arranged their schedules to allow private meetings whenever possible and frequently exchanged reports, with Arnold cautioning Creelman to keep such information "at home or some safe place since this is very much against RF policy."[33] This underground information exchange helped them to avoid "stubbing [their] toes" when meeting with governmental officials,[34] by providing Arnold and Creelman with frank assessments of "the real political situation."

Occasionally, the WHO's chief nursing officer asked her Rockefeller colleague to provide an independent evaluation of a specific WHO program or staff member. Such was the case in Turkey in 1961. Creelman told Arnold privately that she "had heard rumours" that the WHO nurses Faith Hodgson and Susan Sontag Anderson may "have pushed too hard and fast."[35] Afterwards, Arnold sent a note to Creelman's home, "for obvious reasons," thanking her for the copy of Hodgson's report on Turkey. In this instance, Arnold's letter confirmed the WHO nurses' portrayal of their difficulties: "The situation sounds pretty grim but I do remember when I was there I was not overly impressed with the nurse who had recently been appointed in the ministry and I knew that the WHO nurses were having a very bad time with her."[36]

Creelman's relationship with Arnold was a double-edged sword that, if not deftly handled, could jeopardize future requests for assistance. The Portuguese WHO nurse Tito de Moraes was a case in point. According to Arnold, Creelman initially had reservations about Tito, but evidently she changed her mind, for in 1962 Tito replaced Elizabeth Hill as deputy chief nurse. Creelman had given Arnold the heads-up on Tito's pending appointment in order to preclude a request from the Rockefeller Foundation to second Tito for a two-year period. The news of the appointment surprised Arnold, who found it difficult "to believe that LC had a change of heart about MPT de M." Believing that "our effort to get MPT de M. last summer has shaken LC,"[37] Arnold alleged that Creelman had undercut the foundation's earlier efforts with respect to Tito de Moraes for personal reasons: "It is a fairly well known fact that Lyle Creelman does not like MPT de M. and has blocked her on previous occasions when interesting assignments were available or there were opportunities for promotion."[38] She added later, "I agreed to do nothing since this position is far better than we could offer MPT de M. at this time."[39] From Arnold's perspective, the appointment was a success: Arnold remarked that Tito had slipped into the position "with ease and has apparently helped LC to relax." Arnold predicted that there would "be much greater co-ordination in the future with EH out and MPT de M. in."[40] The incident speaks to the Rockefeller's influence within the WHO.

Unlike Hill, Tito had never been a regional nursing adviser. She joined the WHO in 1950, serving in Syria, Iran, Guatemala, and Brazil, and, prior to her appointment as deputy chief nurse in 1962, she was the director of the Higher Institute of Nursing at Alexandria. In 1966 she would exchange positions with Alves Diniz, serving as the regional nursing adviser for the European Regional Office until 1972. Right from the beginning, Alves Diniz, who had developed a close friendship with her chief while the ERO was still located in Geneva, spent many weekends at Lyle's chalet before purchasing her own close by. Tito was a less frequent weekend guest, perhaps because the two Portuguese nurses did not get along. Once the ERO relocated to Copenhagen, Alves Diniz and Creelman kept in touch and visited each other whenever their schedules allowed.

Creelman, adept at quiet diplomacy, continued to rely on the Rockefeller Foundation's Nursing Division for advice and financial support. In 1962 she again dropped by Arnold's office while on home leave to discuss problem areas and to seek the RF's financial assistance to help launch nursing schools, in this case in Nigeria and Ghana.[41] That same year, Creelman approached Arnold to undertake a study for the WHO on the effects of the European Common Market on nursing.[42] Arnold, for her part, regularly kept Creelman informed on other developments that might affect the profession internationally, such as the 1958 American congressional proposal for a National Institute for International Medical Research in the USPHS. That proposal was a direct response to a development at the 11th WHA, held in Minneapolis instead of Geneva.[43] There, the director general had been asked to evaluate the WHO's role in stimulating and coordinating research. In this instance, Arnold sent a letter to Creelman "on a personal basis only to keep [you] informed and express my faith in, and desire for leadership in all fields by the WHO."[44] Specifically, she urged Creelman to consider the establishment of a research position within her office for a nurse with experience. Creelman's guarded reply indicated the difficulties that the Nursing Section confronted in getting a foothold in the newly established Division of Medical Research. Despite the section's aggressive lobbying efforts with "one of the members of the Secretariat whom we felt would be our greatest supporter," its proposal to consider the role of the WHO in nursing research was turned down. Creelman admitted that, although she did not expect the proposal to be approved, she had finally made a submission to have it on the record.[45] Creelman encouraged Arnold to keep her informed: "All information on and suggestions which will serve as ammunition for the right moment will be appreciated."[46] At this juncture, Creelman was especially sensitive to the need for new ammunition to penetrate the medical oligarchy's control of the WHO's administration. Her request for an additional position within the Nursing Section at headquarters – which had a "great deal of support" – had also been denied.[47] Not even determined, shrewd nursing leaders such as Creelman and Arnold could work miracles.

Believing that nurses at all levels of the health-care system needed to collaborate more effectively across borders to influence its policy formation, at home and globally, Creelman increasingly sought opportunities to utilize the ICN and the expert committees both as important leadership foci within the international nursing network and as platforms for the WHO's further expansion and democratization. The 1965 ICN meeting that Creelman attended in Frankfurt on 13–25 June was an important milestone in this direction. The presence of about five thousand nurses at this congress, in Creelman's mind, signalled that "nursing was more organized and powerful" than ever, as demonstrated by the admission of Spain, Peru, Sierra Leone, Hong Kong, and Gambia to membership. Contending that "it was the best meeting yet," she applauded the adoption of a new ICN constitution and the decision to move the organization's headquarters to Geneva. Ever the pragmatist, she remained impatient at the waste of time and sheer hyperbole surrounding the proposed new definition of nurse.[48] Yet she was delighted that Alice Girard[49] was elected president of the new ICN board. She both respected and shared many views with the well-regarded dean of the Faculty of Nursing at the Université de Montréal. In 1965, as dean, Girard established the first French-language master's-level nursing program in the world – a program that benefited Creelman in her search for well-qualified French-speaking nurses. While some found Girard's frank, outspoken, and decisive manner intimidating, Creelman thought it refreshing. During Girard's term, the ICN would undertake a number of studies, including one on working conditions for nursing, and prepare an ICN publication on nursing legislation that facilitated local nurses' advocacy role within their own countries. The studies on working conditions and legislation were both issues that Creelman had long pursued.

Knowing that she would retire in 1968, Creelman began laying the groundwork to pass the leadership torch a half-dozen years ahead. Convening the fifth expert committee on nursing in 1966 was her final attempt to strengthen nursing's voice at both the national and intergovernmental levels and to broaden the horizons of the international nursing community. She deftly quarterbacked the preparation of background studies and committee proceedings to set the

Nursing Section's future direction and to articulate a new vision of modern nursing.

Creelman had her own agenda for striking another expert committee: she was determined to incorporate some of the recommendations of the recent study of the WHO's Nursing Section by Dr Ruth Freeman, a professor of public health administration at Johns Hopkins University and the rapporteur for the fourth expert committee.[50] In asking Freeman to undertake that study, Creelman confided that "lately Elizabeth [Hill] and I have been unhappy about the contribution of nursing in WHO when we contrast what we are able to do with the potential."[51] Even though it had been favourably received and was proving a useful common document for the regional nursing officers, Creelman knew full well that a report from an expert committee, approved by the WHA, would carry more political weight than an internal study.

Creelman's letters surrounding the Freeman study, which were "off the record and not for the official file," vividly depict the administrative isolation in which the Nursing Section functioned. Freeman's simple request to obtain organizational charts proved embarrassing. The Nursing Section did not have any charts, and those eventually provided were only of a "typical" organization. On further investigation, Creelman told Freeman that she had learnt that in some cases no charts were available and that others were out of date. On the existing ones of the African Regional Office and American Regional Office, there "was no indication of where Nursing fits."[52] The sense of growing isolation, as Creelman confided to Freeman, was exacerbated by the decision to relocate the Nursing Section's offices: "We received a real blow last night when we were told that our Division has to move to the other side of the lake. This is the first of the professional groups they have had to move ... We, of course, regret this very much because our contacts with people of the other Divisions means so much to our work and being here to drop in on expert committees, etc. However, it seems that our division was the only one that was the right size."[53] The relocation boded ill for the Nursing Section's future.

Freeman's study provided a systematic and comprehensive evaluation of the Nursing Section's performance – and it was sorely needed. The number of nursing staff skyrocketed during the 1960s, making it increasingly difficult for Creelman to exercise effective oversight or receive adequate feedback from staff nurses. Perhaps remembering the suspicion and distrust that she had encountered in conducting field studies for the Baillie-Creelman Report, Creelman made certain that everyone involved understood that Freeman's study was designed not as an evaluation of individuals' past performance but as a planning tool to increase future effectiveness.[54] The decision to discuss the draft report at a meeting of the regional nursing advisers allowed the document to function as a form of in-service education for senior staff. Together, they assessed its feasibility and implications for programming and identified areas of concern requiring further study.[55]

Again, bureaucratic politics coloured the study's agenda and delayed its progress. Regional nursing advisers exerted pressure for direct contact.[56] Creelman wrote Freeman to explain the further delays in sending out the questionnaires to over five hundred WHO nurses, both active and former, worldwide: "This makes me vexed. The questionnaires have not yet arrived in my office so I don't know the nature or extent of the comments ... All this has arisen because of the Spanish translation; we must have the DG's approval ... I wanted to say ... 'why can't we leave the questionnaire to the experts?' but refrained."[57] Upon being informed that the regional directors would also have to approve the questionnaires, Creelman told Freeman that she would write to all of nursing advisers "to give them some assistance in discussing the matter with their Regional Director."[58] Judging from her later comment that no further changes were required at the regional level, her strategy proved effective.[59]

The nurses' responses to the questionnaire identified several significant issues that the fifth expert committee would need to address. In general, their replies indicated satisfaction with the WHO's nursing program but underlined the need for increased staffing (especially nursing auxiliaries), leadership, clinical specialists, and research. They also underscored the importance of greater cultural sensitivity to accommodate national needs and capabilities in future WHO nursing projects. Many nurses claimed that they were able to do this but "half the nurses and about a fifth of the non-nurses respondents felt that this was only partially true." Defining professional relationships proved equally challenging for the WHO nursing staff. Only six of the twenty senior nursing personnel indicated that "their judgments were fully utilized in relationships to the utilization of nursing staff" and another eleven stating that this was done "on a partial basis." At the field level, 30 per cent stated that the medical staff had little or no understanding of nursing and another one-third felt that the physician usually saw nurses as "handmaidens" or less than full-fledged team members. In turn, non-nursing colleagues complained that nurses focused on maintaining standards instead of getting the work done or "sometimes saw nursing a separate empire." Finally, 37 per cent of those surveyed described their working relationship with other international aid agencies as "collegial" but "unproductive."[60] None of their responses came as a surprise to Geneva's CNO; the survey merely reinforced Creelman's determination to strengthen nursing's position within the WHO before she left.

Whatever its pretensions at being an independent review, the Freeman study carefully delineated the issues that Creelman and Hill saw as inhibiting the

Nursing Section's effectiveness. Given that about half of the nurses employed by WHO were assigned to projects over which the Nursing Section acted only in an advisory capacity, its recommendations, if enacted, would have given the Nursing Section more control over all aspects of nursing in the WHO. Nursing, the report argued, "cannot represent an isolated activity within the Organization – it must permeate and contribute to the many programmes, which include nursing." It was also clear that the "functions and objective of the WHO imply acceptance of a leadership role in nursing affairs and the exercise of initiative in dealing with trends and forces that affect nursing throughout the world."[61] Staking out the Nursing Section's claim to be a co-architect of global health were recommendations governing the recruitment and promotion of highly qualified international nurses; the involvement of nursing in all aspects of the planning process to ensure that programs were tailored to the specific socio-economic conditions of each country; and the expansion of the scope of the section's activities, particularly in research.

The study provided a roadmap to guide the Nursing Section's future work, especially in developing countries. Its recommendations, echoing Creelman's well-established position, supported the development of nursing services countrywide and posited the need to meet the legitimate quantitative demands for nursing services, "even at the cost of some dilution of quality." This came with a caveat: at the same time, preparations should be made for the creation of a nucleus of fully prepared (professional-level) nurses capable of advancing to positions of leadership as clinical nurses, teachers, or administrators.[62] In Creelman's view, the immediate steps to improve the population's health must be accompanied by the development of public health infrastructure; otherwise the disease was treated but its root causes were ignored. Likewise, the Freeman study advocated the development of nursing services geared to existing social, cultural, and economic conditions but "calculated to make it possible for a country to adapt quickly and economically to higher levels of nursing care as resources increase."[63] It also called for greater coordination with other international agencies to support the country in the development of its "own goals and plans for nursing care."[64] This was a tacit acknowledgment of one of Lyle Creelman's guiding principles: effective global-health governance more and more required forming coalitions across borders, both national and institutional, to direct sustainable health improvement.

To build on the Freeman study, Creelman retained Marion Murphy in August 1965 to write a background study for the fifth expert committee. A former WHO fellow whom Creelman had met in South America in 1951, Murphy was a professor-director of the public health nursing unit of the University of Minnesota's School of Public Health. Once again, Murphy's selection allowed

Creelman to incorporate the insights from an earlier WHO specialized publication on public health nursing. Murphy had been one of the contributors to a 1961 WHO technical report, "Aspects of Public Health Nursing," that looked at the challenges to improving public health nursing in various parts of the world, especially in light of the increasing demands for nursing personnel.[65] Creelman used that report to raise controversial professional issues, particularly the role of auxiliaries: "One has the impression that nurses were so intent on defending their professional status that they forgot that health services exist to meet health needs."[66] The papers included in the cutting-edge report showcased a variety of systems of public health training and practices around the world, and documented the need for culturally sensitive frameworks to determine the type and quality of nursing personnel tailored to the individual country's health requirements and current capacity. Significantly, the report ended by exploring the difficulties of designing nursing services in cross-cultural situations.[67]

Murphy's background study for the fifth expert committee provided an important framework for subsequent regional nursing conferences to chart the future development of WHO nursing assistance and sustain nurses' demands for a greater voice at all levels of policy formation, a larger allocation of staffing resources, and funding for nursing research.[68] "Copying the patterns of other countries" was rejected in favour of "multi sectoral planning" that looked "at the particular nursing situation which exists, finding out what patterns of problems and health needs and planning for nursing in a constructive and realistic manner within the national or local health plans now being evolved in accordance with the socio-economic and cultural needs and resources of each country or local area."[69]

Murphy's study, prepared under Creelman's editorial oversight, departed from the traditional view of nursing education and nursing practices that "stressed the role of the physician's assistant." Instead, it portrayed the nurse as "operating independently within the knowledge of the plan for medical management." In this scenario, the nurse had a therapeutic partnership role with the patient, designed "to ensure the patient maintained a state of equilibrium, thereby reducing tension and freeing energies for the process of recovery." On the societal level, the nurse had a unique contribution to make to the patient and family life; the nurse's role included "contributing to the comfort and recovery through interaction in the milieu of which the patient is a part." In brief, "the well prepared nurse was expected to make a 'nursing diagnosis' in which nursing care or 'intervention' is determined."[70] The concept of a nursing diagnosis directly challenged the medical community's sole propriety right in this area. The language in Murphy's study was far stronger than that in Freeman's study.

Significantly, Murphy's background study reiterated the first expert committee's emphasis on "doing with" rather than "doing for" people but, unlike the earlier report, called attention to the need to "demonstrate respect for the individual and awareness of individual differences."[71] It clearly set out the frame of reference for the next expert committee: "It is probable that empiricism characterized early development in all fields now regarded as scientific; thus it may be regarded as a natural, essential phase of nursing but one that must be questioned in light of the developing knowledge on many fronts." More provocatively, it asked, "Why should nursing education in developing countries follow traditions which dictate a curriculum containing fixed experiences of certain length and almost exclusive orientation to biological/medical rather than social approach to nursing?"[72] Although all the four previous expert committees had stressed the importance of research, Murphy confirmed this point by including the recommendations of the WHO's first Scientific Group on Research in Nursing (1963) regarding the links between service, nursing education, and research.[73]

Following upon the Freeman and Murphy studies, the fifth expert committee, meeting in Geneva from 26 April to 2 May 1966, was told that "the present age is one of social, industrial, and scientific revolution, of rapidly increasing populations and of widespread poverty. It is also an age that is seeing a revolution in medicine and nursing, with attendant hazards for the individual."[74] The twelve years since the fourth expert committee on nursing had witnessed profound changes in the nursing services that were required to meet the increased demand worldwide for improved health care. The advent of new technologies ushered in intensive-care and coronary-care units, and new drug therapies dramatically altered the treatment of tuberculosis and polio. These and many other medical advancements revolutionized the scope of nursing practice and the type of specialized education required. The practice-boundary expansion experienced during the 1960s, calling for nurses to make complex, rapid clinical decisions, required new education and models grounded in scholarly inquiry. Within Western societies, the feminist movement of the 1960s would inspire a new generation of nurses to challenge the gender-based roles in nursing and medicine. Nursing leaders in industrialized countries articulated a new professional strategy to legitimize nursing as a profession and academic discipline.[75] As before, Lyle Creelman would have the job of brokering the divergent interests of nursing in a world where the North-South economic development gap had only widened in the intervening years since the last expert committee.

As Creelman had predicted, with Freeman's overview and Murphy's background paper in hand, the committee deliberated on the education and provision of sufficient nursing personnel to meet the new health-care demands and also considered the importance of research aimed at better patient care.[76] The report noted that "a complex group of forces – social, cultural, economic, and political – that affect progress in many other aspects of life have also been brought to bear on nursing. Changes in the status of women; population increases and the increased numbers in some age-groups, particularly the older ones as certain diseases come under control; rapid transportation; educational opportunities; economic and social mobility; increased demands for health services; automation – are all having an impact on nursing in most countries of the world."[77] Accordingly, much of the discussion centred on the importance of focusing "efforts on current and future needs and problems rather than those of the past," with the recognition that "in the next decade nursing will probably be faced with some of its greatest and most exciting challenges. With the trend towards mass medical care and the changing pattern of health service, the nurse of tomorrow will have to accept unprecedented responsibilities."[78] The committee warned that "fundamental rethinking will be necessary." Echoing Murphy's paper almost word for word, it questioned the wisdom of following a nursing "curriculum dictated by tradition and continuing set experiences at fixed length, with an almost exclusive orientation to a biological rather than a social approach to nursing."[79] The committee took the stand that "nurses should, from the start of their education, be given a broad preparation in preventative, curative, and rehabilitative services"[80] and that, in any determination of changing roles and responsibilities, the needs of the patient should be paramount – a position long held by Geneva's chief nursing officer.

The expert committee's report combined the "back to the patient movement" with the proposition that improvements in nursing education had direct benefits for improved patient care. Creelman stood firmly alongside those nurses who had taken the view that the "unique contribution to nursing lies in patient care with its underlying implications for cure."[81] It was, however, the inclusion of the discussion of "teacher-practitioner" – as "a demonstration of the means through which nursing knowledge is continually kept vital" – that most closely embodied Creelman's own leadership and cross-cultural brokerage roles within the WHO:

> Inherent in the teacher-practitioner role is the systematic, contemplative, skillful gathering of significant data about patients, thinking about it, asking questions about it, doubting it, relating it to other information gleaned from observations made by oneself, one's students, one's colleagues and struggling to find in it evidence upon which decisions could or should be made, and then evaluating the outcomes based upon those discussions ... It is incumbent upon this ideal-type of practitioner to share observations made about patients, to talk about them, to

seek the meaning of them from colleagues and students alike, thereby providing a role-model to demonstrate it is the very nature of the professional to engage in a continuous search for refinement of knowledge needed for constant improvement of the practice.[82]

It posited a nursing model of compassionate authority that championed shared learning and enabled the participation of patients and caregivers alike in contrast to the earlier model of unquestioned authority of power over patient care.

The report's recommendations integrated Creelman's experience gained in the field over almost two decades. Indeed, several of its cautionary notes echoed concerns clearly articulated on numerous occasions by Creelman during her duty travels. First, it criticized "the tendency to take a pattern of nursing education (basic and post-basic) developed to fit one country's needs and transplant it *in toto* in another country without due regard of such factors as the extent of industrialization, the level of general education, or the stage of the development of education."[83] Second, the report drew attention to the necessity of providing further professional-development opportunities to nurses trained under the old apprenticeship system to prevent a schism from developing within nursing's ranks. Third, it chided "those who had difficulties in accepting auxiliary workers as an integral part of an organized nursing personal system."[84] Finally, while the report acknowledged that each nation must determine the quantity and quality of nursing services and the kind of education required to fulfil those needs, it restated the long-term goals of establishing nursing education within a university setting and ensconcing nursing leaders within policymaking circles to direct the future development of nursing services and education. Neither Creelman nor the committee questioned that improved educational standards would directly improve the quality of patient care and attract more and better-qualified recruits to the profession.

Assessing the impact of the committee's report is difficult. Creelman's ability to reference the report helped to fund and legitimize the future working documents that followed. The 1968 "Guidelines for the Development of Post-Basic Education for Nurses"[85] called for a "new and imaginative approaches to the public health component of nursing services" that championed primary health care, especially within developing countries.[86] The document reiterated the importance both of understanding the cultural determinants of health care and of developing a national plan for nursing education that would eventually fashion a well-educated, highly skilled nursing force responsive to change and the needs of the patient.[87] "Nurses in every country must receive the kind of preparation that will enable them to teach groups of people, to plan and work effectively with them, and to understand and apply health education principles that will result in the active participation of the community in the improvement of health." Preparing such a document engaged nurses across borders in dialogue on important nursing issues. In completing the circle of knowledge required for its production, Creelman had sent out a survey to eighty-eight selected post-basic schools in forty countries.[88]

The existing evidence sheds some light on the limitations of policy formulation within the WHO and, conversely, the reach of the WHO's recommendations within the international community. Creelman consistently used the expert committees to increase the Nursing Section's effectiveness, institutional profile, and budget. But the committees' recommendations were never accepted automatically. For example, the fifth expert committee's recommendation to create two new positions in Geneva, one a nurse-midwife and the other a research nurse, provoked "considerable argument as to where these nurses should be assigned – the Nursing Section under Lyle Creelman or the section concerned, e.g. – the nurse midwife to MCH."[89] The controversy over this recommendation underscores the Nursing Section's isolation within WHO decision-making circles, even as Creelman's tenure was drawing to a close.

That said, the fifth expert committee was not without accomplishments. The report provided an important reference for WHO nurses in the field. Creelman's fellow Canadian Margaret McLean,[90] a former WHO consultant and vice-president of the Canadian Nurses Association, shared her reactions to the committee's report in a paper presented at the International Congress of Nurses held in Montreal on 25 June 1969. McLean, who had extensive international experience as a hospital consultant in the United States, Mexico, Costa Rica, and the eastern Mediterranean, told her audience, "The more I study the W.H.O. Expert Committee on Nursing Fifth Report, the more impressed I am that eight nurses from eight countries and two international representatives were able to prepare a document that is at one and the same time excellent and progressive and has application and value to nursing in every country."[91]

During the 1960s, as the WHO grew in size and extended its programming to more and more countries, the selection of regional nursing officers became increasingly crucial for maintaining administrative cohesion at the ground level. While Creelman had good relations with her regional nursing officers, there continued to be exceptions. Louise Bell, the British regional nursing adviser of the African Regional Office from 1958 to 1964, became a challenging colleague. Renowned among her colleagues for her mercurial temper,[92] Bell frequently used correspondence to her chief as an opportunity to express her frustration with the administrative inefficiencies of AFRO, as in a letter of 1960: "I am rather tired by this MCH-UNICEF kingdom, they seem to usurp the place of the full health programme for a country; I think it is mainly because UNICEF has been very powerful, it will gradually change, already the outlook is better."[93] Even though she often agreed with the substance of Bell's arguments, Creelman came to question her ability to provide reliable and consistent leadership for AFRO's nursing programs. Despite the civilities exchanged, Creelman, along with others on the WHO staff, found Louise Bell a difficult person, who seldom accepted criticism or suggestions graciously. Even after Bell had unnecessarily affronted WHO colleagues and a government official on an official visit to Mauritius – calling the former "woolly headed" and implying that the principal matron was unqualified for her position[94] – she remained unrepentant. Bell's curt response in 1960 to Creelman's letter attempting to placate her did little to improve their relationship. "You say that from my letter to Losonczi you realize there 'is not much justification for his criticism,' one wonders what has led you to believe that there was any?"[95]

In 1962 Creelman judiciously sought Virginia Arnold's opinion about Bell. During a meeting at Arnold's office, Creelman told Arnold that she was worried about Bell, "who was showing unpredictable swings in moods" that were being manifested "in sudden changes of plans and dislike of individuals."[96] On a visit the following year, Creelman again raised her growing concern about Bell, who, according to Arnold, "showed sign of deterioration" – a situation that was compounded by the fact that "no one in Geneva knows much of what LMB is doing and LC doubts the program can get underway this year."[97] It is clear from Arnold's diary that Bell was at times somewhat of a maverick, whose zeal to establish a university-based nursing program at Ibadan caused her to ignore official WHO channels and keep her national counterparts out of the information loop.[98] Creelman's opinion of her was substantiated a week later when Arnold learned that Isabel Fimister, director of the Hospital School of Nursing at the University of Ibadan, and Matron Richmond of the hospital, both of whom were recipients of RF travelling fellowships, "had never been included in on conversations on plans and knew little or nothing about the scheme." Fimister in particular "was concerned that the program might be pushed too fast."[99] Arnold alerted Creelman privately to the situation before re-routing Fimister through Geneva en route home to "talk frankly with LC." Afterwards, Arnold took care that Geneva's CNO was copied on any correspondence with Bell to avoid any further miscommunication.[100]

One can only surmise how Creelman would have reacted if she had known of Bell's clandestine efforts to get Ibadan chosen as the site for the English-speaking post-basic nursing-education program. Behind the scenes, Kofoworola Abeni Pratt, or Rola,[101] then deputy matron at the University College Hospital in Ibadan, was exerting considerable pressure on Bell to support Ibadan's selection. The two had a long-standing friendship that dated back to Pratt's training days at St Thomas Hospital, where Bell was then a sister tutor. According to Pratt's biographer, "Miss Bell was the most influential force behind her professional rise to eminence in Nigeria and the World."[102] At critical junctures of her professional development, Bell opened the door for Pratt's future success in nursing in Nigeria. Pratt was the first Nigerian nurse to break the colour bar and be appointed as a sister tutor at University College Hospital in Ibaden, where Bell was then serving as the first principal before her appointment to the WHO. Most recently, in 1959, Bell encouraged Pratt to apply for both a WHO fellowship and a Carnegie Travelling Grant. The Nigerian returned convinced of the necessity of creating a university-based nursing program in Nigeria. "Mrs Pratt's trusted friend and mentor, Miss Bell, committed herself to the cause being championed by her favorite nurse."[103] Pratt, recognizing that there was considerable resistance within British nursing circles to university-based programs, orchestrated the invitation for Bell to visit Ibadan and hold confidential meetings with the minister of health at his private residence: "The secrecy which surrounded the exercise was important because of the danger that the [British] Chief Matron might oppose the developing initiative."[104] At the official meeting the following day, attended by the chief matron, no mention was made of the project. It would therefore be erroneous to view the subsequent founding of a university-based nursing-education program at Ibadan as solely a WHO, UNICEF, and Rockefeller Foundation initiative. The local politics were more complicated than Geneva knew; Nigerian nurses were beginning to exert their own sense of agency. The daughter of an influential chief, Pratt was held in high regard within her own country and abroad. Her path and Creelman's would become more intertwined as the 1960s unfolded.

Tensions between Creelman and Bell, meanwhile, had been building for some time, centring on a fundamental difference over the future direction of nursing projects in Africa. "The point on which I feel," Bell wrote, "we have been pulled in opposite directions, in the first instance ... [was] regarding the implementation of the post-basic programs in general." Bell saw no need to hold up the development of post-basic education until a national survey had been completed. As she and Creelman grew estranged, Bell criticized her chief for failing to respond to inquiries and for her lack of trust and support: "Please know there are difficulties enough on the horizon & your real assistance is so much needed, but you must try to believe that I know what I am doing and that you cannot plan for the needs of AFRO in HQ. It is just this year that I have found a lack of understanding from you; I am so sad about this."[105] A month later, in a letter outlining the tensions within the office and describing the political manoeuvring that was infringing on her plans for nursing within the region, Bell lamented that she had not received a response to her previous letter: "Lyle why don't you write? … I get worried and upset about something & write freely and openly – as indeed to a friend – & letters such as these you don't usually answer at all … I am quite prepared to take your candid comments and long so much to know what exactly is in your mind. That is why I wanted to come to Geneva when it was such a real possibility. I know as things turned it was just as well, but I would just about give anything to have a good talk with both you and Elizabeth [Hill] – to gain your support again … There is something wrong – which it seems will not be perhaps be righted except by real discussion – or have you given up on a bad job … Oh for a telephone to Geneva."[106] Whether Creelman was waiting for Arnold's report to gain perspective or merely distancing herself personally remains unclear.

Arnold admitted that, during the first few days of a visit to Nigeria and Ghana, she thought that Bell "would drive me mad," but she subsequently saw her "in quite a different light and learned to respect her knowledge of Africa and her ability to handle top level people. I learned that she is highly respected by Africans, a fact that should not be ignored. If you decide not to renew the contract, it will come as a great shock to them … I think she is undoubtedly 'slipping but far from slipped.' "[107] In fact, Bell's prominence in AFRO meant that, on another occasion, Creelman sought Arnold's assistance to circumvent Bell's known opposition to the WHO nurse whom Creelman wanted to head the Ibadan team.[108] In the end, Bell remained as regional nursing adviser in the African region for another two years. Her replacement was the Canadian WHO nurse Dorothy Potts (1967–76), whose views on the importance of developing regional universities as a preferable alternative to international fellowships, and whose staunch belief in the necessity of involving national counterparts, more closely aligned with the direction espoused by her chief in Geneva.

Building sustainable and balanced health-care systems remained a priority for Creelman, who displayed her allegiance to these principles both in her daily work in Geneva and on her duty travels in the developing world. In March 1963 she toured EMRO to evaluate the progress nursing had made since her last visit in 1954. She found the regional office in Alexandria virtually unchanged. In Cairo, the nursing scene was filled "with many strange contrasts": sophisticated graduates from the Higher Institute alongside the horrible conditions of some of the hospitals.[109] By the end of her tour, when she had the opportunity to evaluate the contrasting philosophies of the three nursing schools in Egypt, Sudan, and Ethiopia – the Higher Institute, Khartoum College, and Asmara – she concluded that Khartoum was probably the best but that the Higher Institute was producing some impressive nursing leaders, while Asmara was training community nurses "who are having a real influence for better health."[110] Creelman was a strong advocate of improving educational standards, but she never lost sight of the importance of community-based public health for improving health care within newly independent countries. Each was a vital component required by all countries to improve health services.

Creelman made every effort to see the WHO's community public health programs; these visits provided her with a fuller appreciation of the factors inhibiting the development of public health nursing within EMRO. For example, Sudan had been riddled with civil unrest since its independence on 1 January 1958 and its current government would be overturned the following October. In many respects, the country proved disconcerting from a nursing perspective. Despite the fact that female circumcision had been illegal for quite some time, Creelman knew that the majority of women were still subjected to the brutal procedure, and "all this because it gives more pleasure to the male." Visits such as this underscored, for Geneva's CNO, the interconnectivity of health and the fundamental human right to economic and personal security.

No matter how time-consuming the burgeoning number of WHO conferences and seminars became, Creelman always believed that they remained a vital part of tailoring the Nursing Section's work to local conditions. Much of Creelman's career had been dedicated to helping nurses organize themselves as professionals and communicate more effectively with one another. And so, in 1966, with her time at the WHO drawing to an end, it was especially fitting that Creelman, accompanied by a distinguished Canadian nursing educator, Helen Mussallem, and Sheila Quinn of the ICN, led a three-week "travelling seminar" in Russia. Mussallem had already acted as a WHO consultant, and, like Creelman, she believed "that the old image of nurses as devoted aides must give way to new images" that demanded new educational patterns based upon a broad liberal education.[111] The possibility of a Russian seminar had started percolating in Creelman's mind in 1964, when she attended a "very successful"[112] conference on midwifery services and education in that country.[113] She noted the health system's negative aspects: nursing practice was procedure-based and lacked clinical teaching opportunities, and all the teaching was done by doctors. But she also acknowledged its strengths: many facilities were well equipped and run; the *feldshers* (a category between doctor and nurse) made a noticeable improvement in maternal and child health, especially in rural areas; and there were no difficulties in attracting students.[114] Privately, Creelman recorded her Soviet colleague's nervousness during their visit to the health ministry. The privileged position of doctors within the highly centralized Soviet medical system made it plain that nursing was regarded not as a separate profession but as a subservient service.[115]

For the 1966 seminar, Creelman visited Moscow from 9 to 12 March to finalize arrangements.[116] The financial side of things was quickly worked out.

Considerable political tact and careful negotiation, however, would be required to open the door for an unfettered exchange with a large international nursing group that might raise "the professional profile of nurses within the country."[117] Eventually, a satisfactory compromise was reached: the key USSR representative would be a physician but the chief nurse of one of the hospitals would be assigned as the secretary. While Creelman had quietly insisted on her inclusion, it turned out that doctors would carefully monitor the group's activities.[118]

In October, nursing leaders from twenty-two countries around the world met in Moscow for six days before beginning a carefully orchestrated program of lectures and visits to selected hospitals, educational facilities, and community-care facilities in the Ukrainian Soviet Socialist Republic, the Georgian Socialist Republic, and the Abkhasian Autonomist Socialist Republic. In the opening days of the seminar, Creelman remained apprehensive about her official counterpart, Dr R.A. Lebedeva: "At first I thought she would be difficult but now seems very pleasant and agreeable. However, she may assert herself before the end."[119]

Colleagues recalled how Creelman set the tone for the camaraderie that evolved among the participants, despite the vagaries of their travel arrangements in a country where tourism was a novelty. Always remaining upbeat, she was unfazed by travelling on rickety and overcrowded aircraft, being housed in cold dirty hotel rooms with faulty plumbing, or having to consume Ukrainian delicacies that tested the strongest constitutions. Good-humouredly, she advocated Scotch for teeth brushing instead of the local water and withstood the rough handling of the local beautician in a filthy Moscow beauty salon to emerge with "quite" a hairdo.[120]

At every facility, the international visitors were lavishly feted and inundated with small broaches depicting Soviet national heroes; sometimes local residents waited for hours to present the visitors with bouquets of flowers. The mood at evening banquets was "reminiscent of Roman days," as everyone drank, made copious toasts, and danced the night away – even doing the "Twist," which was all the rage at the time.[121] Mussallem's letters home captured a typical day for Creelman's travelling brigade:

Well after breakfast ... it was off to meet officials of the Ministry of Public Health of the Georgian Socialist Republic ... a lecture from 9:30 to 11 then off to visit the Polyclinic No. 27 and the feldsher unit at a plant ... happened to be a champagne plant – so there we were having a discussion period as the champagne flowed ... Lunch at 3 pm then writing the report – then off to an official reception at 8 pm – tables groaning with exotic foods – stuffed marrow, caviar – cucumber done up special – fish – hot, cold, medium, bread, pastries, jellied things etc, etc, etc, and then all the champagne, cognac, white wine and vodka kept being poured into glasses ... The medical students did some old Persian dances – very fascinating – and then speeches that left us cold. The first time the propaganda came so thick and fast. We were not amused ... Our driver got drunk so we had to go down on a cable car. What an experience![122]

Before returning to Moscow for the final two days of the seminar, most delegates enjoyed swimming at the beach resorts on the Black Sea – the exceptions were Helen Mussallem and Lyle Creelman, who were too busy writing reports.

Time had been allotted during the concluding sessions for an exchange of ideas on nursing services in the USSR and the countries represented. Mussallem, Quinn, and Creelman all presented papers during this part of the conference, and these were included in the final published report. Creelman's paper outlined the influences changing the delivery of nursing services and the various methods employed around the world to educate various categories of health workers. She consciously chose to convey her point of view within the politically protective language of the WHO's expert committees' reports and Ruth Freeman's recent study of the Nursing Section.[123] Creelman left no doubt that the general trend in nursing education was "towards upward mobility in educational opportunity," with the goal of producing "a more highly skilled nurse with a broader background of general and professional education for the many positions necessary in a more highly organized society."[124] Yet she warned that higher education alone would not allow nursing to meet the challenges implicit in the expansion of medical services. Nursing leaders must be provided with ongoing educational opportunities that would equip them with the research tools they needed to assess health needs and resources and participate in policy development at all levels of the health-care system.[125] Many of these ideas contravened the current practices of the highly centralized Soviet health-care system, where "the key person in the health services is the physician and middle medical personnel are trained as his assistants."[126] Moreover, senior "nursing positions" were often held by *feldshers* or junior doctors and "there was no direct line of authority from the chief nurse to other levels of nurses."[127]

Upon seeing the final report on the seminar, Creelman "was a little concerned ... [to] discover that so much of my paper was included in this particular section." She embraced the report, however, believing "that there is a purpose in it and that it might be worthwhile."[128] Creelman remained intrigued by the Russian model of nursing education, in which nurses graduated from a medical school not obligated to providing service in any hospital, and she acknowledged the strides taken to improve the quality and quantity of medical services, especially from the preventative side, within the USSR. She had few illusions, however, that nurses would soon be partners on the health-care team or positioned to effect change in the provision of nursing services at either the administrative or the policy level.

Creelman happily explored Russia's cultural heritage and vibrant performing arts scene with Helen Mussallem. Strong, determined women, the two Canadian nurses shared a deep mutual respect. The two corresponded regularly, exchanging gifts or sharing confidences, social pleasantries, and sometimes even favourite recipes between personal visits.[129] On their last night in Moscow, at Creelman's insistence, she and Mussallem abandoned their driver and struck out alone to explore Moscow's sights via the subway system. Mussallem described the experience:

> So down we went into the bowels of the earth with the incredibly jammed mobs of people ... Well that was an experience! The Metro is a fantastic series of escalators running about 10 times as fast as I have ever seen – the hordes of people squeeze you into one of these ... When we did get out at the station it was a beautiful sight to behold. Sparkling mosaics at the time of Christ in a very spacious and spotlessly clean station ... Well we did go back and walked across the Red Square to watch the changing of the guards at Lenin's tomb ... The Red Square was lighted with soft lights; it never looked more beautiful I thought ... the golden bubble domes, gilded crescents and crosses and the red, red five pointed stars of the Kremlin ... After that we dashed over to Gum's [sic] the big department store and we tried to spend some rubles – my it is difficult.[130]

Moved by the way in which the Russian adventure strengthened their bonds of friendship, Mussallem afterwards wrote to Creelman, "There are so many things that I would like to thank you for – your hospitality, your leadership, your concern for my welfare, and many other things. All I can say is thank you for everything and most of all, thank you for being you."[131]

In an unwelcome postscript to the seminar, Creelman was soon putting out bush fires at headquarters that Mussallem had unintentionally ignited. Dr John Albert Karefa-Smart, who received his medical degree from McGill and who had been the acting prime minister of Sierra Leone before his appointment as the assistant director general of the World Health Organization in 1965, was up in arms. Mussallem's account of the travelling seminar, submitted as an article for the *Canadian Nurse*, had not been approved by Soviet authorities. Creelman attempted to assure Karefa-Smart that Russian officials said it was not necessary to indicate that the article had not been cleared by the ministry of health. But it was to no avail. "Maybe this was to punish me," Creelman wrote. "I learned that I could not make a transatlantic call without the approval of the Assistant

Director General."[132] The incident was a sign of the storm clouds approaching that would lead to further heated discussion during the transition of leadership as Lyle Creelman prepared to leave the WHO in 1968.

Being Geneva's foremost nurse came at considerable personal cost. The need for political discretion inculcated within the WHO's organizational culture, combined with her extensive administrative responsibilities and heavy travel schedule, reinforced Creelman's reserved nature and imposed significant barriers to maintaining relationships in Geneva and back home. In particular, she became increasingly guilt-ridden about the long stretches of time between visits with her aging, widowed mother.

Lyle struggled to reconcile her own career aspirations with her mother's loneliness and failing health. Years earlier, in 1952, Creelman had found it "hard to leave here [Geneva] for even that short time"[133] for study leave at the University of British Columbia – a move she deemed vital to prepare her for promotion within the WHO or before seeking a position elsewhere.[134] She made the trip back home, only to suffer pangs of guilt over the happiness she felt on her return to Geneva. Her sense of remorse increased over the years as her mother's health declined.[135] After her visit in January 1956, she wrote, "Mother remained well all year and was very brave over breaking up the apartment and my going. First experience in a nursing home was shattering for both of us. Hope she adjusts where she is now. It was a very hard break and I certainly have not recovered yet. Have returned to Geneva without any enthusiasm – hope that it comes as it will be hopeless without it. Can only rationalize that here I can earn the money to keep Mother in comfort, while I could not do otherwise."[136] While she knew that her mother's health had "failed some," Creelman took small comfort "that my visit gave her a new lease on life. Said she enjoyed being alone and just waiting for me to come home."[137] But in 1958, after much discussion at Christmas and many more letters after she returned to Geneva, the idea of relocating her mother to Geneva was permanently set aside: "My desire to have her here to stay was selfish I know. I feel that I should go home to stay but know that would not be the thing to do now. Neither of us would be happy."[138] In December 1961 she took emergency leave to return to Vancouver to arrange extended care for her mother. Knowing that her mother was upset by the move, Lyle was particularly uneasy on leaving for Geneva.[139]

As the 1962 year opened, life seemed "to be one mad whirl," as "every minute something new comes to mind"[140] that she felt she should get done before departing for Canada on a three-month leave. Creelman left Geneva "in a very depressed state. Political pressure entering selection of nurses. After left learned that Tito [as deputy chief nurse] selected on second go. Seven weeks study leave given me a new lease on life. Found Mother better than at xmas [sic]. More comfortable about leaving her ... Not so much talk of retiring as when home at x-mass [*sic*]."[141] The unsettled atmosphere awaiting in Geneva – as well as her continued guilt over her long absences from her mother – weighed upon her mind as she made a stopover in Ottawa en route to Switzerland. She was there to explore the possibility of assuming Penny Stiver's position when the executive director of the Canadian Nurses Association retired in 1963. But she quickly rejected the idea: "Financial sacrifice too great for me to consider in any case. Besides more interesting to remain with W.H.O."[142]

Her February 1962 leave in Canada allowed her to spend some precious time with her mother. Their time together lifted both women's spirits and eased somewhat the news of Lyle's mother's death soon afterwards, on 24 July 1962: "I owe so much to her and wonder if my contribution can ever be good enough to make up for the loneliness she felt. But, in my heart, I know it would not have been better for her or me had I been home."[143] In the end, she chose not to return home for her mother's funeral. Hers had been a private goodbye. For women of Creelman's era, international leadership brought to the fore her conflicting duties as an unmarried daughter and the sole breadwinner expected to be the caregiver in familiar settings with her professional aspirations to be an agent of social change outside the female domain.

When time permitted, she relished, as she always did, the anonymity experienced on her road trips. That feeling frequently disappeared, though, as she succumbed to loneliness or felt stigmatized when queried about her marital status, as happened on a road trip outside Geneva in 1964: "About five days of being only single person ... really had enough of that life although I enjoyed it very much ... It is certainly not customary for a woman to travel alone in this country."[144] On the same trip, she left another establishment with a bad taste in her mouth when the proprietor informed her that she was bad for business because she was too maternal. Back in Geneva, she felt somewhat inhibited when attending the endless rounds of dinners and cocktail parties as a single woman.[145]

It was at Sam Suphy, her chalet, that Lyle Creelman spent her most enjoyable times, again for the most part with other nursing colleagues from around the world. She had explained her reason for purchasing the chalet to her friend Ruth Freeman, writing, "I am going to need it for my mental health the next five years."[146] Her weekends at the chalet began on Friday at noon. Colleagues from the International Red Cross and the Swiss Schools of Nursing joined Canadian nursing leaders, such as Helen McArthur, Helen Carpenter, Jean Wilson, Trenna Hunter, Helen Mussallem, and Alice Girard, as guests at the rustic chalet. For Creelman, personal and professional relationships were inextricably linked. Yet friends rarely crossed her barrier of aloofness – one that was reinforced by the professional and societal expectations inherent in being the WHO's chief nursing officer. An intensely private woman, she enjoyed a range of social friendships but seldom found, or indeed sought, emotional intimacy. Nursing was her life. Keeping in contact with friends and colleagues, however, assumed new importance as her retirement drew closer.

Chapter Eleven

A Chance for Retrospection, 1968

Changes in leadership, Lyle Creelman discovered, came with opportunities, challenges, and increased anxiety. In 1968, on the eve of her retirement from the WHO, Creelman continued to prepare the Nursing Section for the upcoming transition. The Freeman report and the fifth expert committee on nursing had been strategic pieces of that succession planning. But her successor had not been appointed and there was no assurance that Creelman's preferred candidate, Lillian Turnbull, would be confirmed. For the moment, she was busy making plans for a trip to Africa, specifically Kenya, Congo, Nigeria, Ghana, Niger, and Senegal, from 26 February to 30 March. Whatever the reason, be it WHO budgetary considerations, her pending retirement, or internal politics at the regional or headquarters level, permission for the trip was unusually slow in coming.

During the 1960s, the WHO had helped launch a number of university-based post-basic nursing-education programs in Africa. The first such project opened in Ghana (1963), followed by Nigeria (1964), and Senegal and Kenya (1967). A major purpose of Creelman's carefully orchestrated trip in 1968 was to visit those projects. As always, her discussions with the African Regional Office would provide important political intelligence on the future direction of nursing services in the postcolonial era as well as the opportunity to sort out more tangled administrative and staffing matters. During conversations at the regional office, Creelman would explore possible appointments of African nurses to the WHO's expert panel on nursing and discuss the questionnaire sent out to obtain feedback from the field on the guide to post-basic education then under preparation. Other sensitive issues, such as the submission prepared by the Nursing Section for the UN Commission on Human Reproduction, would be addressed as well. Although Candau had gained acceptance for the controversial family-planning initiative by establishing a special program for research and training in human reproduction, the issue still required careful handling.[1] The right to health includes sexual and reproductive health; again, a UN convention could potentially strengthen the WHO's position in negotiating new programs to improve access to reproduction information and services.

As always, duty travel would be unpredictable; delayed or cancelled aircraft would further complicate an already exhausting schedule, leaving Creelman to admit, "In the brief time spent at each of the four [post-basic WHO-assisted] educational programs, one can only have impressions which may or may not be valid."[2] Despite the limitations inherent in duty travel, the 1968 African trip would afford Creelman a final retrospective – one she could pass on to her successor – on the Nursing Section's efforts in these politically turbulent African countries, while also being a personal litmus test to assess her contributions as CNO.

While discussions of nursing issues would fill her days on this trip, Lyle Creelman relished having one last opportunity to capture Africa on film. The sights and sounds of Africa from her 1964 tour were still vivid in her mind – "the songs of the pygmies, the birds singing in the African bush … the tom-toms, the African telegraph, the tensions, the great need."[3] The lens of her camera, as ever, served as an analytical tool to record, understand, and share the diversity of world cultures with her WHO staff and nurses around the world. Leaving Geneva on 20 February, she looked forward to a weekend getaway with Faith Hodgson,[4] the public health adviser to the Kenyan Ministry of Health, at Kilaguni Lodge, located in the Tsavo West National Park. She was not disappointed. The two British Columbian nurses were in their element observing the movements and antics of elephants, rhinoceros, hyenas, owls, and impalas. Yet, even here, the conversation often turned to the challenges confronting African nursing and to the government officials whom Creelman might count on for support. Discussions of the civil turmoil surrounding the Kenyan government's approach to Africanization – which inhibited non-citizen British Asians from holding gainful employment – provided an early indicator of the postcolonial political complexities engulfing the WHO's African nursing programs.

Throughout Africa, international health aid had become entangled in the politics of decolonization.[5] Would it develop along a politically democratic model or along communist lines? An astute international civil servant like Lyle Creelman understood the negative legacy of colonial expansion: she knew that independence would be "fraught with many difficulties and even revolutions." Senior administrative posts had been filled during colonial rule "by foreigners," with "little opportunity given to nationals to learn to assume responsibility … Those responsible now have enormous problems in relation to health, education, the development of industries [and] education." These new bureaucrats lacked experiences and would require assistance. "But they will be in charge."[6] Normally, Creelman's diaries and official reports remained circumspect, seldom commenting on the impact of local politics on the WHO's nursing programs, lest an inadvertent remark become ammunition against her recommendations. Still, the "confidential" section of her report on Kenya did not mince words: "There is great insecurity in the Ministry. It is apparently a very weak one ... There is insecurity on the part of the Europeans because of rapid Kenyaization. Miss Koinange told me that all nursing posts will be held by Africans by 1970 and 1972 at the latest."[7] Creelman was left wondering whether Margaret Koinange, "one of the soundest matron-in-chiefs in the developing countries," would keep her position.[8] Eunice Muringo Kiereini replaced Koinange shortly thereafter and served as Kenya's CNO from 1968 until 1986.

After so many years of duty travel, Creelman looked beyond the whirl-wind of social engagements and official visits to form her own assessment of nursing's future within African countries where regime changes frequently meant starting the planning process at ground zero. Often the new govern-ments' dependence on military power meant that new health initiatives were put on the back-burner. On 8–9 March, accompanied by the French Canadian Marie-Andrée Vacherot, Creelman briefly visited the Democratic Republic of the Congo; the former French colony had adopted "scientific socialism" after gaining independence in 1960. Others were concerned to contain the country's apparent move into the Soviet sphere of influence, but Creelman focused on the widespread corruption that undermined the training of medical personnel. The government used state authority to maximize its own benefit, not that of its citizens, as had been naively assumed by Western international aid agencies. Centralized national-scale economic planning, it was believed, was required to propel newly developed countries to fast-track the nation through the stages of economic growth. Erroneously, it was believed that "by treating the economy as an engineering problem, planning would remove ideology or even history from the development equation; it was the moral equivalent of anti-colonialism."[9] By the end of the 1960s, it was clear to Creelman from her personal observa-tions that Africa was not a blank slate where cultural modernization would reinforce economic development.

Post-independence politics certainly complicated the delivery of the WHO's African nursing programs. But, at times, Lyle Creelman attributed the lack of progress to problems within WHO teams: conflict, unfilled positions, and ill-ness or other family issues that led to the recall or resignation of several WHO nurses and the inability of others to adjust to the rigours of international nurs-ing. As Creelman appraised one nurse's experience in Congo, "She has had a very difficult time in adjusting. However, she seems to be catching on now.

Her worst handicap is feeling that she is a very important advisor!"[10] In some cases, the WHO nurses were reassigned through no fault of their own: one WHO nurse experienced "some difficulty" because "the people value the light colour of their skin ... Miss ... is somewhat darker. She has therefore experienced a little racial prejudice."[11] Before returning to Geneva, Creelman would review staffing requirements with AFRO's regional nursing advisers, the veteran Dorothy Potts and the recently appointed Vacherot. There seemed to be "a good feeling" within AFRO, and Creelman believed that Vacherot had "been a good appointment" who had taken "hold of her responsibilities very quickly." The need, however, to recruit twenty-two French-speaking nurses and to make available more support for the fourteen French-speaking countries than could be provided by one nursing adviser led Creelman to recommend appointing zonal nursing advisers within AFRO. As always, the demand for assistance far outstripped the WHO's resources.

The West African nation of Ghana had been plagued by coups and economic instability since gaining independence in 1957.[12] But, in Creelman's view, the frequent turnover of WHO staff and lack of decisive leadership lay at the heart of the WHO's difficulties in launching a post-basic nursing education there: "There is almost a complete lack of communications between the nursing education project and the Ministry people and the College. I think that this is due to the change in leadership of the WHO assisted project and the clash between the methodology taught there and the old sister tutor. Undoubtedly on the part of a few of them there is some sabotage."[13] Creelman had recruited well-respected Canadian nursing educator Rae Chittick[14] to assist with the establishment of the post-basic diploma program. In fact, four of the initial five WHO consultants had received nursing degrees or held positions at McGill University.[15] The McGill approach to nursing education, pioneered by Chittick and predicated upon developing problem-solving skills in their students, signalled a significant departure from the prevailing British-based system that promoted rote-based learning. Unfortunately, Chittick's brusque personality and impatience with the rate of progress only intensified tensions within the Ghanaian nursing community.[16]

Creelman's insistence on having national counterparts appointed as soon as possible triggered controversy within many African countries but especially strained the WHO's relationships with Ghana's health officials, who "considered the WHO nurses as additional staff."[17] Geneva's CNO concluded that well-qualified Ghanaian counterparts were needed "to salvage the post-basic nursing education program and to assist those who have been prepared in it abroad to use their new learning to advantage, otherwise they will simply fall back on the routine ways of classroom teaching."[18] Unfortunately, the approach of the first

Ghanaian chief nursing officer, Docia Angelina Naki Kisseih, mirrored the clash of professional views between the Ibadan nursing director, trained in the old apprenticeship system of nursing education, and the new university-trained faculty that Creelman encountered there: "The conflict of the old and new in regard to educational methodology is very marked and until this is overcome the success of the post-basic program is in jeopardy."[19] After meeting with Kisseih, Creelman noted that "she has been very upset by our insistence on counterparts. It is obvious that Louise Bell never requested and in fact stated that they would not need to have counterparts for the post-basic program for five years." If true, Bell's action seems at odds with her past efforts in Nigeria on behalf of Kofoworola Abeni Pratt. In any event, even though Kisseih agreed to the appointments, Creelman privately characterized her colleague, "who did not see the need for the co-ordination between service and education," as the typical old British matron – "commanding obedience and subservience from all."[20]

The tensions between the two chief nurses went beyond a mere personality clash. During her 1958 visit, Creelman had formed a negative view of the British influence on nursing's development and the Ghanaian government's decision to maintain reciprocity in training with the United Kingdom; her views remained unchanged: "The ultramontane attitude which has tied nursing closely to the British system lest standards be lost, has not given sufficient flexibility, stimulation and scope for the development of a pattern of nursing education and service to cope effectively with the unique health problems of a tropical country."[21] Interestingly, Kay Dier – the Canadian nurse-educator tasked with integrating social sciences, public health, obstetrics, and psychiatry into the basic curriculum and shifting nursing services away from the hospital to the broader community – developed a deep respect for Kisseih's personal and professional integrity.[22] Starting in her UNRRA days, Creelman often made caustic comments about "autocratic" or inept British-trained matrons. She never questioned that university-trained North American nurses were better equipped to adapt nursing principles to the local setting. This conflict of perspectives between North American university-trained nursing experts and their British-trained counterparts attested to the complexity of the competing influences that shaped the development of nursing within postcolonial Africa.

After a delayed flight, Creelman was met in Lagos by Pratt, now the chief nursing officer of Nigeria's Ministry of Health, to begin her three-day mid-March visit.[23] At that time, Nigeria was engulfed in a bitter civil war triggered by the attempted secession of the southeastern provinces of Nigeria known as the Republic of Biafra. However, neither the failure to appoint national counterparts nor civil unrest fully accounted for the difficulties encountered in establishing a three-year nursing program at the University of Ibadan leading to a BSc.[24] The program, led since 1967 by the Scottish nurse Mary Abbott, had experienced significant problems. Although small in stature, and gentle-natured by disposition, Abbott had been pushed towards brinkmanship diplomacy by the general lack of acceptance concerning the nature of the program within the university community.[25] While Creelman's official report merely noted that the WHO senior educator was acting as director for another year, there was no hint of the controversy ignited within AFRO by Abbott's decision to assume the directorship. Nor did Creelman's report reveal her personal sentiment that it was good to have "a team leader with a British accent" after a series of American nurses. Moreover, her subsequent reports and private journal did not mention the personality and professional conflicts among the WHO team that were still festering when she returned in June to attend the inaugural graduation ceremonies.[26] She left believing that, despite the turmoil in the country, the program was now established on a firm basis and that, with its public health component, a good start had been made in improving nursing services.[27]

  Despite all the substantial obstacles to the improvement of nursing within these countries, Creelman remained optimistic about the future. The WHO's post-secondary nursing programs were not Creelman's only yardstick for measuring a country's progress. At the time of her Kenyan visit, plans for a post-basic nursing course under the Faculty of Medicine, University College, Nairobi, were still in the embryonic stage, without either adequate facilities or qualified Kenyan national counterparts, but the first twelve students were to be admitted the following fall. More important, Creelman thought that, overall, nursing had experienced "great development since 1956."[28] Crediting Hodgson's "close working relationship" with Margaret Koinange, Creelman praised Hodgson's "extensive" contribution to Kenyan nursing,[29] particularly her initiatives to introduce public health – a key element that had been missing during her 1956 visit.[30] Her report highlighted the fact that 70 per cent of the total auxiliary personnel employed at health centres throughout Kenya had taken the two-month refresher course. It showcased Hodgson and her Kenyan counterpart's efforts to hold a series of provincial nursing conferences for all registered nurses in government and mission hospitals, as well as in municipal and district health services, in order to discuss the changes needed in nursing services and training and how they could participate in their implementation. Combined, their approach contained all the key components of the model of community-health services long espoused by Geneva's chief nurse: health promotion to reduce the need for curative or rehabilitation services; ongoing professional development to disseminate appropriate skills; and increased intersectoral cooperation to meet local needs with local resources. Yet, despite her admiration for Hodgson's accomplishments, Creelman concluded that she was not the best candidate to guide the advanced nursing-education projects planned for Kenya in the future – a conclusion that set the stage for her subsequent reappointment.[31]

Elsewhere, there was encouraging evidence that the Nursing Section's efforts to move beyond the hospital-based curative training that had characterized the colonial era were beginning to produce results. In Ghana, where the nursing project had been plagued by problems, Creelman reported that the WHO-assisted community-nursing programs in Tamale, Oda, and Ho were "very successful" and "it is understood that the community nurses are making a very good contribution to health services."[32] After visiting "the very fine set-up" at the community nurses' training school, Creelman was encouraged by the "many indications of the adaptation to the particular situation and culture of the country."[33] As always, Lyle Creelman looked for signs of an increased public health perspective to prevent illness and promote health. She viewed that approach as the most effective way to deliver health services that were better tailored to local conditions, more affordable, and therefore more accessible to larger segments of the community.

In Niger, where progress was slower than hoped for, Creelman was still prepared to recommend assistance beyond the planned five-year period because "it is a program which is really being adapted to the needs of the country."[34] Her report acknowledged, "Nursing is largely composed of techniques here but with the conditions as they are, it is difficult to see how it could be different."[35] Finding the school of nursing to be much better than expected, she credited the hard-working WHO team, which laboured "under difficult conditions" and in a "trying climate" to establish the groundwork for a system of nursing education geared to producing more midwifes as well as nurses with baccalaureates.[36] Despite the WHO's increased attention on post-basic nursing education programs in Africa during the 1960s, Creelman never lost sight of the need to increase all types nursing personnel within developing countries.

In contrast, her appraisal of the school of nursing in Dakar, Senegal – targeted to become a centre for advanced training for the French-speaking region – was the most negative one given during this duty tour. "For many reasons, their efforts were not as successful as it was hoped."[37] She described the wards attached to the school of nursing as "really very sad, absolutely no nursing care, in fact they do not understand what nursing is. The French nurse does not set an example for the Africans."[38] The first stage of the project was now complete but had failed to make a difference.[39] Still, even though "it will take a long time for this program to make an impact" and "the clinical facilities are poor," she recommended starting the Dakar project: "I do not see any other way that an improvement can be encouraged."[40] Her official report trusted that "the starting of this project will be a stimulus to improve and gradually it is hoped the graduates ... will be given the opportunity to effect change."[41] Privately, she was more circumspect; the WHO nurses in Dakar had a "hard task ahead of them" before they could initiate significant change.[42]

Creelman's overall assessment of the WHO's assistance to post-basic nursing-education programs in Africa sounded familiar refrains. Advanced nursing-education programs, she warned, required the support of the whole nursing profession so that university graduates did not "constitute a threat to the older experience of nurses." A sufficient number of qualified students should be available before the program was launched. Ideally, university-based nursing-degree programs should be built upon sound basic nursing education, or, if that was not possible, assistance to improve the basic programs should be given at the same time. Where clinical facilities were inadequate, attention should be devoted to their improvement as a foundation for nursing education. Plans to prepare national counterparts should be finalized before the project started. While Creelman remained an exponent of regionally based university nursing education, she was fully cognizant that time would be required for national counterparts to assume control of such a system and thus ensure its widespread acceptance among the African health community. Fundamentally, she remained a pragmatic visionary who believed that a start had to be made towards improving the quality and quantity of nursing services but that there should be a long-range plan that would allow for the gradual evolution towards higher standards as resources became available. These were not new problems. Many times before, both on visits within other regions and through letters and field reports exchanged with her field staff around the world, she had encountered the same obstacles. It was why she had had them raised both in the fifth expert committee's report and, two years later, in the 1968 "Guidelines to the Development of Post-Basic Nursing Programs" prior to her departure from the WHO.

After a month on the road, Creelman retuned to Geneva on 30 March, her mind whirling with conversations, people, and places and believing that the trip had been very worthwhile. While in Ghana, she had been presented with the "Gold Coast Crest" emblem and was the guest of honour at a tea given by a branch of the Ghana Registered Nurses Association – a tribute that sustained the nurse and the woman. Nonetheless, physically exhausted, she looked forward to the refuge from work that awaited – her "humble" chalet, Sam Suphy, tucked in the mountains. Other anxieties, as recorded in her diary, deepened her fatigue and uncertainty upon her return: "I don't know what is happening in WHO but I'm planning on finishing in August."[43]

By temperament, Creelman preferred to initiate major changes in her life circumstances. As the 1964 diary entry indicated, the timing of her departure from the WHO – set for August 1968, when she would reach the WHO's mandatory retirement age – was planned well in advance: "Hated to leave Vancouver. It has been a lovely holiday. Did not miss Geneva but perhaps that is because I knew I would be going back. Vancouver is the place I want to retire to. Have told my friends – in 4 years & 8 mo[nths]!"[44] As her 1967 home leave ended, she continued to be "very happy at the thought of returning home within a year."[45] The purchase of a new car in Geneva meant that she had to delay her departure for Canada several months; the interval gave her time to travel in Europe and to prepare mentally for the transition to retirement and a new life back home. Perhaps the hardest goodbye was to Sam Suphy; her diary records the bittersweet emotions she felt on her final visits there: "The cow bells are tinkling down in the valley and the clouds are clearing … I shall always remember the peace of this place but will find peace by the sea." Creelman took change in stride, determined to "enjoy the freedom which retirement brings."[46] The Geneva years had offered a richly rewarding career, but her achievements had demanded enormous commitment and energy for almost two decades.

At the time of Creelman's retirement, the executive director of the ICN offered a moving tribute to Geneva's CNO: "In those fourteen years she probably has achieved more for nursing throughout the world than any other nurse of her time." She had "propelled the nursing program to new heights."[47] This tribute was echoed by many others that poured in from around the world. In response, Creelman correctly credited her WHO nursing colleagues for whatever success she had achieved: "I feel that they have been too generous to me personally; any progress, which has been made in nursing through WHO's efforts, has been due largely to the hard work and devotion of the Regional Nursing Advisors and field staff."[48] Creelman's contemporaries, for their part, believed that her contribution was never properly acknowledged at WHO headquarters before her departure.

While Creelman was touched by all the tributes and thoughtful gifts, only her close friends were aware how difficult she found her last months in Geneva – especially not knowing who her replacement would be or when she would be named: "My successor has not yet been appointed – this is difficult to understand." Sometime, she promised Helen Mussallem, "I will share my thoughts about this with you, but this could not be done in writing!"[49] Her diary, however, does record her distress in the month prior to her scheduled departure: "Lil [Turnbull] in Geneva in early Aug. Karefa-Smart told her that I was staying to end of Dec. Nothing said to me. Hans Johnson tried to help. I told K.S. what I thought about the situation. Left. Never want to go through again another month like that."[50] This was the final stand-off in a series of scrimmages over the past two years between Creelman and Karefa-Smart, who seemed determined to rein in the CNO.

As Lyle Creelman prepared to leave Geneva, she had every reason to look back with considerable satisfaction on her WHO career. She left a complex legacy to the world of nursing in an era revolutionized by technological and scientific advancements. The difficulties that she and Olive Baggallay initially confronted in establishing a voice for nursing within the fledgling international health organization were intimidating. Much of Europe, the Middle East, and Asia still lay in ruins after the Second World War; infectious diseases and poverty threatened global health within countries where virtually no organized health care existed. Subsequently, Creelman's tenure as the chief nursing officer of the WHO from 1954 to 1968 – a period often heralded as the golden age of international nursing – presented her most daunting challenges: first, to promote "a social approach to nursing" that looked beyond the increasingly expansive functions of hospital care and took into account the underlying socio-economic determinants of health care through public health systems; second, to institutionalize nursing's presence within the WHO's decision-making circles; and third, to advance nursing's broader agendas worldwide.

While the WHO would build on the work begun by UNRRA, the Rockefeller Foundation, and other pre-war health agencies,[51] the scope of its activities and interests surpassed those of any previous international health organization. In the early post-war period when reconstruction and recovery were the priority, the WHO's initial programs focused on malaria, tuberculosis, and venereal disease, women's and children's health, nutrition, and environmental sanitation. The Nursing Section set out to improve basic nursing education and services within countries seeking the WHO's assistance. But right from the start, Creelman articulated a broader perspective on health. Public health nurses, including Lyle Creelman, had long identified the wider influence of low standards of living, inadequate housing and nutrition on poor health, and the inequalities between and within countries. That perspective would eventually be embodied in primary health care.

By the time that Creelman took over from Baggallay, the scores of new nations emerging from their colonial past had created unprecedented global challenges for curative and preventative health care. As the Cold War deepened, it undermined the resolve of the international community to address these new health challenges collectively, diverted financial resources from global health care towards the arms race, and made global health a strategy of alliance building. As significantly, the change of directors general heralded a major departure in the WHO's global health priorities and a move to further decentralization. Even as the idealistic hopes for a collective approach to peace and security in the early post-war era faded, the international nursing community still looked to the United Nation's technical agencies, such as the WHO, to contribute to the more equitable and humane treatment of people throughout the world. Under Candau, however, the WHO largely abrogated its role as international gate-keeper for the right to health, opting instead for a vertical, technology-driven approach to global health. As the WHO's chief nursing officer, Creelman also had the added complication of considering how ethnicity, race, gender, and professional rivalries within the health-care community and between international aid agencies, as well as the revolution in medical technologies in the age of automation, moulded the role of modern global nursing.

All of these factors made it more imperative to strengthen nursing's voice in formulating health-care policy, especially within newly independent nations. During the 1960s, an era of rapid decolonization, the Nursing Section had to focus on preparing national leaders and services to replace those of the former colonial administrations. Accordingly, greater attention was paid to developing post-basic nursing programs and the development of national nursing services. It would also necessitate adopting new administrative strategies to connect the Nursing Section with nurses at all levels across borders.

But was the nursing profession prepared for a key role in the ambitious endeavour to improve global health care, defined in the WHO's constitution as "not merely the absence of disease" but "a state of complete physical, mental and social well being"?[52] The ability of nursing leaders to influence policy development within the WHO or their own countries remained untested. In many countries, nursing as a profession was just being established or administered by colonial authorities, and even in those countries with more advanced health-care systems the national nursing organizations wielded limited influence over health-care policy. Further, even the more mature national health-care systems, created to provide nursing service during the war and in post-war reconstruction, allowed for little carry-over to the nascent international health body.[53] That said, the clear evidence of a worldwide shortage of nurses and the valuable contribution that nurses and nursing leaders made during the war and in the post-war relief efforts with UNRRA provided a vital impetus for strengthening nursing within the new organization. Others led the way well before Creelman arrived in Geneva, but she and her colleague Olive Baggallay were determined to build on that legacy.

Creelman's style of leadership at the WHO, while reminiscent of her UNRRA years, evolved as she gained experience with nursing issues in a global context. She and Baggallay began by nurturing their contacts with established nursing leaders, and then, as CNO, Creelman acted as a catalyst to broaden the transnational dialogue within all levels of the global nursing community. Ultimately, she pioneered a transcultural approach that planted the seeds to change the face of international nursing. Navigating the politics of global health policy at headquarters and beyond to liaise with professional nursing organizations, other UN technical agencies, and non-governmental health-care foundations required vision, diplomacy, and dedication. With experience, she proved up to the task.

To achieve her goals, Creelman eventually acted as a cross-cultural broker connecting three functionally distinct but intellectually interrelated nursing networks: a transnational leadership network, an underground intelligence network linking the WHO's nursing staff, and a trans-governmental informa-tion and advocacy network connecting nursing personnel across national and professional boundaries at a more grass-roots level. Within them, Creelman acted as the international gatekeeper, connecting nurses at all levels in their search for new sources of power and authority in the turbulent post-war world. She used the networks to navigate the competing bureaucratic cultures – a bio-logical versus a social approach to population health – within the WHO and the schisms dividing the nursing world itself. During Candau's directorship, this became a more critical strategy to advance a community based health-care approach. Creelman's career, then, offers an important window on the Nursing Section's contested role in transforming nursing throughout the world, and especially within the newly independent countries, during its first two decades following the Second World War.[54] Her career sheds light on the historical tensions between the Global North and South over nursing knowledge, skill, and professional identity. It deepens our understanding of the accommoda-tion, assimilation, and agency of nurses on both sides of widening cultural and economic divide. Lyle Creelman became a vital conduit between the new face of nursing then emerging outside the industrialized nations and Western-based nursing.

The transnational network of interlocking personal and professional relation-ships connected a generation of professionally ambitious nursing leaders and offered them exciting opportunities to raise nursing's international profile while advancing their national agendas. Membership within this nursing-leadership network gave Creelman access to decision-making circles, thereby enhancing her stature as the voice of nursing worldwide. It kept her abreast of the rapid post-war developments in nursing education and practice. It also allowed her to distribute the Nursing Section's increasingly heavy administrative burden and extended her recruiting reach. As the demand for assistance to develop nursing programs skyrocketed, the private-public partnerships developed within this network allowed scarce financial and personnel resources to be pooled.[55] As important as all the above, these relationships provided a personal support net-work. Nursing leaders in the ICN, the USPHS, the International Red Cross, and the Rockefeller Foundation – to name a few – became Creelman's confidants in a way that her own staff, for political reasons, could not.

Creelman's brokerage role within all of the expert committees on nursing convened between 1950 and 1968 is critical for understanding the process whereby ideas about practice, professional identity, and agency circulated among networks. This important subgroup of nursing leaders functioned as an epistemic community, broadly understood as a transnational network of knowledge-based experts who were able to leverage their skills and specialized knowledge to gain entry into decision-making circles.[56] While membership within the group became more geographically diversified, these nursing leaders continued to be bound by a shared community of ideas, such as the belief in the scientific method as a way of generating truth, and shared core values, such as "caring and sharing," "service," "professionalism," and the "universalism of nursing principles." The expert committees provided an important forum for nurse-experts, motivated by a variety of goals, to negotiate differences, crystallize and rank policy priorities, and engage in a common policy enterprise to exercise power within the hierarchical medical community. Their recommendations on the health problems facing decision-makers underscored their mutual interest in and ability to address the global shortage of nurses and to improve health care. But, equally, nursing leaders framed policy issues within these international forums to advance their professional agendas nationally as well as globally.

All five expert committees served a vital function in reinventing nursing's professional identity. The rapid transformation of medicine triggered by the explosion of new technologies and drug therapies and the shift of patient-centred care to the hospital blurred professional boundaries, forcing nursing to define and defend its space within the differentiated structure of its workforce (both professional and lay practitioners). Especially within developed countries, nurses attempted to reconcile their traditional core value of caring and service with their desire for a more autonomous and satisfying role for nursing within the gendered realities of increasingly medicalized healthcare systems. In conceptualizing a social approach to nursing, Creelman and others stressed that nursing brought added value beyond the bio-medical approach, which focused on disease rather than implementing a holistic treatment plan for the individual patient. Comparing the more radical language of the background papers to that of the final reports, it is evident that the nursing experts embraced the male-defined models of scientific rationality to re-envision the ideal nurse as a teacher/practitioner/researcher in a fashion that would gain the modern nursing profession greater credence within the medical community.

Nursing leaders knew that the expert committees' reports, once approved by the World Health Assembly, purportedly became the standards guiding the conduct both of the WHO and of its member governments. They believed that policies ratified at the WHO would have a favourable "boomerang effect" on national policy development.[57] These reports provided a common set of documents to buttress their demands to improve nursing education and services within their home countries and for inclusion within health-care policymaking circles. Similarly, their recommendations strengthened nursing's authority within the WHO bureaucracy and other international nursing bodies, such as the ICN, and other UN technical agencies, such as the ILO, that shaped nursing worldwide. Creelman relied heavily, but not exclusively or entirely successfully, upon the expert committees to enlarge the Nursing Section's jurisdiction over the nursing aspects of the WHO's work and to insinuate its influence into broader international health-care politics. More specifically, she used the committees to challenge the view that the development of nursing in the newly independent countries should follow Western curriculums and methods, and to raise contentious issues that divided nursing, such as its gender exclusivity, its ambivalent relationship with collective bargaining and labour organizations, and the boundaries of professional practice within the health team. As Creelman gained a greater appreciation of midwifery and ancillary nursing services – often the sole providers of rural health care in developing countries – she used the expert committees on nursing, public speeches, and various WHO publications to confront the "the psychological resistance of nurses to accept the auxiliaries as members of the nursing team with a distinct and valuable role to play."[58] From Creelman's perspective, the expert committees were also invaluable in her broader efforts to strengthen nurses' ability to communicate more effectively across borders. The treatment of auxiliaries within the reports mirrored a broader shift. They became less directed at control and regulation of the profession; instead, the barriers that inhibited nursing's contribution to health promotion worldwide became their central focus.

Although the reports were widely distributed and publicized within the WHO and beyond, their usefulness was limited by the fact that they were available only in English.[59] In some cases, however, the committees' reports were the only resources available to WHO nurses in the field.[60] They were discussed within the WHO's regions, and individual nurses wrote Creelman citing their usefulness in curriculum development or for organizing regional workshops.[61] Creelman contended that the true value of the reports was that they "[were not] an American textbook or an English textbook – here was something that was international."[62] It would have been more accurate to say that they became increasingly international in character as time progressed.

Perhaps, though, the wider involvement of the nursing world in the course of the reports' preparation and implementation was as important as the reports themselves. Creelman used the expert committees to launch a different kind of information and advocacy network, especially among the developing countries – one that is overlooked in the historical literature. The entire process justified the striking of specialized technical nursing committees, regional conferences, or intra-country research seminars – a move necessary to overcome resistance within the WHO and developing countries, where the voices of the medical community were louder and where the funding required for nursing forums to exchange ideas and share experience, knowledge, and skills was scarce. It also allowed her to focus discussion on the development of public health systems and their underlying determinants, even as the WHO global health priorities shifted way from a social approach to global health.

The expert committees were an important element in the work of the Nursing Section, especially in the early years. In the end, however, Lyle Creelman championed regional seminars and conferences and intra-country research and nursing-education programs as more effective mechanisms for translating her vision into action than either the expert committees or fellowships held outside the region. "Helping people to help themselves" provided the bedrock for Creelman's campaign to evolve a transcultural approach to international nursing that respected cultural diversity, built local competencies and sustainability, and encouraged community participation in identifying the health needs of countries and in evaluating the merits of alternative approaches to address those needs. Regional conferences of health professionals, like that held within the WPHO regional conference, were convened to discuss the main problems of maternity care within the region and how these could be "approached in light of local circumstances.[63] As Creelman's public speeches stressed, both the "quality and quantity [of nursing services] must be considered and each country must decide that relationship for itself."[64] The WHO's desire to empower the local nurses as the key decision-makers within regional forums sometimes triggered the animosity of other powerful international agencies deliberately excluded from participation.[65] The nursing network also helped refine Creelman's views, most notably leading to her acceptance of the idea that meeting health needs might necessitate the lowering of professional standards in the short term and of the value and permanency of auxiliary workers within health-care teams. Long gone were the days when regional conferences that determined nursing's future direction were attended only by doctors representing imperial powers – as had been the case in the early years of the WHO in Africa. This trans-governmental information and advocacy nursing network was central to balancing the competing needs of hierarchy and democracy, efficiency and inclusivity, and consensus and disagreement within the nursing world.

Finally, for the workforce Creelman led, this network brought together nurses to find solutions for common problems at the regional level, thereby facilitating the dissemination of the critical knowledge and research skills that local nurses required to empower them as agents of change. Seminars, conferences, and intra-country projects offered a collaborative environment in which to develop professional and personal self-respect, self-awareness, and sensitivity to the needs and feelings of other people – all of which Creelman believed to be critical components for the maturation of nursing as a modern profession. "Nurses within developing countries," she contended, "are used to being told what to do and like the security of that. Must help [them] to realize that they must take an active part in developing the nursing profession."[66] Breaking down authoritarian thinking was a step towards removing the vestiges of colonialism and embedding a democratic approach.[67] Indeed, as Creelman once told her fellow Canadian nurses, in some countries where entering nursing represented a "rebellion on the part of women against their conditions, and [where nurses] have shown an interest in becoming better educated and in making a contribution in service to their people," WHO nurses were charged with the task of empowering women by "helping to develop this spirit."[68]

When viewed together, these networks illustrate nurses' diverse ways of acting, identifying issues, and exercising agency, often outside formal political structures. Within them, Creelman's practice of traditional leadership was transformed: "The relationship between leaders and followers shifts from command-obedience structure based on fear or loss of protection towards a more consensual egalitarian model." The transformation of leadership style from "power over" to "enabling power,"[69] predicated upon shared learning, paralleled a similar shift in the approach to nursing care, embodied in the nursing/teacher model discussed earlier.

Creelman encouraged her nurses to be agents of change, but with a significant caveat – that they take time with the local nurses to understand the country's culture and to evaluate its nursing needs and resources. It was a tall order. Not all of the WHO nurses either understood or possessed the temperament or desire required to achieve the ideal. Moreover, the calls for a collaborative and culturally appropriate approach were not always welcome, to say the least, either within the local medical community or among health officials. Showcase projects distorted the equitable delivery of primary health care within developing countries. On occasion, WHO nurses complained that national nursing associations' curricula ignored the practice and needs of local hospitals.[70] Duty travel alerted Creelman to the many obstacles that WHO nurses confronted in developing effective and mutually respectful working relationships with their national counterparts – sometimes through no fault of their own. She repeatedly warned her staff that often national counterparts felt threatened or alienated because they were completely removed from the planning process; as soon as possible, she involved national nursing leaders in discussions with the top governmental levels or WHO regional staff.[71]

Creelman always recognized that the tendency to promote "adoption" rather than "adaptation" among the international community of health workers inhibited the development of a more practical and culturally appropriate pattern of nursing within what she called the "fast developing countries."[72] Field reports made it clear that some WHO nurses were "understandably reluctant to impose changes," while others grew impatient with the lack of progress.[73] That realization inspired speeches and comments in expert committees about conditions in WHO posts around the world where, as Creelman put it, "to help people help themselves was one of the hardest things to do ... when there was so much to do and so few to do it."[74] Unlike many of her contemporaries, who emphasized only the roadblocks to closing the gap in medical services between developed and developing countries, Creelman pointed out the opportunities to avoid the previous mistakes made by Western industrialized nations, such as specialization in health services.[75] She fervently believed that, while life was different in developing countries, "there was something fine in their cultures and it should not be sacrificed to western technology and civilization."[76] She stressed again and again that Western nations had much to learn from other countries. Creelman's attitude was a logical extension of her belief that the hospital should function as a community-health centre – a view that Western countries had been slow to adopt – so as to forge closer links between health-care services inside and outside its walls. Equally, it reflected her own background as a teacher and public health nurse. The roots of her vision of public health as the linchpin within the health-care continuum can be traced back to her work and writings in the interwar era.[77]

Creelman expected her nurses' professional conduct to be governed by local circumstances. To direct their activities, she needed accurate information on conditions at WHO postings; the carefully scrutinized field reports, however, were succinct, dry, and without names. "Lyle's secret service" provided franker strategic assessments of the WHO's nursing programs and alerted her to shifting political priorities and fortunes within the receiving countries. It extended her administrative reach and partially circumvented the administrative roadblocks and political intrigue enmeshing the WHO's selection process at every level. It served as a key intelligence corridor to orientate, support, and evaluate her field staff's cultural adaptability and leadership. Lyle Creelman consistently credited the dedication and hard work of the WHO nursing staff. Nurses of all ranks within the worldwide nursing network were essential to her leadership of the WHO, as well as to her attempts to define her personal and professional space within the male-dominated medical community that controlled policy-making in both the WHO and its member countries.

Creelman's ability to forge a multi-tiered gendered network where female professional and personal allegiance were closely interwoven only partially explains her successful leadership. Her intelligence, self-confidence, determination, sociability, and integrity all contributed to the perception of her being an exceptional nursing leader. Creelman's keen intellect and extensive knowledge of nursing worldwide strengthened her international prestige. Her sound judgment and extensive knowledge of nursing worldwide prevented her from posing unrealistic ideas. Physicians were both her advocates and her adversaries. At times, she exhibited great diplomacy, courtesy, and wit, all of which made her dogged determination acceptable and, indeed, earned her the respect and friendship of medical colleagues and government representatives worldwide. In other situations, Lyle could be demanding, intellectually intimidating, or difficult as a colleague. Dedicated, decisive, and a perfectionist by nature, she set high professional standards and was not shy about calling others to account.

Creelman always defined herself first and foremost as an educator. Personal observations in and reports from the field confirmed her long-standing personal belief – one embodied in the report of the first expert committee on nursing – that only by raising nursing's educational standards would the profession be able compete with the other careers then rapidly opening up to women.[78] Sterile professionalism was never her primary goal. Her ideals were formed against the harsh realities she observed nurses confronting around the world. Indeed, her approach to reforming nursing education identified and attempted to address problems that still bedevil the profession in many countries: shortage of personnel, minimal involvement of nurses in planning at all levels of health care, lack of career opportunities, poor working conditions, and inadequate resources. To address these concerns, she endeavoured to place nursing education on a basis equal to that of other professions, but she never considered that this alone was sufficient. Believing that nurses and their professional associations needed to be less insular to reach their goals, she promoted partnering with the ILO and other collective-bargaining units to improve nurses' wages and working conditions around the world.

A leading advocate of a broad liberal education for nurses, Creelman remained adamant that there "could be no one pattern for schools."[79] Recognizing that nurses had to be prepared for different levels of responsibility that met local needs and resources, she never prescribed a monolithic approach to the development of nursing education.[80] The Nursing Section campaigned to broaden the educational opportunities for auxiliary personnel on the same basis. Creelman took the view that auxiliaries should not be viewed as an inadequate or expedient substitute for nurses but as an integral part of the health team. The issues relating to auxiliary personnel – their training and supervision and quality of care – remain a concern today. Her extensive public health experience and innate open-mindedness encouraged experimentation with and adaptation of Western models of nursing education.

At the same time, while she acknowledged that there were no universal standards of nursing education and practice, she also believed that certain common conditions were required to foster nursing excellence: "good educational background; well qualified teachers, good training methods (including close integration of theory and practice, at least a minimum of equipment; a reasonable work-load and good human relationships, as important as any other)."[81] Knowing, however, that the majority of nurses would be trained within a hospital setting for many years to come, she advocated that they be treated like students rather than as hospital employees. She championed a progressive vision of nursing education, built upon a participatory and problem-solving approach to nursing and imbricated in a wide variety of clinical experience and research. Only then, she believed, would nurses be prepared to meet the future challenges of improving the delivery of health services.[82] She endorsed a vision of nursing education that embraced the core competencies of self-knowledge, strategic vision, risk-taking, and innovation, and paid heed to interpersonal and communication effectiveness. Although it was certainly not a straight-line trajectory, the antecedents of contemporary nursing education were clearly visible in Creelman's thinking.

She never had any illusions about the degree of resistance that either the WHO nurses or new graduates faced within newly independent countries. While she understood that advanced study abroad would be required for some time to come, she simultaneously supported the development of national and regionally based university programs or workshops precisely because she believed that these facilities would produce curricula that would be more relevant to local conditions and would reduce the cultural shock experienced by nurses upon their return to their own countries. Her early recognition of the limitations of international fellowships and their potential to be exploited to recruit cheap labour were exposed in the WHO's 1959 technical report[83] and led to more diligent oversight of nurses studying abroad. Whenever she could, she visited students holding WHO fellowships, including her own staff, during her North American visits. More significantly, she encouraged Canadian universities, such as McGill and the Université de Montréal, to exchange faculty with other African university-based programs on a continuing basis to develop a better appreciation of the needs of their international nursing students – the forerunner of WHO's collaborative arrangements with nursing centres around the world. Creelman's actions stand as a corrective to the view that the WHO's educational programs simply mirrored the experience of U.S. aid agencies or foundations.[84]

For Creelman, the goal of improved nursing education at all levels remained improved patient care, in both its curative and its preventative aspects. Creelman maintained that the purpose of nursing education was to prepare nurses for service. As late as 1964, she could note that the essence of nursing was best expressed by Virginia Henderson's *Basic Principles of Nursing Care*: "To assist the individual, sick or well, in the performance of those activities contributing to the health or its recovery (or to peaceful death) that he would perform unaided if he had the necessary strength, will or knowledge. And to do this in such a way as to help him gain independence as rapidly as possible."[85] However, nursing's core value of compassionate care giving, as well as its professional boundaries, had to be realigned to modern practice. Like the expert committees' reports, her own field reports, speeches, and articles promoted the unique role of the nurse as the integrating force within the health team, stressed that nurses' education must adapt to a wide variety of circumstances, and advocated that nursing education be patient-centred not technique-oriented. Accordingly, Creelman cautioned that professional advancement must not take the nurse "further and further from the patient" – a continuing concern for nurses today. She believed that the primary goals of nursing – "the alleviation of suffering, rehabilitation, and teaching of health" – were the same all over the world; it was "the conditions under which and for which nursing care is given and to which it must adapt that differ."[86] There were limitations to her vision, however. She never questioned that better-trained nurses would translate into better nursing care and remained confident that university-prepared nurses were capable of providing superior care because they were more perceptive in meeting patient needs.

The heavy emphasis she placed upon raising educational standards always went hand in hand with her early recognition of the need to develop more fully the preventative function of community-based or primary health care. At every opportunity, she encouraged the integration of public health into hospital schools' curriculum, where the majority of nurses would continue to be trained for the foreseeable future. During her extensive duty travels, she consistently stressed the need to integrate public health services with other aspects of social-development policy. A strong proponent of a social approach to nursing, she constantly demanded that staff and consultants consider the underlying determinants of health – the social and economic structure, the status of women, and particularly the educational opportunities available to them and their conditions of work – in constructing a well-thought-out plan for the long-term development of nursing services in the country concerned. Creelman's trans-cultural approach to international nursing evolved from her fundamental belief that "all citizens of the world need to realize that all [are] equal – no one race is born inferior or superior intellectually to another."[87] All were entitled to universal health care as a fundamental right of human security. The antecedents of the WHO's contemporary human rights based on global health, so clearly articulated by Geneva's chief nurse, can be traced back to a nascent Canadian welfare state that came of age as Creelman launched her international career.[88]

This rights-based approach to global health allowed nurses like Creelman to reconcile their core values of "caring" and "universalism" with their life-long professional aspirations for self-direction and self-regulation. Yet there was more to it than simply arguing the now recognized correlation between the availability of nurses, coverage of services, and improved population health. She urged the nursing profession to cast aside its "silo mentality" to join forces with other social activist groups to strengthen its voice within the global health-care system. Globalization has only reinforced the importance of strong link-ages between national, regional, and international nursing and non-nursing organizations. Equally, Lyle Creelman remained a fervent believer that global access to fundamental health care would never improve as long as health was treated as a separate silo. The now-accepted linkage between health improve-ment and sustainable social and economic development became an enduring hallmark of Creelman's leadership of the WHO's Nursing Section, as did its underlying philosophy of community involvement, more appropriate tech-nologies, and health-care staffing models with a countrywide basis. The next decade would hear new voices calling for more radical changes along lines long championed by Creelman.[89]

Her approach remains a critical framework for WHO primary-care nurs-ing initiatives to achieve health for all in the twenty-first century. In 1978 the International Conference on Primary Health Care in Alma Ata, Kazakhstan, issued a declaration, which stated that primary health care is the key to pro-viding health for all by the year 2000,[90] a concept that in turn requires that the health system "reflects and evolves from the economic and social cultural and political characteristics of the country." The Alma Ata Declaration also identi-fied eight essential elements of primary health care that, in turn rest on five basic principles: health services should be universally accessible, organized around people's needs and expectations, integrated into public policy reforms, com-mitted to collaborative models of policy dialogue, and based on stakeholder participation. All of this is premised upon the belief that developing primary health care requires not tearing down existing structures but rather building and expanding upon them, so that the new services are community-based and part of an integrated and comprehensive health system. The Declaration of Alma Ata "stands as a vision of health that has lost none of its urgency."[91] All eight essential principles were clearly evident throughout Creelman's years with the WHO. Her later contention that nursing under her direction had been advocating this approach all along, but that the doctors just were not listening, was well founded.

Creelman's leadership and vision of a social approach to nursing were not without limitations, contradictions, or – not the least important – opponents. Of course, the WHO was but one of many international agencies and foundations whose nursing programs shaped the delivery of nursing within newly independent countries. There was always an inherent tension of using Western trained nurses to implement a more transcultural approach to nursing. Creelman's own experience, and her exchanges with her frontline staff, however, suggest the need to admit the notion of learned cultural sensitivity within any given contact zone, based both on these nurses' own experiences and their interactions with indigenous nurses, whose activities and agency clearly shaped Western nurses' attitudes.[92] Scholars should not ignore the diversity or experimental nature of the WHO's nursing initiatives, which, in their focus on the local community, were designed to offer a more affordable and effective option for the delivery of health-care services than the existing model of centrally run hospital care.

More so than previously believed, the kaleidoscopic flow of power and authority was multi-directional and contested. The WHO's nursing programs were not entirely donor-driven in a top-down process but rather evolved within a framework of negotiations with local officials and communities. Nor should the wide-ranging discussions surrounding nursing's role within developing nations that occurred within transnational nursing networks in the decades following the Second World War be overlooked. Finally, Creelman's career suggests that nursing was increasingly open to the changing political currents, social movements, international migration trends, economic globalization, and technological revolutions that defined the post-war global health landscape.[93]

Creelman earned a reputation as an adept administrator and as an authoritative voice for nursing worldwide. Her leadership style evolved within an increasingly complex transnational context that went well beyond traditional intergovernmental or interagency relations to include non-state actors. But nation states still remained powerful actors. Efforts of the WHO leadership to forge strategic alliances with various governmental and non-governmental movements as part of a broader effort to foster greater equity in health care across and within nations was uncharted territory. Creelman's style of leadership anticipated a more modern leadership model, one that in her case used effective communication and interaction to connect with front-line staff and nurses around the world. An inspirational leader, she created an environment that encouraged individuals to take on responsibilities and challenges and to experiment in effecting change in their country's health-care system or in the larger organization's nursing programs.

Creelman's leadership strategies displayed some weaknesses. Her strategy to carve out an increased organizational presence for nursing within a physician-led and decentralized, sprawling administrative structure was never entirely successful. Years later she acknowledged that her attempts to recast nurses as key actors and interpreters within the scientific community failed to gain the acceptance of physicians. Her strategy did highlight the need for nursing practice to be based upon a sound scientific basis that took into consideration the socio-economic and cultural factors shaping the delivery of nursing services and practice. But her leadership was highly personalized, relying on an extensive informal intelligence network of professional and personal relationships. It was never institutionalized. Lacking her political finesse or extensive nursing connections, her immediate successors were not as successful in negotiating the political corridors within the WHO's decentralized bureaucracy or in exercising influence within the broader international nursing community. Nursing's battle to gain a seat at the health policy table continues today.

As she prepared to leave Geneva for the last time in 1968, Creelman had much to think of – friendships and rivalries, successes and failures, professional achievements and personal disappointments. She had been thrust onto the international stage during the UNRRA years, opening the door to a key leadership role in the WHO for fourteen years. Her life, in short, had long been one of unremitting work, and of daunting responsibility. The question now was: What would she do next?

Epilogue, 1968–2007

Some change is hard. Not surprisingly, for Lyle Creelman, leaving Geneva, the centre of her exhilarating professional and personal life for almost two decades, triggered considerable emotional ambivalence. After years full of clear purpose, her pending retirement felt void of direction; her future plans remained uncertain. But gradually, although "sad to leave Geneva,"[1] an "international centre where people from so many countries are passing through," she convinced herself that she had "missed being part of a local community."[2] Retirement in Canada also offered the prospect of re-establishing closer ties with family and friends. Did it signal the start of an exciting new phase of her professional life, or would, and indeed could, she simply slow down and relax?

Nursing colleagues speculated about their friend's future contribution to international nursing.[3] They did not "like to contemplate Hq without [Creelman] running interference for nursing": "Your departure will leave a great gap ... the absence of your support and commonsense objectivity will be missed beyond measure."[4] Her field staff felt "as though the Organization just wont be the same when you leave."[5] But they "could not imagine ... that nurses are going to let you hide away."[6] Like Virginia Arnold, many hoped that "once you have had a chance to rest your weary bones and get away from the silly pressures, you will decide that you want to be busy again. You are so full of energy and have a tremendous wealth of knowledge of the nursing world which we need."[7] It remained to be seen whether Director General Candau's "hope that WHO can continue to count on your active interest"[8] would be realized.

Several times during home leaves, Creelman had contemplated teaching after retiring. Yet, when she learned that Helen Mussallem, the executive director of the CNA, had approached Dean John F. McCreary at UBC's Faculty of Medicine about prospective employment on her behalf, she confided to her friend that a job "at such a high level would frighten me."[9] The response was uncharacteristic of the WHO's normally confident CNO. As she prepared to leave Geneva, Creelman shared a confidence with Mussallem: "Just between you and I, I have had two enquiries from the USA re future employment. I am making no decision at this point. Except that I am sure that I don't want full-time work and that I want a full year off."[10] She did agree to allow Mussallem to nominate her to the Membership Committee of the ICN for 1969–73.[11] Her election to that committee, however, did not portend any long-term involvement in either the ICN or the CNA.

Disposing of Sam Suphy, the purchase of a new car, and packing her Geneva apartment took most of the month of November, leaving little time for Lyle to speculate about future directions. It was only as she bid a final farewell to close WHO colleagues Clair Melson, Fernanda Alves Diniz, and Helen Martikainen that "I knew parting with Geneva & all it had come to mean had really come."[12] To ease the adjustment to the post-work world, she left for San Francisco on 29 November and visited family and friends in California and Arizona. She simply needed time "to know that I have retired and that it is not just a holiday."[13] After she returned to Vancouver on 1 February 1969, the next few months flew by as she set up house and enjoyed renewing old acquaintances – some of whom delighted her by holding a party and showering her with gifts.

Soon, an interesting job prospect surfaced. Despite her earlier determination to take a year off from nursing activities, Creelman changed her mind after Dorothy Hall, the regional nursing adviser, requested her to prepare a report on the recruitment and training of auxiliary personnel for the next SEARO Regional Committee meeting.[14] Having already refused two previous WHO assignments, Creelman decided that "I could not keep on being negative if I ever wish to do further international work."[15] As it turned out, however, the three-month assignment – involving visits to India, Thailand, Nepal, Burma, and Indonesia – only strengthened her disenchantment with WHO politics and policies.

Once she was back in Geneva, the political pressures of international nursing quickly resurfaced. Arriving on 15 April, she found her first few days "upsetting." At headquarters, the office appeared disorganized under interim CNO Alves Diniz (Lillian Turnbull had only recently arrived in Geneva to take up the post permanently). Moreover, while happy to see old friends in a town that seemed like home, Creelman soon grew impatient listening to colleagues' professional issues: "Helen [McArthur], national director of nursing services with the Canadian Red Cross Society, talked all the time. Maybe if I had her problems I would also."[16] Clearly, she was relieved not to be in either chief nurse's position. It was an ominous warning for what lay ahead.

Her uneasiness grew as the assignment proceeded.[17] Two days after her arrival in Jakarta, Creelman, fed up with the "politics – confusion – more than any other country I have ever visited," declared that, if she "had plenty of money," she would take the first available plane to Delhi. "I would there return all the money spent on me, tell them what I thought of this assignment, and return home. I really wonder why I accepted this assignment. I will certainly consider more carefully before accepting another with WHO."[18] She criticized the briefing that she and Dr Hugh Russell[19] received in Delhi as "ineffective" and proof that those "responsible were glad to leave the matter to us." On top of that, the arrival in Jakarta of Dr A. Malaterre, the SEARO representative for Indonesia,[20] emphasized the limitations of her role as a consultant. To her chagrin, Malaterre had promptly announced that "he represents the organization at diplomatic functions!" She found this particularly jarring after he subsequently referred to the wrong operations plan during their meetings with Indonesian officials. The last straw was her poorly organized itinerary. In Bangkok and Rangoon, Creelman was "taken on the tourist route of rural health centres," during which she "did not actually see one centre in operation," and then was provided with questionable statistics as the basis on which to make her recommendations.[21]

Oppressive heat, gruelling days, and lack of safe food or, at times, of any toilet facilities resulted in Creelman leaving Indonesia exhausted and suffering from an intestinal infection. A diary entry upon arriving in Singapore on 14 May captured her final, conflicted impressions: "Now that the Indonesian experience is over, I am glad that I had it but what a country!"[22]

The rest of the trip proved equally challenging. Returning to the heat of Delhi (109° Fahrenheit), Creelman began what would be the physically hardest part of the assignment: first Bombay, then Poona and Najpur, and then back to Delhi – all within a week. Unable to fly to their final destination because of an airline strike, she and Russell declined the option of taking a train without air conditioning or any first-class accommodation.[23] After visiting Nepal, she returned to India to visit Najpur in early July and write her report. But there was little respite from the heat and humidity; it was as she wrote, "a hell of a place to be in summer."[24]

But the real source of Creelman's growing despondency lay elsewhere. As on earlier trips to SEARO, she again observed the confluences of factors hindering the improvement of these countries' health services: civil unrest, poverty, gender discrimination, and the lack of support from the medical community all contributed to the low status of the nursing profession. In Burma she was told that the family of a nurse permitted to leave the country on a fellowship had to be prepared to go to jail if she did not return. The state nursing superintendent there confided to Creelman, "Girls who enter the BSc nursing do so as second choice – if parents had money they would go into medicine." In Nepal, Creelman heard that often nurses walked for days to take short courses. In India, the caste system along with the requirement for a dowry upon marriage – although both were now technically illegal – still shaped nursing's development. "Many chose nursing because their parents could not afford a marriage dowry." When she finally was able to visit Najpur's health facilities, she concluded that "nursing is being ruined by the Drs; no amenities provided for the p.h.n. [public health nurse] when she goes on supervisory visits." Once again, officials had failed to consider the country's conservative culture: "In this country – very difficult for girl to travel alone."[25]

As important, in her view, was the fact that many of the countries had the wrong health priorities and had little to show for all the international aid efforts. Following a visit to the Academy for Health Controllers and the School for Sanitarians in Jakarta, Creelman concluded, "Complete nonsense. Add & add useless subjects to curriculum & no regard for what they have to do."[26] No stranger to India's poverty or its lack of adequate medical facilities, she nevertheless found it difficult to accept the lack of progress in centres that the WHO had worked so long to improve. Even more difficult for her to comprehend was India's apparent indifference to the "poverty and misery of their own people."[27] She believed that a country that was more concerned about the lack of kidney machines than about the public health threat posed by the presence of 2.5 million rats had its "priorities all wrong!"[28] Health promotion and protection, she believed, required states to take concerted action through national health policies directed at alleviating the risks to health. She was disturbed when an Indian member of Parliament, N.R. Malkani, author of *Clean People and an Unclean Country*, was driven from politics and had his book banned.[29] Simply put, it was hard for nursing to make progress unless these governments were willing to take an active role in addressing the grinding poverty of their people. Lyle Creelman left Delhi on 15 July feeling glad that she had taken the assignment and believing that it "has brought me closer to reality." But she was happy "to be going home."[30]

Creelman never accepted another WHO assignment. In part, sensitive to the VIP treatment she had received in Geneva, she wanted to avoid overshadowing Turnbull, the new CNO. Yet there were other factors at work too. The assignment had reinforced Creelman's view that physicians' focus on specific medical care and technological projects within the WHO and developing countries, often to the exclusion of basic public health, compromised the right of everyone to the enjoyment of the highest attainable standard of physical and mental health. Her conversations with nursing colleagues on this assignment graphically illustrated that the improvement of population health also required addressing fundamental human rights. And there was no indication that either primary health or cooperation with other UN agencies to codify human rights, including the right to health, would be the WHO's global health priorities in the near future. Her views on public health policy ran counter to the dominant approach to development since the Second World War, which focused on economic growth as a Cold War strategy to the exclusion of social and human development.[31] As the decade progressed, others were questioning whether vertical health programs, such as the malaria or smallpox eradication campaigns, could be successful without adequate supporting health infrastructures.

Creelman's initial impression of Candau's successor, Dr Halfdan Mahler, confirmed her views. She was affronted by his condescending attitude towards nursing. After hearing his address to the 1973 ICN Congress, she characterized the speech as "shameful": "Had I been a nurse [I] would have shrunk away. All the nurses sad – ICN has tried so hard. I feel the future of international nursing rests with the ICN without the support of the WHO."[32] Her successor would also conclude that the organizational changes made at WHO Headquarters in 1978 appeared to the nursing world "to be part of a whole plan to destroy the visibility of nursing at all levels."[33]

After so many years of arduous and incessant travelling, Creelman found that life in the field was becoming much less attractive. The years had exacted a toll; she exhibited signs of what modern nursing terms "professional compassion fatigue." It is noteworthy that her successor, Turnbull, would make a similar decision "to cut the cord and not go on dangling as a miscarriage." After only seven years as CNO, Turnbull felt "drained like a sponge that has been run over and backed up over by a bulldozer and there's no more juice left. They have wrung it all out of you. It's gone. I was dry as a chip."[34] More fundamentally, in Creelman's case, she was unwilling to spend any more time negotiating the contested politics of international health without being able to influence future policy.

In the fall of 1970, she turned down an offer from an old friend and WHO colleague, Bea Solomon, to teach in New Zealand.[35] In her 1970 Christmas letter to friends, she noted that, in planning her trip to attend the ICN meeting in February 1971, she realized "that during 1970 I haven't been in an airplane! It has been good to stay close to home."[36] Her attention had shifted towards creating a new sense of community for her retirement years. She appears never to have regretted the decision.

Visits to Verna Huffman Splane,[37] Canada's first principal nursing officer (1973–81) and vice-president to the International Council of Nurses (1973) increasingly provided an essential focal point to keep Creelman abreast of contemporary developments in nursing during her retirement. On many occasions, when Lyle joined nurses from around the world who gathered in the Splanes' Vancouver home,[38] she often left feeling that "it is ... good to talk to her."[39] A telling 1974 diary entry, written after such a gathering, Splane recently returned from Geneva, simply observed that "the professional talk did not make me nostalgic – the thought of Geneva did, however."[40] Splane always regretted that Creelman elected not to engage in a more serious and sustained way in the UBC nursing community.[41]

Creelman received tributes from nurses' association at the provincial, national, and international levels. She received an honorary doctorate in 1992 from the University of British Columbia. For Creelman, the UBC ceremonies proved memorable. The presenter of her degree observed, "Occasionally we encounter someone in life whose dedication to his or her calling is an inspiration. To thousands of Canadian nurses, indeed to nurses all over the world, Lyle Creelman is such a person ... no other Canadian nursing professional has surpassed the international reputation she has established."[42] In 1967 Creelman was awarded the Centennial Medal and in 1971 she received the Medal of Service of the Order of Canada. On becoming a member of the Order of Canada, she wrote, characteristically and with considerable reason, to friends, "I am proud of this honour from [my] country: I recognize it as a tribute to nursing and to nurses of the World Health Organization with whom I was privileged to be associated for so many years."[43] In 1972 she received a lifetime honorary membership from the Canadian Public Health Association. In June 1974, along with her friends Alice Girard and Electra MacLennan, she was given the Jeanne Mance Award, the highest honour of the Canadian Nurses Association.[44] Yet, despite these public accolades, Creelman claimed that the majority of Canadian nurses remained disinterested in her past international work and that she was seldom approached to speak or share her experiences.[45]

While formal professional nursing contacts were gradually severed, the personal friendships endured. Nursing "remained a part of them in a way that other women's work simply does not."[46] Although scattered around the world, Creelman and her friends celebrated each other's significant milestones, comforted each other in time of illness or death, and provided a shared sense of kinship that enriched their retirement years. At reunions of former WHO colleagues or her UBC graduating class, Lyle enjoyed reminiscing about their adventures, challenges, and considerable accomplishments. She would find a warm welcome from her nursing colleagues on her travels at home and abroad. And, as always, she herself remained the gracious hostess, now welcoming friends to her new house on Bowen Island, off the southwestern coast of British Columbia, a property that she began negotiations for just prior to her 1969 WHO assignment and that would be her home for the next sixteen years. There she would continue to mentor nurses from around the world who stopped by to relax, reminisce, or reflect on their international endeavours. Others, nursing colleagues with whom she worked in Vancouver and abroad, either worked or resided after their retirement in British Columbia, and they, too, became inextricably woven into Lyle's retirement years. They enjoyed "great talks" while eating lunch perched on the stone steps of her chalet.

Finalizing the purchase of the property on Bowen Island, and then hiring a builder and architect for her new home, consumed most of her time after returning from Geneva in early September 1969. Building Cedar Chalet proved immensely important in easing her transition from the cosmopolitan life of Geneva to the intimacy of a small island community. Still, a discerning and demanding client, she experienced "lots of problems in handling both the builder and architect."[47] She insisted on supervising construction while living in a trailer on the property, and she had definite design ideas. In planning the chalet, she placed great emphasis on open spaces that were both functional and aesthetically pleasing and gave careful consideration to their future upkeep as she aged. The chalet's eavestroughs were located unusually low so that she could clean them; her gardens mimicked the native vegetation to minimize upkeep. Cedar Chalet and its gardens epitomized her self-reliant attitude towards life.

Overall, the Bowen Island years brought contentment, an opportunity to renew friendships, and the freedom to travel and undertake new hobbies and interests. Typically, Lyle assured friends, "I will be reminded frequently of the happy times with friends at 'Sam-Suphy,'" but, as always, she was not one to dwell on the past: Bowen Island, she said, "has a lovely coast-line, i.e. heavily wooded and, as yet, delightfully quiet."[48] Determined to be the architect of her retirement, she rekindled family ties and created new community connections. Her nieces Hazel and Kay and nephew Arthur Creelman, with whom she had grown up in British Columbia, figured prominently in Lyle's retirement years. After assuring Hazel and her husband, Elliott Dawson, that money would not be a factor in their discussions, Lyle was delighted when they finally agreed to purchase a lot she owned directly across the road in 1970. Hazel and Elliot were an important anchor for daily life on the island, offering companionship, engaging in lively political discussions on their regular walks, and providing great bridge partners several times a week. Just as important for a woman who loved children, they and their children included her in their family activities.

In retirement, Lyle demonstrated as much enthusiasm for her new pursuits – gardening, preserving, cooking, even sewing and knitting – as she had in direct-ing the WHO's expert committees. She maintained an extremely hectic social schedule, making regular weekly trips to Vancouver to play bridge, attend book club meetings, and take in concerts, plays, or lecture series at UBC. An avid bridge player, she did not "play" bridge; she "waged" the game as though it were a battle. Her regular bridge partners recalled that "small talk" ceased when Lyle was at their table; she was there to win, not socialize.[49] After one unsatisfactory bridge outing, Lyle confessed, "Couldn't keep my mouth shut when they made such blatant errors. Stuffy room. Small talk!"[50] This was a typical comment: she remained a serious, no-nonsense woman. A voracious reader with a discerning intellect, she characterized the women in her university women's book club as a "nice group but not all good reviewers."[51] As she herself once candidly admitted, "I could never be a club person."[52] She craved a sense of belonging to a community and developing closer ties with family, but she desperately needed constant activity and the intellectual stimulation that neither could completely provide. On those rare occasions when illness forced her to slow down for a week, she quickly became "bored," "lonely," or "depressed."[53] She wanted friends to engage in a wide variety of social activities with her but remained a fiercely independent woman.

Creelman became an active participant in a wide range of community activities. She told friends that she "found participating in local community affairs very rewarding, since for so many years abroad this was not a possibility."[54] It would have been more honest to say that she enjoyed leading community initiatives. When she served as secretary of the Bowen Island Historians (BIH), founded in 1969, she vowed that this would be "the last time I'll be secretary of a group."[55] Quite simply, in her opinion, the group was not business-minded enough. Her diary entries frequently noted that meetings were "disorganized as usual. Must keep quiet."[56] Elected president in June 1975, she was excited by the group's discussions about building a museum but acknowledged that "it was not going to be easy" since she "felt resistance" among the membership.[57] Creelman's drive and ability to envision a major capital campaign to build a museum created tensions with the more "conservative" members.[58] As president, Creelman arranged the financing and obtained the key to the cottage on what was known as the Orr property.[59] With only $10,000 in their account, the BIH were probably somewhat overwhelmed when past-president Creelman, as chair of the planning committee, retained the architect and presented the September 1977 meeting with plans for the museum that would necessitate raising $150,000![60] Plans for the museum were postponed twice, first to support the coming of a bookmobile to Bowen Island and then by the campaign to save the Union Steamship Store, known as the "Old Store."[61] Despite the setbacks, she served a second term as president in 1979–80 and continued to support the group's fundraising activities. Even after moving to Vancouver, she still attended BIH functions. She returned in 1992 for the 25th Anniversary Annual General Meeting of the BIH in the "Old Store," which had come to house the community library by 1981, and to speak at the opening of the group's museum archives in May 1995. Her view of the BIH as a "nice group of women, although sometimes some are exasperating," remained unchanged.[62] Enamoured with the ideal of being integral part of a small community, Creelman found the parochial aspects of island life sometimes frustrating but still rewarding.[63]

Throughout the Bowen Island years, Creelman remained an adventurous wanderer, travelling across North America and to Hawaii, Europe, New Zealand, and China. Travel became an important way to reconnect with family and old friends, and retirement allowed her to set her own itinerary for longer annual vacations in search of new vistas and cultural experiences. On many of these trips, Anne Beech, a fellow UBC graduate and recent widow, became her constant companion and confidant. They came to each other's aid in times of illness or injury. Anne was always a willing participant in the bustle of gardening, preserving, and entertaining at Cedar Chalet, and Lyle frequently stayed at Anne's Vancouver home when her social engagements ended after the last ferry back to Bowen Island.

A new travel chapter opened for Creelman in August 1972, when she purchased a mini camper van, the perfect second vehicle for wilderness adventures, whether it involved being awakened by bears knocking the lids off their garbage cans or hiking across the alpine meadows. On one such outing, in December of that year, Lyle, accompanied by Anne and her beloved poodle, Tiki, now fourteen years of age and nearly blind "but still enamoured of the vagabond life," set out on 9,000-mile drive. It had been Lyle's "dream to see more of North America." They spent Christmas with Lorna Creelman Nauss (Prescott's daughter) and her family, just south of San Francisco, and New Year's with friends at San Juan Capistrano before exploring Arizona, New Mexico, and Texas. With "neither fixed address nor date of return," they experienced all types of weather on the journey – even a snowstorm in Corpus Christi, Texas – but Lyle observed that Texas's "wild life refuges … more than compensated for any discomfort."[64] Always an avid photographer, hiker, and birdwatcher, she continued to enjoy these activities on the island and during her world travels.

The following year, once again accompanied by Anne and Tiki, Lyle set out to cross Canada on the Trans Canada Highway from coast to coast – over 10,000 miles. Their "venture was made highly enjoyable by the friends we visited along the way. The memory of warm hospitality, the beautiful homes, the obvious enjoyment of work and retirement, will long remain. The snow capped mountains, the gold of the prairies, and the red and golds of the eastern autumn foliage will be recalled frequently when we show our slides to friends at home. We saw and we 'felt' the vastness of Canada." After so many years abroad, Lyle derived "great pleasure in re-discovering my native land."[65] By the time she sold the camper van, "her trusted friend of five years," she and her two travelling companions had covered some 44,000 miles. "It was an interesting five years and will remain a special segment of our lives."[66]

The following year, sadly, what should have been a delightful trip for the two friends ended in tragedy. On their second night on the garden island of Kauai, Hawaii, Anne Beech died after suffering a cerebral haemorrhage. Some found it strange that, after making the necessary arrangements to return her close friend's body home, Lyle, seemingly unaffected, completed the trip. Others, who knew both women well, believed that it was simply Lyle's way of dealing with a deeply felt loss.[67] Her circumspection made it difficult for others to gauge her emotional state, explaining in part why she remained such a quandary to her friends.

While Creelman aspired to live independently as long as possible on Bowen Island,[68] as early as 1981 she had briefly considered moving. Hazel and Elliott "told me off re. going to Sr. Cit. [senior citizen] Housing. What I needed. When time will sell house and buy apart. in West Van."[69] Now more crippled by arthritis,[70] she was increasingly concerned about her own declining health. The previous year, she had been told that the prolonged bouts of dizziness and problems with her vision during the past few years were symptomatic of cerebral arteriosclerosis, requiring that she take medication to decrease the likelihood of a stroke. Finding the Bowen Island winters somewhat depressing,[71] in 1983 she purchased a small apartment in West Vancouver. Typically, she also considered the purchase "from soundness of investment, not just convenience."[72] She believed it was "a good buy."[73] The next year, she moved into a larger apartment in the same building; offering an outstanding view, "glorious sunsets over the Gulf of Georgia and to the north mountains," it provided the ideal home away from home. Finding "four nights at apartment too much,"[74] she divided her time between Bowen Island and the Vancouver apartment over the next three years.[75] But increasingly she considered selling her island home: its upkeep and the travelling back and forth had begun to take their toll on her health.[76] In the spring of 1987, she made the difficult decision to leave Bowen Island and relocate to a condominium in West Vancouver, within a six-minute walk to the ocean shore.

In 1995, shortly after returning from "a very pleasant trip to England and Scotland" to attend a reunion of retired WHO nurses in Edinburgh, Lyle suffered a stroke. After two months in hospital, where she celebrated her eighty-seventh birthday, she was able to return home, eventually recovering to the point where she walked assisted only by a cane. Characteristically, she commented to friends, "It seems very slow to me but I guess some progress is being made." During her recuperation, letters of encouragement poured in from around the world: "The W.H.O. nurses have a wonderful network, the news travelling trans-Atlantic, trans-Pacific, across Canada, England and New Zealand. And perhaps a few other places."[77]

In early December 1996 she moved to Hollyburn House, "a very nice retirement home centrally located near the library, a very active seniors' centre and the sea wall."[78]

Lyle fitted well into the Hollyburn community and was an active participant in the full range of activities offered at Hollyburn House for many years. She had two further strokes. After the first one, she used a walker – and she used it, as she did with most things in her life, "with style, firmness and sense of dignity." Even after her second stroke confined her to a wheelchair, she remained an active participant in her rehabilitation program, resolute as always to be as independent as possible. Inevitably, as she aged and her health failed, her world at Hollyburn became more insular – despite the impressive support system that was put in place to assist her to be out and about as much as possible.

On 27 February 2007 Lyle Creelman died, at the age of ninety-nine. She had made careful arrangements for her memorial service and disposition of her estate to the UBC nursing school that she believed had made a vital contribution to her career. The Lyle Creelman Research Endowment Fund to further research by the UBC School of Nursing in the area of public health and the prevention of disease was entirely fitting with her lifetime interest in public health and in improving nursing education based upon sound scientific foundations.

Although raised in a devout Presbyterian family, Creelman, disenchanted with religious institutions she had seen around the world, had chosen not to have any religious service at her funeral. Instead, family, friends, and nursing colleagues celebrated her life at a "warm, caring, and friendly" memorial tea held at Hollyburn House in March 2007. Family members remembered trying to keep pace with Aunt Lyle on many rigorous hiking outings. Friends from Hollyburn recounted her independent and fiercely competitive spirit during bridge games. Nursing colleagues paid homage to a respected nursing leader's lifetime achievements. They recalled her strength of character, her candour, and her forceful personality, while simultaneously noting her gracious hospitability and fun-loving side. Everyone seemed "busy fitting new pieces into the delightful puzzle that was Lyle."[79] But few knew her complete story or fully understood the complexity of her character.

Lyle Creelman had been an active force in the transformation of twentieth-century nursing. Starting, in rural British Columbia, as the messenger of the state for cleanliness, citizenship, and morality, she went on to champion a more modern view of community-based, holistic, and multidimensional public health nursing worldwide. Her philosophy was forged within the nascent

Canadian welfare state, which enshrined citizens' rights to health and human security. It was further refined during her first international assignment with UNRRA, a pioneering post-war international welfare organization that, like its successor, linked peace, prosperity, and democracy, and viewed health as the foundational pillar for realizing these goals. It came of age during the WHO years.

Primary health care, social justice, and compassionate care remained the core values underpinning her philosophy of nursing. Lyle Creelman became the voice of international nursing, pioneering a transcultural approach that valued sustainable and culturally appropriate health care and nursing-education programs. Her views and leadership style were not without their limitations, contradictions, or fierce opponents. Nor would her accomplishments have been possible without the dedication, activities, and agency of the thousands of nurses of all ranks and nations with whom she worked. Lyle Creelman, and many WHO nurses, attempted to put forward a different vision of global health care, one that rejected the primacy of the vertical biological approach predicated on medical technologies and based on American developmental models envisaged by WHO physicians. Creelman advocated shifting global health priorities away from expensive, curative medical approaches to those that emphasized disease prevention and health promotion. The complex, often conflicted, and intriguing story of WHO nursing cannot simply be understood as a saga of secular missionaries or agents of cultural imperialism. Theirs is a far more telling story of the structural weaknesses that continue to inhibit nursing's voice in global health care.

Lyle Creelman campaigned for an approach to global health that considered the social determinants of health that ameliorated risks and fostered equity of care. She believed that governments had a responsibility to provide adequate health and living conditions but argued that nurses at all levels must be educated to negotiate a wide array of issues – social, political, and ethical – that shape health policy debates. Accordingly, she championed nurses' participation in program and policy development across the range of essential health-care services. Internationally, she believed nurses had a unique opportunity to fulfil their social responsibility as health promoters by collaborating with political leaders, foundations, international agencies, health-care workers, and community stakeholders to create sustainable solutions to identified needs. She spent her career helping nurses to communicate more effectively across geographic and professional boundaries to gain a more powerful voice for nursing in the struggle to improve health care. Consequently, her concept of leadership moved beyond the elitist notion of civic or faith-based duty to one of social advocacy and intersectoral collaboration to strengthen health equity globally and nationally. Accordingly, she preferred and used a new "flatter" style of administrative leadership that delegated authority to well-chosen lieutenants. This administrative style was to become widely used in health care in Canada and the United States in the 1970s and 1980s.[80] Her efforts to open up new political spaces for nurses that bypassed discriminatory health-care systems, globally and nationally, in order to permit them to represent themselves in less mediated ways were not totally successful. But she helped set the stage for an approach that championed primary health care and social advocacy networks as the preferred pathway for improving global health.

Creelman's career provides a salient historical lens with which to view the interaction of institutional, religious, educational, legal, and economic impediments that discriminate against not only nurses' but women's participation and access to decision-making and global power. Creelman was a woman of her day. Her leadership journey occasioned an ongoing struggle with her internalized gender stereotypes: the respectable feminine behaviour required of a nursing leader and a self-supporting, attentive daughter. It was complicated by the resistance to nurses as political actors in health-care formation that the stereotypes of nursing as an extension of maternal care engendered. She addressed institutional barriers – the inequalities of power, authority, and resource distribution – by seeking greater representation in policymaking, increased educational opportunities, improved compensation, and greater professional recognition and authority in the workplace. This legacy has been long-lasting: more resources, better-educated nurses, and the participation of nurses as leaders, focused on health and health-care systems, and as valued clinicians are still considered foundational for improving health care.[81]

True, the WHO after Creelman remained physician-dominated, which in practice meant a "man's world." But one should not ignore the diverse collegial ways in which nurses, during Creelman's tenure and subsequently, identified common goals, acted to negotiate differences of views, or exercised agency outside formal governmental or institutional structures to advance their agenda. Nursing networks remain important actors shaping health-care expectations, standards, and delivery. Feminist perspectives and analysis have changed over time. Today the hard-fought battle for gender equality is directed ultimately at de-gendering world politics through renewed polices of representation and redistribution.[82] Yet contemporary feminist critics of humanity's failure – despite the increased traction that gender equality has gained in the global community – to achieve security or social justice in the twenty-first century would find common ground with an earlier generation of nurses who believed that these issues could not be addressed independently of each other and with solutions imposed from above.

Nursing's struggle during the Creelman era foreshadowed its battle today to be regarded as a co-architect of the WHO's vision of "Health for All"[83] and the dramatic failure of the WHO, more than sixty years after its founding, to take the lead in establishing an effective global-heath governance system to ensure human security.[84] In an era before the term had been invented, when, as Akira Iriye writes, "globalization, as a state of mind and as an international expression, was dawning,"[85] Creelman understood that nursing must form coalitions across borders to influence both global and local health policy. If we accept one prominent formal definition of global public health as "the collective ability to conduct healthy public policy at a global level through a network of public, private, non-governmental, national, regional and international organizations by regime formation,"[86] we must also recognize the continued need for skilful cross-cultural brokers, like Lyle Creelman. Nurses functioning across multi-tiered networks that forge alliances with other social-justice advocacy groups remain a key precondition of sustainable worldwide health care and social justice.[87] At a time when nursing leaders are challenging nurses to enter the global-health dialogue by supporting global-health advocacy movements, such as Nightingale Initiative for Global Health[88] and the People's Health Movement,[89] Creelman's voice still resonates.

Appendices

APPENDIX A

Metropolitan Health Committee of Greater Vancouver, 1938

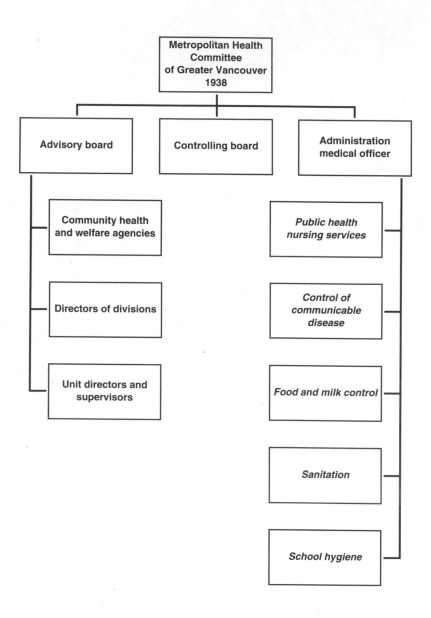

APPENDIX B

Ratio of Public Health Nurses to Population, British Columbia, 1942–3

UNIT	1942	1943
Vancouver	1:8000	1:8093
Burnaby	1:7500	1:6306
North Vancouver	1:6000	1:9000
Richmond	1:5000	1:5148

Source: Compiled from CVA, "Public Health Nursing Division," *Medical Health Officers Annual Reports*, 1941, 1942, 1943

APPENDIX C

Functions of the World Health Organization

The WHO's definition of its work included responsibility for the field of mental hygiene, nutrition, medical care, and environmental sanitation – indicating a much wider concept of public health than previously envisaged. The WHO was authorized:

- to assist governments, upon request, in strengthening health services;
- to promote improved standards of teaching and training of the medical and related professions;
- to provide information, counsel, and assistance in the field of health;
- to promote, in cooperation with other specialized agencies where necessary, the improvement of nutrition, housing, sanitation, recreation, economic or working conditions, and other aspects of environmental hygiene;
- to promote cooperation among scientific and professional groups that contribute to the advancement of health;
- to promote maternal and child health and welfare and to foster the ability to live harmoniously in a changing total environment;
- to foster activities in the field of mental health, especially those affecting the harmony of human relations;
- to promote and conduct research in the field of health; and
- to study and report on, in conjunction with other specialized agencies where necessary, administrative and social techniques affecting public health and medical care from the preventative and curative points of view, including hospital services and social security.

APPENDIX D

Headquarters Organization, July 1946

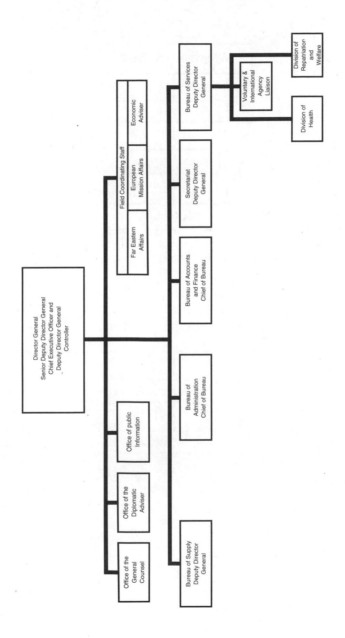

APPENDIX E

The Nursing Section within WHO

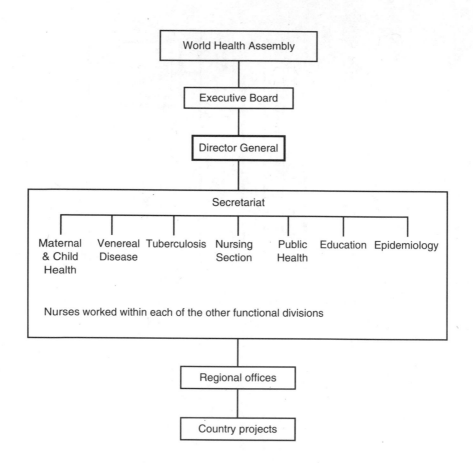

Notes

Preface

1 Lyle Creelman, interview with the author, Vancouver, 10 Aug. 2004.
2 See Lerner, "Placing Women in History"; and Grypma, "Critical Issues in the Use of Biographic Methods in Nursing History."
3 Grypma, "Critical Issues in the Use of Biographic Methods in Nursing History," 66.

4 World Health Organization, *Strategic Directions for Strengthening Nursing and Midwifery Services*.

5 International Council of Nurses, "Going, Going, Gone: The Nursing Presence in the WHO" 155. See also ibid., "Who Is Missing at the WHO?"

6 Boschma, "Writing International Nursing History," 11.

7 "Othering" relies on a binary dyad that divides a population into "us" who belong and 'them" who do not belong. The process of "othering," constructing negative identities often in binary opposition to Western ideals, creates "power over" relationships that sustained imperial hierarchies predicated upon cultural superiority.

8 Irwin, "Nurses without Borders," 78.

9 See Healey, " 'Seeds That May Have Been Planted May Take Root.' " Healey's assessment of the WHO is based upon secondary sources and makes no mention of Lyle Creelman's views or role.

10 Eschle, *Global Democracy, Social Movements and Feminism*, quoted in Peterson and Runyan, *Global Gender Issues in the New Millennium*, 236.

11 See, for examples, Healey, " 'I'm the Gal That Can Do It If They Let Me' "; and Healey, " 'Seeds That May Have Been Planted May Take Root' "; Jones, "Heroines of Lonely Outposts or Tools of the Empire?"; and Sweet, " 'Wanted: 16 Nurses of the Better Educated Type.' "

12 Sylvia D. Rinker, "Introduction," in D'Antonio, Baer, Rinker, and Lynaugh, *Nurses' Work*, 167.

13 Patricia D'Antonio, "Preface," in D'Antonio, Baer, Rinker, and Lynaugh, *Nurses' Work*, xvii. See also Elliott, Stuart, and Toman, *Place and Practice in Canadian Nursing History*.

14 D'Antonio, "Thinking about Place," 767.

15 See Farley, *Brock Chisholm*; and Irving's earlier biography, *Brock Chisholm*, where nothing is said about Lyle Creelman beyond a mention of her professional relationship with Chisholm.

16 See Armstrong-Reid and Murray, *Armies of Peace*; Brush, Lynaugh, and Boschma, eds., *Nurses of All Nations*; Toman, *An Officer and a Lady*; Grypma, *Healing Henan*; Choy, *Empire of Care*; Flynn, *Moving beyond Borders*; Lynaugh, Grace, Smith, Sena, and Duran de Villalobos, *The W.K. Kellogg Foundation*; and Solano and Rafferty, "Can Lessons Be Learned from History?"

17 A notable exception is Irwin, "Nurses without Borders."

18 Grypma, 65.

19 Each generation of global health scholars has posed questions relevant to the concerns of its era. For an excellent discussion of the literature, see Kirton and Guebert, "The Field of Global Governance."

20 This definition, first enunciated by Anne W. Goodwich, dean of the Army School of Nursing, in 1932 (*The Social and Ethical Significance of Nursing*) is quoted in Henderson, "The Development of a Personal Concept," 308.

21 Keohane, "Introduction."

22 Ibid., 1.

23 Ibid., 10.

24 The paradigm of "complex interdependence" – based on rationalist theory and drawn from models of economic behaviour – was developed in conjunction with Joseph Nye.

25 Keohane, ed., *Power and Governance*, 2.

26 Ibid., 3.

27 Ibid., 4–6. See also Keohane and Goldstein, *Ideas and Foreign Policy*.

28 See, for example, Fennimore and Sikkink, "International Norm Dynamics," for a discussion of how changing ideas channel and frame issues as a prelude to the convergence on institutions.

29 International-relations scholars' work identifying the importance of "epistemic communities" and "transnational advocacy coalitions," as increasingly important modes of operation for contemporary advocacy groups in global politics, illuminates the tensions Creelman experienced as a cross-cultural broker within the various nursing networks as the WHO's CNO. See Keck and Sikkink, *Activists beyond Borders*.

30 Keck and Sikkink contend that networks are both structured and structuring, with a focus on what they call the boomerang pattern: when power-holders use power or repression, local groups appeal to citizens of another country, through a transnational advocacy network, to lobby their own government to pressure the offending regime. See Keck and Sikkink, *Activists beyond Borders*, 16.

31 Bandy and Smith, "Factors Affecting Conflict," 231.

32 My views were stimulated by Keck and Sikkink's examination of the tactics used by networks to "bring new ideas, norms, and discourses into policy debates and serve as sources of information and testimony." See *Activists beyond Borders*, 16.

33 Ibid.

34 D'Antonio, "Rethinking and Rewriting of Nursing History," 299.

1. The Formative Years, 1908–1936

1 "Creelman-Creelman: A Pretty Home Wedding," 1907, newspaper clipping, box 1, Lyle Creelman Private Papers (LC), University of British Columbia (UBC).

2 Mrs MacRae to Jessie C. O'Brien, 8 Apr. 1954 (not catalogued), LC, UBC.

3 Dave Creelman, *Stewiacke Valley Sketchbook*.

4 Kay Creelman, daughter of James Creelman, interview with Susan Armstrong-Reid, 9 Apr. 2010.

5 City of Richmond Directories, 1924–8, City of Richmond Archives.

6 Lyle Creelman, interview with Audrey Stegen, West Vancouver, 3 July 1987, College of Registered Nurses of British Columbia (CRNBC).

7   Kay Creelman, interview.
8   Ibid.
9   Diary, 19 Dec. 1942, 1942–5, file 2-3, box 2, LC, UBC.
10 B.D. Boden, secretary of Board of School Trustees, Richmond Municipality, 4 July 1930, file 2-3, box 2, LC, UBC.
11 Roy, "'Due to Their Keenness regarding Education,'" 212.
12 Diary, 19 Dec. 1942, 1942–5, file 2-3, box 2, LC, UBC.
13 See Melchior, "Feminist Approaches to Nursing History," 348.
14 For a fuller discussion of the discrimination against Asian women either entering nursing education programs or practising afterwards, see Zilm and Warbinek, *Legacy*, 76–8.
15 Connolly, "Nurses: The Early Twentieth-Century Tuberculosis Preventorium's 'Connecting Link,'" 179.
16 Calhoun, "Public Health Activities," 336.
17 See Gray, "Nurses' Undergraduate Society," 1935, 1936; Zilm and Warbinek, *Legacy*, 60.
18 Riddell, "Curing Society's Ills."
19 Calhoun, "Public Health Activities in the Province of British Columbia." See also Davies, "Competent Professionals," 59.
20 For an elaboration of this viewpoint, see ibid., 62–3.
21 Dr Esson Young studied within North America at the McGill Medical College and then under William Osler at the University of Pennsylvania before completing further studies at London and Guy's Hospitals in England. Prior to his appointment as provincial health officer, he had been the minister responsible for education, health, and welfare from 1907 to 1915. His belief that "it is a very unfavourable comment on our intelligence when we compare the amount of money we are spending on curing people with the small amount that is spent in Canada by way of prevention of disease" spurred the expansion of public health nursing services within the province. Ewan and Blatherwick, *History of Public Health in B.C.*, 2.
22 For a more extensive discussion of Premier Duff Pattullo's political views on the social-welfare state, see Ormsby, *British Columbia*, chap. 15.
23 For a fuller discussion of the unique aspects of public health policy in British Columbia, see ibid., 56–83. Davies argues that Young's influence on public health diminished somewhat when younger men appeared on the scene at the beginning of the Depression. Davies, "Competent Professionals," 59.
24 Davies, "Competent Professionals," 72.
25 Ibid.
26 Quoted in Zilm and Warbinek, *Legacy*, 75.

27 Davies, "Competent Professionals," 63.
28 Kinnear, "Professionalization of Canadian Nursing," 169. Kinnear argues that the political alignments between physicians and nurses were more complex than recognized in the historical literature and also suggests that nursing leaders may have concluded that an adversarial relationship would not advance their professional agenda.
29 Quoted in Davies, "Competent Professionals," 33.
30 See D'Antonio's discussion of this trend in *American Nursing*, 32.
31 Kinnear, "Professionalization of Canadian Nursing." See also Calhoun, "Public Health Activities in the Province of British Columbia," 341.
32 Kinnear, "Professionalization of Canadian Nursing," 156.
33 Ellis, "Review of the Modern Trend of Nursing and Nursing Education," 61.
34 The Goldmark Report became one of the most influential documents of its day and influenced the development of nursing not only in the United States but Canada and elsewhere for years to come. It supported the claims of nursing elites that the quality of existing nursing programs was inadequate.
35 For examples, see 59–62; Meiklejohn, "How to Provide a Sufficiently Broad Training and Experience for the Pupil of the Small School," 124–6; "Editorials: Why a Nursing Survey," 660.
36 Johns, "Canada Looks at the Neighbours."
37 Zilm and Warbinek, *Legacy*, 72.
38 D'Antonio, *American Nursing*, 28.
39 Kinnear, "Professionalization of Canadian Nursing," 206.
40 Copy of Gray, "The Department of Nursing and Health," 4, file 7-20, School of Nursing Fonds, UBC.
41 Fairley, "Report of Conference on University Courses in Nursing," 141. See also "The Trained Nurse as a Storm Centre for Discussion," 359.
42 Russell, "The Canadian University and the Canadian School of Nursing," 630.
43 UBC undergraduate calendar, 1932, 204, Rare Books and Special Collections, UBC.
44 Copy of Gray, "Department of Nursing and Health," 3.
45 Fairley had obtained her initial nursing training from Swansea General Hospital in Wales before taking postgraduate studies in Glasgow. She served as the superintendent of nurses at Montreal's Alexander Hospital (1912–19), the Montreal General Hospital (1919–24), and the Victoria Hospital in London before her appointment to VGH in 1929.
46 Ellis, "Grace M. Fairley"; file: Grace M. Fairley, vol. 158, I-248, MG 28, Library and Archives Canada (LAC).
47 "Grace M. Fairley," *Canadian Nurse* 65, no. 5 (1969): 18; see also file: Grace M. Fairley, vol. 158, I-248, MG 28, LAC.

48 Zilm and Warbinek, *Legacy*, 86.
49 Kinnear, "Professionalization of Canadian Nursing," 158.
50 This comment was made by Helen Mussallem, a former student and distinguished nursing educator, on Fairley's fight to admit Japanese and Aboriginal students in 1942. "Names: Grace M. Fairley," 18.
51 Fairley served as president of both the Registered Nurses Association of British Columbia (RNABC) and the CNA, and she was also appointed the third vice-president of the International Council of Nurses, a position she held until 1953.
52 *Vancouver General Hospital Annual Report*, 1937, 25, Vancouver General Hospital Archives (VGHA).
53 Mabel Gray had taught prior to entering training at the Winnipeg General Hospital, where she rose through the ranks to become the superintendent of nurses and principal of the School of Nurses on the eve of the outbreak of the First World War. She received a certificate in public health nursing from Simmons College of Public Health Nursing in Boston in June 1920.
54 "Miss Gray Retires," *Canadian Nurse* 37, no. 11 (1941): 755.
55 "The Future of the Nursing Profession," 6, Speeches, file 1-9, box 1, Mabel F. Gray Fonds, UBC.
56 Zilm and Warbinek, *Legacy*, 62.
57 Ibid., 81. See also copy of Gray, "Department of Nursing and Health," 4.
58 "Preparation for Community Work," 2, Speeches, file 1-9, box 1, Mabel F. Gray Fonds, UBC.
59 See D'Antonio, *American Nursing*, 35.
60 "The Nursing School and the Community," 1, Speeches, file 1-9, box 1, Mabel F. Gray Fonds, UBC.
61 Ibid., 7.
62 Zilm and Warbinek, *Legacy*, 72.
63 "Services Commemorate Passing of National Nursing Figure," news release, 30 June 1976, file: Margaret Kerr, vol. 248, I-248, MG 28, LAC.
64 Kerr, "The Importance of Post-Graduate Public Health Training," 135.
65 Ibid., 136.
66 "A Tribute to Our Editor and Executive Director on Her Retirement," 707.
67 Dodd, "Nurses Residence: Using the Built Environment as Evidence."
68 *Vancouver General Hospital Yearbook*, 1936, 24, box 1, LC, UBC.
69 Diary 1936, 8 Jan. 1936, file 2-1, box 2, LC, UBC.
70 Ibid., 15 Jan. 1936. See also ibid., 21 Jan. 1936, where Lyle Creelman is critical of her abilities to give immunization.
71 Ibid., 17 Jan. 1936.

72 Mabel F. Gray, "The Department of Nursing and Health, the University of British
    Columbia," repr. from *Methods and Problems of Medical Education, Twenty-First
    Series* (New York: Rockefeller Foundation, 1932), Speeches, file 1-9, box 1, Mabel
    F. Gray Fonds, UBC.
73 Mabel Gray to Miss Kerr, "Memorandum regarding Routine Matter," n.d., file 7-20,
    School of Nursing Fonds, UBC.
74 Diary 1936, 3 Feb. 1936.
75 *VGH Nurses Annual Report*, 1933, 16, VGHA.
76 R.G. Ferguson, "M.O. Tuberculosis among Nurses," *Canadian Nurse* 31, no. 12
    (1936), qtd in Ester I. Paulson, "The School of Nursing at R.C.H. and Nursing
    Education in Canada 1901–1976," 14, Ester Paulson Fonds, School of Nursing
    UBC, the B.C. History of Nursing Society (BCHNS).
77 Diary 1936, 28 Jan. 1936, file 2-1, box 2, LC, UBC.
78 Ibid., 4 Feb. 1936.
79 Chodat graduated from the UBC degree program in 1935. Zilm and Warbinek,
    Legacy, 108.
80 Diary 1936, 12 Feb. 1936, file 2-1, box 2, LC, UBC.
81 Ibid., 14 Feb. 1936.
82 Ibid.
83 Zilm and Warbinek, *Legacy*, 112.
84 Diary1936, 17 Jan. 1936, 28 Mar. 1936, file 2-1, box 2, LC, UBC.
85 A graduate of Dalhousie University (BA), Electra MacLennan completed nursing
    training at the Royal Victoria Hospital School of Nursing in Montreal in 1932 and
    obtained a certificate in teaching and supervision from McGill School for Graduate
    Nurses (1933).
86 Diary, 28 Apr. 1936, Apr. 1936, file 2-1, box 2, LC, UBC.
87 See "The Nurses Undergraduate Society," *Ubyssey*, 15 Oct. 1932, 2 Mar. 1938,
    9 Nov. 1933, 2 Mar. 1934.
88 Diary 1936, 25 Feb. 1936, 1936, file 2-1, box 2, LC, UBC.
89 Ibid., 3 Mar. 1936.
90 Ibid., 4 Mar. 1936.
91 Ibid., 5 Mar. 1936.
92 Ibid., 11 Mar. 1936. See also ibid., 10 Apr. 1936.
93 Ibid., 6 Mar. 1936.
94 Ibid., 17 Mar. 1936.
95 Ibid., 23 Mar. 1936.
96 Ibid., 6 Apr. 1936.
97 Ibid., 9 Apr. 1936.
98 1936 VGH Diploma and UBC graduation program, file 1-5, box 1, LC, UBC.

99 "A Tribute," 705.

100 Ibid., 707.

101 "Announcement for the *Canadian Nurse*," file: Margaret E. Kerr, vol. 158, I-248, MG 28, LAC.

102 Diary 1936, 7 June 1936, file 2-1, box 2, LC, UBC.

103 See, for example, ibid., 6 Mar., 4 Apr., 2 May, 8 June 1936.

104 "A Tribute," 708.

2. New Beginnings, 1936–1939

1 Esson Young, as quoted in Green, *Through the Years with Public Health Nursing*, 9.

2 Klassen, "Camp Alexandra: A Brief History," 10.

3 Diary 1936, Apr. 1936, 1936–7, file 2-1, box 2, LC, UBC.

4 Ibid., 12 June 1936.

5 Ibid., 27 July 1936.

6 Ibid., 25 June 1936.

7 Esson Young, provincial health officer (BC), to Lyle Creelman, 14 May 1936, file 3-2, box 3, LC, UBC.

8 Diary 1936, 27 Apr. 1936, 1936–7, file 2-1, box 2, LC, UBC.

9 Ibid., 8 May 1936.

10 Ibid., 30 June 1936.

11 Ibid., 15 July 1936.

12 Ibid.

13 See, for example, her diary entry of 27 Aug. 1936, where, after a visit with Dr Amyot, she records that even though she found his suggestions "daft," "it would not hurt her to read along the lines he suggested." Ibid.

14 Ibid., 1 Aug. 1936.

15 Ibid., 1 Oct. 1936.

16 Ibid., 6 Aug. 1936.

17 "Notes on the Development of Public Health Nursing in British Columbia," 3, Directors 1952–82, file 7-20, School of Nursing Fonds, UBC.

18 Henry Esson Young, *Public Health Nurses' Bulletin* 1, no. 1 (1924): 1.

19 Creelman, "Revelstoke Reflections," 11.

20 Agnes Thom, "Health Pursuits in Revelstoke," *Public Health Nurses Bulletin* 3, no. 3 (1936): 44.

21 Creelman, "Public School Health Report," 19.

22 Creelman, "Revelstoke Reflections," 12.

23 Qtd in Lewis, "'Creating the Little Machine,'" 57.

24 Creelman, "Revelstoke Reflections," 13.

25 Ibid.

26 "The Nursing School and the Community," 4, Speeches, file 1-9, Mabel Gray Fonds, UBC.
27 For a discussion of public health nursing in British Columbia as a "critical component of the social gospel and the missionary zeal that characterized middle-class activism during the late nineteenth and early twentieth centuries," see Riddell, "Curing Society's Ills."
28 For a broader study of the concerns with family, gender, and state that shaped the modernizing nation's medical response to maternal care, a context in which nursing sought to define its place as the gatekeeper of medical expertise within the hospitals and the wider community, see Mitchinson, *Giving Birth in Canada*.
29 Mitchinson states, "The VON nurses separated themselves from the Ukrainian Women on the basis of ethnicity and class, feeling that part of their job was to imbue them with 'Canadian ideals' as represented by scientific medical care." Ibid., 133.
30 See, for example, Geraldine Homfry Langton, oral history interview, Aug. 1988 (tape no. 120 and transcript), biographical file, CRNBC Library.
31 See Lewis, " 'Creating the Little Machine,' " 56.
32 Mitchinson, *Giving Birth in Canada*, 135.
33 A public health clinic that dealt with the total well-being of children and family and provided a safety net for the economically disadvantaged by offering low-cost health care and parent education.
34 Creelman, "Revelstoke Reflections," 12.
35 Creelman, "Protect Your Child from Diphtheria."
36 Diary 1936, 30 Aug. 1936, 1936–7, file 2-1, box 2, LC, UBC.
37 Ibid., 1 Sept. 1936.
38 Ibid., 3 Sept. 1936.
39 Ibid., 9 Sept. 1936.
40 Creelman, "Revelstoke Reflections," 12.
41 Lewis develops this argument in " 'Creating the Little Machine,' " 45.
42 Creelman, "First Monthly Infant Weighing Station Held."
43 Diary 1936, 18 Sept. 1936, file 2-1, box 2, LC, UBC.
44 Ibid., 19 Sept. 1936.
45 Creelman, "First Monthly Infant Weighing Station Held."
46 For a comparison of the range of activities, see Agnes Thom, "Nurse Thom Presents Final Health Report," 26 June 1936; and Creelman, "Public School Health Report."
47 See, for example, the following issues of the *Revelstoke Review*: 23 Dec. 1936, 28 Jan. 1937, 29 Jan. 1937, 26 Feb. 1937, 12 Mar. 1937, 25 Mar. 1937, 29 May 1937, 11 June 1937.
48 Diary 1936, 28 Sept. 1936, file 2-1, box 2, LC, UBC.
49 Ibid., 21 Oct. 1936.

50 Ibid., 25 Nov. 1936.

51 Ibid., 28 Oct. 1936.

52 Ibid., 25 Nov. 1936.

53 Ibid., 28 Nov. 1936.

54 Historians have noted public health nursing's negative side as a paternalist pur-
veyor of middle-class values and as a vehicle for the assimilation of new immigrants into Canadian society, especially within the western provinces. See Dehli,
"Health Scouts for the State?"

55 Elizabeth Breeze to Lyle Creelman, 24 June 1937, 9, telegram, file 3-2, box 3, LC,
UBC.

56 Journals 1939–1952, 19 Dec. 1942, file 2-3, box 2, LC, UBC.

57 "Metropolitan Board Robs Province of Best Nurses," newspaper clipping, file 1-7,
box 1, LC, UBC.

58 "Greater City in Health Unit: Metropolitan Board Becomes Reality on Sunday,"
Vancouver Daily Province, 31 Oct. 1936.

59 Ewan and Blatherwick, *History of Public Health in B.C.*, 2. Its governing body was
composed of representatives appointed by the councils and school boards of each
participating city or municipality, with the provincial government appointing representatives for those areas under its control. Under an agreement signed in 1937,
the medical health officer of the city of Vancouver was appointed the senior medical health officer for the whole area, and the Metropolitan Health Committee was
to have a coordinating function.

60 Elizabeth Breeze, "The Metropolitan Health Committee of Greater Vancouver,"
draft article for the *Canadian Nurse* (May 1938), CVA.

61 Metropolitan Health Committee Minutes, Wednesday, 21 Dec. 1938, 67, CVA.

62 Ibid., 4.

63 Ewan and Blatherwick, *History of Public Health in B.C.*, 60.

64 Evans to Dyball, 16 June 1975, file: Health Services, City of Richmond Archives.

65 Obituary, *Canadian Nursing Journal*, June 1938, 313, City of Richmond Archives.

66 Elizabeth Breeze was a graduate of the Hospital for Sick Children in Toronto
and had obtained a certificate in public health nursing from the University of
California. See file: Elizabeth Breeze, vol. 157, I-248, MG 28, LAC.

67 Journals 1939–1952, 3 Jan. 1942, file 2-3, box 2, LC, UBC. (Note: the dates at the
top of diary pages are to be ignored since Creelman transcribed earlier diaries into
the 1943 journal.)

68 After receiving her initial training and supervisory experience at the Winnipeg
General Hospital, Stewart obtained a diploma in hospital economics (1909), a
BSc (1911), and an MA (1913) from Columbia University before joining its staff.
In 1925 she succeeded Adelaide Nutting as chair of the Department of Nursing
Education at Teachers College. In that capacity she was involved in writing three

classics: *The Standard Curriculum for Schools of Nursing, A Curriculum for Schools of Nursing,* and *A Curriculum Guide for Schools of Nursing.* Stewart co-authored *A Short History of Nursing* with Lavinia Dock and *A History of Nursing* with Anne Austin.

69 Goostry, "Isabel Maitland Stewart," 303.

70 Quoted in ibid., 141.

71 Ibid.

72 Quoted in Donahue, "Isabel Maitland Stewart's Philosophy of Education," 142.

73 Donahue, "Isabel Maitland Stewart's Philosophy of Education," 141.

74 The TC's Division of Nursing Education worked closely with the NLNE. The NLNE, now known as the National League for Nursing Education, traces its origins to the American Society of Superintendents of Training Schools for Nurses in 1893; the first organization for nursing in the United States of America, it was dedicated to the establishment and maintenance of a universal standard of training for nursing.

75 Donahue, "Isabel Maitland Stewart's Philosophy of Education," 90.

76 Christy, *Cornerstone for Nursing Education.*

77 As chair of the Education Committee of the International Council of Nurses from 1925 to 1947, Stewart helped to establish international standards of nursing education and promoted the standardization of nursing curriculum. Her curriculum guide *The Educational Program of the School of Nursing* was distributed in translation to several countries through the International Council of Nurses and the Red Cross Society.

78 A graduate of the Army School of Nursing, Washington, DC, in 1921, Henderson had obtained an MA in nursing education before joining the TC staff in 1934 to teach research and medical surgical nursing.

79 Henderson, "Development of a Personal Concept," 312.

80 Ibid., 316.

81 Ibid.

82 Rose's Foundations of Nutrition and Feeding the Family "linked the findings of the nutrition laboratory with the daily lives of the people." Emerson's contributions to disease nomenclature, vital statistics, epidemiology, and public health administration were widely recognized. Rosenfield, "The View from the Dean's Office," 201. For a fuller description of Emerson's accomplishments, see Bolduan, "Haven Emerson," 1–4.

83 For a further elaboration of Osborne's innovative and interactive approach to teaching, see Hey, "Ernest G. Osborne."

84 Ibid., 135.

85 Osborne and Osborne, "Parent Education and the Nurse," 1258.

86 Ibid., 1259.

87 Mary Elizabeth Tennant obtained her BA from the University of Colorado in 1916 before attending the Vassar Rainbow Division Training Camp for nurses during the summer of 1918. She received her nursing education at Philadelphia General Hospital and Simmons College. Tennant had joined the RF in 1928 and was then serving as a member of the International Health Division staff, specializing in nursing and public health. She eventually rose to become assistant director in 1945.

88 Lyle Creelman, Canada, Fellowship Recorder Cards, Rockefeller Foundation Fonds, RFAC; Mary Elizabeth Tennant, 25 Jan. 1939, 1939, Officers Diaries, 12, Rockefeller Foundation Fonds, RFAC.

89 Creelman, Fellowship Recorder Cards.

90 For a description of the development of the East Harlem Nursing and Health Services, see Christy, *Cornerstone for Nursing Education*, 85.

91 Rockefeller Foundation, *Annual Report*, 1939, 153.

92 Rosen, "Public Health Then and Now," 1631.

93 Ibid., 1620.

94 Creelman, Fellowship Recorder Cards.

95 Journals 1939–1952, 4 Mar. 1939, file 2-3, box 2, LC, UBC.

96 Ibid., 31 Jan. 1939.

97 Ibid., 11 Feb. 1939.

98 Ibid., 12 Feb. 1939.

99 Quoted in Duranti, "Utopia," 666.

100 Ibid.

101 Ibid., 683.

102 Journals 1939–1952, 19 Dec. 1942, file 2-3, box 2, LC, UBC.

103 For example, Ethel Johns had undertaken a major study of the working conditions of black nurses in the United States funded by the RF.

104 Rockefeller Foundation, *Annual Report*, 1940 and 1941, RF, RFAC.

105 Mary Elizabeth Tennant, 25 May 1939, 1939, Officers Diaries, 12.1, RF, RFAC.

106 Journals 1939–1952, 3 June 1939, file 2-3, box 2, LC, UBC.

107 Kirkwood, "Blending Vigorous Leadership and Womanly Virtues," 184.

108 Kerr, "Innovation in Public Health Nursing Education in Canada," 3.

109 For a more complete discussion of Edith Kathleen Russell's relationship with the Rockefeller Foundation and Teachers College during her thirty-year effort to nurture the development of a nursing school within the University of Toronto, see Kirkwood and Kerr as cited above.

110 Kirkwood, "Blending Vigorous Leadership and Womanly Virtues," 181–3.

111 Ibid., 185. Jean Wilson, a long-time instructor in the University of Toronto's School of Nursing; Ethel M. Cryderman, head of the Victorian Order of Nurses; and Jean Gunn, the superintendent of nurses at the Toronto General Hospital,

who was involved in the Canadian Red Cross and was "a leading spokesperson" for the CNA.

112 Although Emory did not have a university degree, she had extensive public health experience with Toronto's Department of Public Health and had spent a year at Simmons College before joining the teaching staff in the fledgling Department of Public Health Nursing at the University of Toronto in 1924. See Kirkwood, "Florence Emory," 32–5.

113 See Journals 1939–1952, 30 June and 5 July 1939, file 2-3, box 2, LC, UBC.

114 Ibid., 9–17 Aug. 1939.

115 Ibid., 7 Jan. 1943, file 2-3, box 2, LC, UBC.

3. The Shadow of War, 1939–1944

1 Miscellaneous newspaper clipping, dated 28 Aug. 1939, file 1-7, box 1, LC, UBC.

2 Aletha MacLellan, the second school nurse appointed in Vancouver in 1911, later became the supervisor of the School of Nursing in the Metropolitan Health Committee in 1936. Lyle Creelman, "Public Health Nursing Division," *Medical Health Officer's Annual Report of the Greater Vancouver Metropolitan Health Committee*, 1941, 17, CVA.

3 Journals 1939–1952, 16 Oct. 1939, box 2, file 2-3, LC, UBC.

4 Ibid., 28 Nov. 1939.

5 Ibid., 19 Jan. 1940.

6 Constitution dated April 1940. Executive and Regular Meetings: The Science Girls Club, University Nurses Club, file 7-30, School of Nursing Fonds, UBC.

7 Minutes of the Science Girls Club, 19 Dec. 1939, file 7-31, box 7, School of Nursing Fonds, UBC.

8 Ibid., 16 Jan. 1940.

9 I am indebted to Glennis Zilm for drawing my attention to this source. Report of the Meetings, etc – UBC Nurses Club, file 7-30, School of Nursing Files, UBC.

10 Minutes of the Science Girls Club, 18 June 1940.

11 See, for example, Minutes of the Science Girls Club, 5 Dec. 1941, file 7-31, box 7, School of Nursing Fonds, UBC.

12 Lyle Creelman, Canada, 29 Apr. 1940, Fellowship Recorder Cards, RF, Rockefeller Foundation Archival Center (RFAC).

13 Journals 1939–1952, 23 and 28 Nov. 1939, file 2-3, box 2 LC, UBC.

14 Ibid., 4 Feb. 1940.

15 Ibid., entry written on 19 Dec. 1942 but entered on pp. 8 and 9 Jan. 1943.

16 Ibid., 5 Sept. 1940.

17 Ibid., 13 Mar. 1940.

18 Ibid., 27 June 1940.

19 Ibid., 29 Aug. 1940.

20 Ibid., 1 Sept. 1939.

21 Ibid., entry written on 19 Dec. 1942 but entered on p. 9 Jan. 1943, UBC.

22 Ibid., 8–9 Jan. 1943.

23 Ibid.

24 Creelman, Canada, 23 Feb. 1942, Fellowship Recorder Cards, RF, RFAC.

25 Journals, 1939–1952, entry written on 2 June 1943 but entered on p. 5 Feb. 1943, file 2-3, box 2, LC, UBC.

26 Ibid., 10 Jan. 1943.

27 Creelman, Canada, 23 Feb. 1942, 8 June 1942, Fellowship Recorder Cards, RF, RFAC.

28 Mary Elizabeth Tennant, 9 June 1942, 1942, Officers Diaries, 12.1, RF, RFAC.

29 Creelman, "Public Health Nursing Services," *Medical Health Officers Annual Report of the Greater Vancouver Metropolitan Health Committee*, 17, 1941, CVA.

30 A 1939 graduate of VGH, Hunter completed a diploma course in public health at UBC.

31 Sheila Zerr, "Interview with Trenna Hunter, BAScN, 1944 March 1987 and transcribed by Ethel Warbinek, 26 March 1993," 3, oral history interview, CRNBC.

32 Journals 1939–1952, entry written 2 June 1943 but entered on Feb. 1943, file 2-3, box 2, LC, UBC. Both Creelman and Dr Murray praised Hunter's work when they met with Tennant. See Mary Elizabeth Tennant, 7 June 1942, 1942, Officers Diaries, 12.1, RF, RFAC.

33 Mary Elizabeth Tennant, 25 Jan. 1939, Officers Diaries, 12.1, RF, RFAC.

34 Abrams, "Seeking Jurisdiction," 277, makes a similar argument in discussing the development of generalized public health services in the United States.

35 This theme permeated all Creelman's reports on the Public Health Nursing Division from 1941 to 1943. Medical Health Officer's Annual Reports, CVA.

36 Creelman, "Public Health Nursing Division," *Medical Health Officer's Annual Report*, 1941, 18, CVA.

37 "Names," *Canadian Nurse* 29, no. 10 (1966): 18.

38 Zerr, "Interview with Trenna Hunter," 7.

39 T. Hunter to P. Stiver, 3 Apr. 1956, file: Trenna Hunter, vol. 158, I-248, MG 28, LAC.

40 Ibid., biographical information form dated 22 June 1943 for the *Canadian Nurse*.

41 Zerr, "Interview with Trenna Hunter," 7.

42 Ibid., 19–20.

43 Ibid., 20.

44 Mary Elizabeth Tenant, 9 June 1942, 1939, Officers Diaries, 12.1, RF, RFAC.

45 Williams, "Public Health Nursing in a Japanese Community in British Columbia."

46 Creelman, "Public Health Nursing Division," *Medical Health Officer's Annual Report*, 1941, 18, CVA.

47 Ibid., 19.
48 Ibid., 20.
49 Ibid., 19. New child health centres were opened in the west end of Vancouver at Gordon House, in Richmond at the Mitchell School, and at Lions Gate to serve the local Wartime Housing Development.
50 Ibid.,16.
51 Ibid., 19.
52 Ibid., 20.
53 Ibid.
54 Preliminary planning was begun in cooperation with the Division of Tuberculosis Control to have students from the five nursing schools in British Columbia spend a week of their TB practicum with the Metropolitan Health Committee.
55 Creelman, "Public Health Nursing Division," *Medical Health Officer's Annual Report*, 1943, 22, CVA.
56 Creelman had worked with Langton in the Richmond Unit and they both had served on the executive committee of the Science Girls Club. More important, in March 1939, Creelman, then at Teachers College, had arranged for Langton, while on a study leave in the United States, to observe the generalized nursing services operated by the Henry Street Visiting Nurse Society.
57 Mary Elizabeth Tennant, 27 Jan. 1939, 1939, Officers Diaries, 12.1, RF, RFCA.
58 Langton and Chodat, "Planning Field Experience," 739–40.
59 See, for example, Creelman, "Public Health Nursing Division."
60 Zilm and Warbinek, *Legacy*, 97–8.
61 See Tennant's earlier diary entries discussing Dolmon's discontent. Mary Elizabeth Tennant, 27 Jan. 1939 and 9 June 1942, 1942, Officers Diaries, 12.1, RF, RFCA.
62 Ibid.
63 The outbreak of war in 1939 forced Henderson, a Florence Nightingale Foundation Fellow, to study administration and supervision at the University of Toronto rather than in Britain.
64 Mary Elizabeth Tennant, 27 Jan. 1939, 1939, Officers Diaries, 12.1, RF, RFCA.
65 Mary Elizabeth Tennant, "Fellowship Program for Nurses: International Health Division, the Rockefeller Foundation," 6, 24, 42, file 351, box 46, 100EC Fellowships Nursing, RG1.2, RF, RFAC.
66 See Saunier, "World of Nursing."
67 Creelman, "Public Health Nursing Division," *Medical Health Officer's Annual Report*, 1942, 17, CVA.
68 Creelman, "Mental Hygiene in the Public Health Program."
69 See Davidson, "Mental Hygiene and Nursing"; Mathers, "Mental Hygiene and Nursing"; Lawrence, "Mental Hygiene from the Standpoint of a Social Nurse"; (no author), "The Mental Hygiene Movement in Canada"; Laycock, "Mental

Hygiene and Public Health"; Mitchell, "The Importance of Mental Hygiene" and "Mental Hygiene"; Harvey Clarke, "Mental Hygiene for Nurses"; Emma de V. Clarke, "Mental Hygiene in Public Health Nursing"; Montgomery, "The Mental Health Clinic"; Mitchell, Mitchell, Rogers, and Peden, "Selection of Students." I am indebted to Dr Geertje Boschma for directing me to these articles.

70 McLaren, *Our Own Master Race*, 28.

71 Ibid., 29.

72 See Clarke, "Sacred Daemons," for a discussion of how eugenics ideology affected the treatment of "mentally deficient children as threats to society."

73 McLaren, *Our Own Master Race*, 110–11.

74 Thomson, "Not an Attempt to Coddle Children."

75 Creelman, "Mental Hygiene in the Public Health Program," 680.

76 Ibid.

77 Ibid., 683.

78 See Emma de V. Clarke, "Mental Hygiene in Public Health Nursing," 457; Harvey Clarke, "Mental Hygiene for Nurses," 71.

79 McLaren, *Our Own Master Race*, 111.

80 Journals 1939–1952, entry written on 28 Nov. 1943 but entered on p. 27 Mar. 1943, file 2-3, box 2, LC, UBC.

81 Creelman, "Mental Hygiene in the Public Health Program," 681.

82 Ibid., 682.

83 Ibid., 684.

84 McLaren, *Our Own Master Race*, 113. The motivation that underpinned the delivery of community mental-health services and institutions was more complex than McLaren suggests. Geertje Boschma offers a more textured understanding of families' ability to contest and negotiate the existing medical and legal norms that structured asylum care. See her article "A Family Point of View."

85 Creelman, "Mental Hygiene in the Public Health Program," 680.

86 Ibid., 684.

87 Creelman, "What Is Public Health Nursing?" 111.

88 Ibid.

89 Ibid., 112.

90 Kerr and Creelman, "Public Health Nurses in Canada," 42.

91 Creelman, "Report of the Public Health Section," 682.

92 Kerr, "Kla-How-Ya, Tillicum," 41.

93 My thinking on the public health nurse's agency role was stimulated by Maxwell's perceptive article "Children and State Intervention."

94 Comacchio, *"Nations Are Built for Care Saving,"* has made a similar argument in respect to maternal health care.

95 Journals 1939–1952, 11 Jan. 1943, file 2-3, box 2, LC, UBC.

96 Ibid., entry written on 15 Nov. 1942 but entered on p. 17 Jan. 1943.

97 Wilson, "Notes from the National Office."

98 The CNA concern to maintain uniform standards of training and supervision is clearly evident in a series of resolutions passed at the Montreal meeting of 1942. See file: Min A1-1/s, vol. 36, I-248, MG 28, LAC.

99 Journals 1939–1952, entry written on 19 Dec. 1942 but entered on 11 Jan. 1943, file 2-3, box 2, LC, UBC.

100 File: Min A1-1/s, vol. 36, I-248, MG 28, LAC.

101 Ibid.

102 The recommendations were reported to the CNA membership in Sept. 1942 through the *Canadian Nurse* 38, no. 9 (1942): 688–9. See also Kerr and Creelman, "Public Health Nurses," *Canadian Nurse* 38, no. 1 (1942): 42–4.

103 Creelman, "What of the Future?," 36.

104 For a more detailed discussion of the growing disconnect between the nursing leadership and the rank and file, who had focused more on economic survival as the 1930s progressed, see McPherson, *Bedside Matters*, 74–114.

105 Creelman, "What of the Future?," 37.

106 Ibid. The data collected on salaries was published in Creelman, " Report of the Public Health Section," 682–4.

107 Journals 1939–1952, 15 May 1941, file 2-3-2, box 2, LC, UBC.

108 Ibid., entry written on 2 Feb. 1943 but entered on p. 1 Feb. 1943.

109 See, for example, Edith Birth, "Report of the Labour Relations Committee."

110 Minutes of the regular meeting of the Registered Nurses Association of British Columbia, 5 Apr. 1944 (no. 209), 2, College of Registered Nurses of British Columbia.

111 Ibid., 3.

112 Zilm and Warbinek, *Legacy*, 106.

113 Ibid., 121.

114 Creelman, "Report on the Public Health Section," 682.

115 Johnson, commissioned in the U.S. Public Health Service (USPHS), had served as the senior public health nurse with the Office of Foreign Relief and Rehabilitation Operations, a subdivision of the State Department responsible for much of the preliminary planning for UNRRA. "Interesting People: Lillian J. Johnston."

116 "Notes from the National Office," *Canadian Nurse* 40, no. 7 (1944): 493–4.

117 Journals 1939–1952, 12 Jan. 1942, file 2-3, box 2, LC, UBC.

118 Ibid., 15 Jan. 1942.

119 Ibid., 16 Jan. 1942.

120 Ibid., entry written on 15 Nov. 1942 but entered on p. 24 Jan. 1943.

121 Ibid., entry written on 13 July 1943 but entered on p. 10 Feb. 1943.

122 "N.F "Dick" Pullen," *Cariboo Observer*, 3 Jan. 1963.

123 Journals 1939–1952, account of trip entered on p. 24 Feb. 1943, file 2-3, box 2, LC, UBC.

124 Ibid., entry written on 12 Oct. 1943 but entered on p. 21 Mar. 1943.

125 Ibid., account of vacation entered on p. 26 Feb. 1943.

126 Ibid., account entered on p. 26 Feb. 1943. The visits from a sister whom Prescott both adored and respected professionally were valued throughout his life. Lyle was the family member to whom he felt most closely connected.

127 Ibid., account of trip home entered on p. 3 Mar. 1943.

128 Ibid., comment entered on p. 4 Mar. 1943.

129 Ibid., entry written on 3 July 1943 but entered on p. 5 Mar. 1943.

130 Ibid., p. 7 Mar. 1943.

131 Ibid., entry written on 3 July 1943 but entered on page 6 Mar. 1943.

132 Ibid., entry written on 25 Nov. 1944 but entered on 31 Mar. 1943.

133 Ibid., entry written on 4 Jan. 1944 but entered on p. 6 Apr. 1943.

134 Ibid., entry written on page 7 Apr. 1943.

135 Ibid.

136 Ibid., entry written on 24 July 1944 but entered on p. 11 Apr. 1943.

137 Ibid., entry written on 24 Sept. 1944 but entered on p. 21 Apr. 1943.

138 Zilm and Warbinek, *Legacy*, 102.

139 Journals 1939–1952, entry written on 24 Sept. 1944 but entered on p. 29 Apr. 1943, file 2-3, box 2, LC, UBC.

140 Ibid., p. 25 Apr. 1943.

4. Soldier of Peace, 1944–1946

1 Although access to UNRRA personnel records is restricted, the surviving out-placement records of some Canadian nurses who remained with UNRRA until it closed its doors provide an indication of why UNRRA salary levels were so attractive. Civilian salary ranges within this limited sample appears consistent with the national averages quoted in a 1944–5 Canadian Military Recruiting Brochure and with a 1941 survey of public health nurses in Canada reported in the *Canadian Nurse*. The average salary for public health nurses was $950 per annum and the highest $1,800: "Report of Studies Made by the Provincial Public Health Sections and in a 1941 Survey of Public Health Nurses in Canada," *Canadian Nurse* 39, no. 10 (1943): 678.

2 Journals 1939–1952, entry written on 15 Apr. 1944 but entered on 17 July 1944, file 2-3, box 2, LC, UBC.

3 Class II employees, recruited from among the nationals in the country receiving aid, were paid in line with local wages and costs of living so as not to distort the local economies. Displaced persons could aspire to only Class II employment status and received considerably lower wages. Class III employees were members of voluntary agencies, who, while not paid by UNRRA, were administratively accountable in practice to UNRRA. To many observers, the treatment of Class II employees breached the organization's mandate not to discriminate according to sex, nationality, race, or creed. Woodbridge, *UNRRA* 1:242.

4 Minutes of meeting of the Executive Committee [MEC], 1 July 1944, 318, file: Min AI- 2/2, Canadian Nurses Association, vol. 36, I-248, MG 28, CNA Fonds, LAC; Minutes of the CNA Executive Meeting, 31 May–2 June 1945, MEC A1.2/4.

5 Ibid., Minutes of the CNA Executive Meeting, 31 May–2 June 1945, MEC A1.2/4.

6 The CNA continued to lobby Ottawa on the salary question. See *Canadian Nurse* 41, no. 9 (1945): 713.

7 Editorial, "God Bless Us, Every One," *Canadian Nurse* 41, no. 1 (1945): 19.

8 Hall to Claxton, 12 July 1945, DEA, RG 25, LAC.

9 This theme is developed at length in Armstrong-Reid and Murray, *Armies of Peace*.

10 1944–1945 Record of Service with UNRRA, 1, file 2-2, box 2, LC, UBC.

11 Journals, entry written on 26 Apr. 1944 but entered on 18 Sept. 1944, file 2-3, box 2, LC, UBC.

12 1944–1945 Record of Service with UNRRA, 8 Oct. 1944, file 2-2, box 2, LC, UBC.

13 Address by James Struthers at the 75th Anniversary Dinner, Faculty of Social Work, University of Toronto, 12 Oct. 1989, PAG 4/4.0:6, UNRRA, United Nations Archives (UNA).

14 For a more detailed analysis of Cassidy's philosophy, see Armstrong-Reid and Murray, *Armies of Peace*, 119–23.

15 1944–1945 Record of Service with UNRRA, 1, file 2-2, box 2, LC, UBC. See Journals 1939–1952, entry written on 28 Apr. 1943 but entered on 8 Oct. 1944, file 2-3, box 2, LC, UBC.

16 Ibid., entry written on 28 Apr. 1943 but entered on p. 8 Oct. 1944.

17 Ibid.

18 1944–1945 Record of Service with UNRRA, 2, file 2-2, box 2, LC, UBC.

19 Journal 1939–1952, entry written on 30 Apr. 1943 but entered on page 8 Oct. 1944, file 2-3, box 2, LC, UBC.

20 1944–1945 Record of Service with UNRRA, 4, file 2-2, box 2, LC, UBC.

21 Ibid., 7–8.

22 Ibid., 7.

23 Ibid., 5.

24 Ibid., 8.

25 The "Anders Army" refers to the Polish armed forces set up in the former Soviet Union in the period 1941–2 and named after its commander, General Władysław Anders. The army provided the bulk of the Second Corps of the Polish Armed Forces, which fought under British command in Italy.

26 1944–1945 Record of Service with UNRRA, 11, file 2-2, box 2, LC, UBC.

27 Creelman, letter to the editor, *Canadian Nurse* 41, no. 6 (1945): 477.

28 Wing Commander McCreary was a graduate in medicine from the University of Toronto and was appointed to Supreme Headquarters Allied Expeditionary Force in 1945. On the condition of civilians in Western Europe at the conclusion of the German occupation, see McCreary, *Empire Club of Canada Speeches 1946–1947*, 228–44. McCreary later became dean of medicine at UBC and was instrumental in trying to coordinate more inter-professional health sciences education.

29 1944–1945 Record of Service with UNRRA, 12, file 2-2, box 2, LC, UBC.

30 Ibid., 15.

31 Ibid., 11.

32 Ibid., 15.

33 Ibid., 17.

34 Ibid., 18.

35 Ibid., 22.

36 Journals 1939–1952, entry written on 15 Apr. 1945 but entered on 5–6 May 1943, file 2-3, box 2, LC, UBC.

37 Ibid., entry written on 15 Apr. 1945 but entered on 8 May 1943.

38 Ibid., entry written on 15 Apr. 1945 but entered on 7 May 1943.

39 Ibid., entry written on 15 Apr. 1945 but entered on 9 May 1943.

40 See the early diary entry where she debated under what circumstances she would stay in Vancouver if Dick were still unmarried when she returned. Journals 1939–1952, entry written 4 Mar. 1945 but entered on 1–2 May 1943, file 2-3, box 2, LC, UBC.

41 Ibid., entry entered on 9–10 May 1943.

42 The remaining record, which covers only part of the period of her service with UNRRA in Germany, makes no reference to Dick. There are no surviving letters from him during this period.

43 1944–1945 Record of Service with UNRRA, 24, file 2-2, box 2, LC, UBC.

44 Ibid., 25.

45 Ibid.

46 Lyle Creelman to Dr Phillips, 3 Nov. 1945, Miscellaneous Nurses' Reports to ERO from Camps and Teams, PAG 4/2.0.6.0:3, UNRRA, UNA.

47 Creelman, "With UNRRA in Germany," *Canadian Nurse* 43, no. 9 (1947): 711.

48 1944–1945 Record of Service with UNRRA, 24, file 2-2, box 2, LC, UBC.

49 Ibid., 23.
50 Wodlinger, "UNRRA Field Supervisor Looks Back," 14.
51 Lyle Creelman to S.J. Haines, deputy chief nurse, ERO, 3 Dec. 1945, S-0523-563, UNRRA, UNA.
52 Steppe, "Nursing in the Third Reich."
53 Ibid., 36.
54 Ibid., 34.
55 Lawson, "German Nursing Services, 1945–1946," 29.
56 Ibid., 28.
57 See Lagerwey, "Third Reich, Nursing and the AJN."
58 On 25 Nov. 1944 Director Herbert Lehman concluded an agreement with General Eisenhower, supreme commander, Allied Expeditionary Forces (SCAEF). Known as the SCAEF Agreement, its terms recognized that while UNRRA would assume control of relief and resettlement in the post-military period, it would participate in the planning and operations only under the authority of the Allied Expeditionary Forces.
59 J. Alex Edmison, "UNRRA's Trials and Triumphs: An Address before the Canadian Club in Montreal," 18 Feb. 1946, file 4, vol. 4, John Alexander Edmison Fonds, Queen's University Archives.
60 For a more extensive discussion of the difficulties UNRRA faced during the early days in the field, see Armstrong-Reid and Murray, *Armies of Peace*, chap. 6.
61 Alex. E. Squadrill, deputy zone director, "Current Status of Displaced Persons in the US Zone in Germany," 25 May 1946, 11, PAG 4/2.0.0.0:44, UNRRA, UNA.
62 Woodbridge, *UNRRA* 3:401.
63 Lyle Creelman, letter to the editor, *Canadian Nurse* 43, no. 7 (1947): 532–3. This letter was titled "With the UNRRA in Germany," and Creelman wrote a series of articles for the *Canadian Nurse* over several years using the same title.
64 1944–1945 Diary of Service with UNRRA in Germany," 1, file 2-2, box 2, LC, UBC.
65 Creelman, "With UNRRA in Germany," *Canadian Nurse* 43, no. 7 (1947): 152.
66 Ibid.
67 For a discussion of the Canadian forces role in the defence of the Nijmegen, see Copp, *Cinderella Army*, 149–73, 178, 188, 203–12; Williams, *Long Left Flank*, 171–5, 181–98.
68 1944–1945 Diary of Service with UNRRA in Germany, 3, file 2-2, box 2, LC, UBC.
69 Ibid., 4.
70 Ibid., 1.
71 Interview with Lyle Creelman, Vancouver, 27 May 1985, KD.
72 According to her fellow Canadian and the chief nurse of the American zone, Madeline Taylor, many European nurses had only hospital experience and were simply overwhelmed: "The result was she either did nothing or left." Taylor,

"History of Nursing Operations in UNRRA Displaced Persons Camps," Historical Monographs, UNRRA, UNA.

73 Sir Ralph Cilento to E.E. Rhatigan, 1 Aug. 1945, British Zone Germany, Health Program, PAG 4/2.0.6.0-14, UNRRA, UNA.

74 Journals 1939–1945, entry written on 1 May 1945 but entered on 16 June 1945, file 2-3, box 2, LC, UBC.

75 Cilento to Topping, 23 July 1945, British Zone Germany, Health Program, PAG 4/2.0.0.0:44, UNRRA, UNA.

76 Creelman, "Diary of Service with UNRRA in Germany," 3, file 2-2, box 2, LC, UBC.

77 Creelman, "With UNRRA in Germany," *Canadian Nurse* 43, no. 7 (1947): 552.

78 Record of Service with UNRRA in Germany, 3, file 2-2, box 2, LC, UBC.

79 See Cilento to Topping, 23 July 1945, British Zone Germany, Health Program, PAG 4/2.0.0.0:44, UNRRA, UNA.

80 Sir Ralph Cilento to Dr Andrew Topping, 22 July 1945, British Zone Germany, Health Program, PAG 4/2.0.6.0-14, UNRRA, UNA.

81 Fisher, *Raphael Cilento*, 202.

82 Ibid.

83 E.M. Thorne, "Report for History Project, British Zone Headquarters, Division of Health, Nursing, History of Nursing Division, D.P., BR #.19," Historical Monographs, UNRRA, UNA.

84 Taylor, "History of Nursing Operations in UNRRA Displaced Persons Camps," 2; "Report – Health DP – US," 53, UNRRA, UNA.

85 Lyle Creelman, interview with Kay Dier, 27 May 1985, Vancouver, KD.

86 See Hulme, *Wild Place*, 28–37. After hearing Canadian nurses' accounts of dealing with these patients, Chief Nurse Rutherford astutely remarked, "These people are alive to-day simply because of their wits, they have special psychology, very difficult to deal with." L.C. Rutherford and O.J. Gobert, "Report on Trip to the Field (American Zone), 6–13 Dec. 1946," UNRRA file, vol. 20, K9, MG 31, FLP, LAC.

87 Harrison wrote to President Truman, "As matters now stand, we appear to be treating the Jews as the Nazis treated them except that we do not exterminate them. They are in concentration camps in large numbers under our military guard instead of S.S. troops. One is led to wonder whether the German people, seeing this, are not supposing that we are following or at least condoning Nazi policy." Report of Earl G. Harrison, United States Memorial Holocaust Museum, http://www.ushmm.org/museum/exhibit/online/dp/resourc1.htm.

88 Doherty, *Letters from Belsen 1945*, 207.

89 Ibid., 146.

90 1944–1945 Diary of Service with UNRRA in Germany, 2, file 2-2, box 2, LC, UBC.

91 "R.W. Cilento, To: Dr. Neville Goodman, Health Division, ERO, August 16, 1945, UNRRA Supervision of the Hospital at Belsen Camp," 1, PAG 4/2.0.6.0-14, UNRRA, UNA.
92 Creelman, "With UNRRA in Germany," *Canadian Nurse* 43, no. 7 (1947): 556.
93 1944–1945 Diary of Service with UNRRA in Germany, 2, file 2-2, box 2, LC, UBC. Doherty wanted twenty nurses but Creelman thought she could manage with eleven or twelve. In the end she found fourteen nurses for the hospital. Creelman, "Diary of Service with UNRRA," 2, file 2-2, box 2, LC, UBC.
94 Doherty, *Letters from Belsen*, 137.
95 Creelman, "Diary of Service with UNRRA," 3, file 2-2, box 2, LC, UBC.
96 Creelman, "With UNRRA in Germany," *Canadian Nurse* 43, no. 7 (1947): 556.
97 Creelman to Dr W.J.E. Phillips, "Nursing Report for January 1946," Nursing Reports from Germany, PAG 4/2.0.6.0:3, UNRRA, UNA.
98 As a consequence, for example, she took the unusual step of ensuring that her trusty Canadian surgical nurse, Janet Vanderwell, was present in the operating theatre to supervise the German doctor whom she neither liked nor trusted. Doherty, *Letters from Belsen*, 99.
99 Ibid.
100 An American military nurse, Lorraine Setzler, described the efforts to de-Nazify the German nursing schools and associations in the American Zone of Occupied Germany in the period before UNRRA assumed responsibility. She downplayed the number of German nurses who were influenced by Nazi ideals, and she also noted that every effort was being made to rehabilitate the German nursing institutions so that German nurses could be mobilized to help with control of epidemics. Setzler, "Nursing and Nursing Education in Germany," 993–5.
101 1944–1945 Diary of Service with UNRRA in Germany, 10, file 2-2, box 2, LC, UBC.
102 See, for example, Sidney C. Wooten, "Inspection Report of Displaced Person Camp," 28 Jan. 1946, PAG 4/3.0.11.3.2, file 25, box 13, S-0435, UNRRA, UNA.
103 Creelman, "With UNRRA in Germany," *Canadian Nurse* 43, no. 8 (1947): 606.
104 Ibid., 607.
105 1944–1945 Diary of Service with UNRRA in Germany, 2, file 2-2, box 2, LC, UBC.
106 Creelman interview with KD.
107 Dr L. Hahn, "UNRRA Team at Belsen Displaced Persons," #Br 26," 7, PAG 4/4.283, UNRRA, UNA.
108 Nursing Reports from Germany, PAG 4/2.0.6.0:3, UNRRA, UNA.
109 Creelman, letter to the editor, *Canadian Nurse* 41, no. 12 (1945): 986.
110 "Performance Evaluation, Copy of United Nations Relief and Rehabilitation Administration Displaced Persons Operations, Germany, Personnel Action,

August 27 1946, C.H. Crammer, Chief Personnel Officer," Edna Osborne Private
Family Papers, held by John Stotts, Oshawa, ON.

111 Creelman interview with KD.

112 Edna Osborne had worked as a public health nurse with the Victorian Order
of Nurses in Ottawa and in Sherbrooke and later (1942–5) as a medical social
worker in Montreal, where she had attended the McGill School of Social Work.
For a biography, see "Edna Osborne," Saskatchewan Association of Social
Workers, http://www.sasw.ca/history.html. The private family papers have copies
of her application to the Canadian Association of Social Workers, which describes
her educational background and work experience in more detail. Biographical
information on Jean Watt is contained in file 57, vol. 160, Biographical Files,
I-248, MG 28, CNA, LAC.

113 1944–1945 Diary of Service with UNRRA in Germany, 3, file 2-2, box 2, LC,
UBC.

114 Creelman, letter to the editor, *Canadian Nurse* 41, no. 12 (1945): 986.

115 See, for example, Lyle Creelman to Dr W.J.E. Phillips, Nursing Report for January
1946, PAG 4/2.0.6:3, Nursing Reports from Germany, UNRRA, UNA.

116 Creelman, "With UNRRA in Germany," *Canadian Nurse* 43, no. 8 (1947): 608.

117 See Mary Dunn's official team history of an assembly centre of fourteen thousand
displaced persons near Hamburg. Mary Dunn, Health Personnel, S-0518-0024,
UNRRA, UNA.

118 Creelman, letter to the editor, *Canadian Nurse* 41, no. 12 (1945): 986.

119 Ibid.

120 Creelman to Dr Phillips, "Report for February 1946," Nursing Reports from
Germany, PAG 4/3.0.11.2.0.2, file 1, box 21, S-0409, UNRRA, UNA.

121 "Review of UNRRA Nurses' Activities in the Hamburg and Wentorf Areas, Mary
Dunn, Public Health Services in Wentorf Camp, British Zone, Schleswig-Holstein
Region," file. 11, vol. 3,. PAG/4/3.011.202, S-040424, UNRRA, UNA.

122 Creelman to Dr Phillips, "Report for February 1946," UNRRA, UN. See also ibid.,
Creelman to Dr Phillips, "Report for November 1945," "UNRRA-ERO,
Miscellaneous Nurses Reports to ERO from Camps and Teams," S-0523-563,
UNRRA, UNA.

123 Creelman, "With UNRRA in Germany: Repatriation of DP's," *Canadian Nurse* 43,
no. 9 (1947): 710–11.

124 "Nursing Reports from Germany, Minutes of the Nurses Conference 53 Welfare
Division," 19 Jan. 1946, PAG 4/2.0.6.0:3, UNRRA, UNA.

125 See, for example, "Lyle Creelman, Chief Nurse, British Zone, Germany to: Miss
S.J. Haines, Deputy Chief Nurse, UNRRA, ERO, December 3, 1945," S-0523-563,
UNRRA, UNA.

126 1944–1945 Diary of Service with UNRRA in Germany, 7, file 2-2, box 2, LC,
     UBC.
127 Dr Goodman, Director of Health, to Lt Col. Hugh R. Leavell, USPHS, 13 Aug.
     1945
     UNRRA Health Country Missions, Germany, S-0523-561-1, UNRRA, UNA.
128 Florence Udell to L. Johnson, 1 Sept. 1945, "Nursing Reports to ERO from Camps
     and teams etc.," UNRRA-ERO, S-0523-S63, UNRRA, UNA.
129 Thorne, "Report for History Project." See also "Nursing Program: Strictly
     Confidential: Miss L. Johnson and Miss F.N. Udell, Chief Nurses, to Dr Goodman,
     Director Health Division," 16 Mar. 1946, S-0520-0399, UNRRA, UNA.
130 Thus, despite the efforts of both of UNRRA's chief nurses, Lillian Johnson and
     Francis Udell, to intercede on behalf of the first chief nurse of the American Zone,
     there was little improvement after their visit. The chief medical officer contin-
     ued to assign and promote nurses without regard to nursing qualifications and
     without consulting the chief nurse. See, for example, "Madeline S. Taylor, District
     Nursing Consultant to: Mr A.C Dunn, Director District No. 3 Regensburg,
     Subject: Bamberg, Team 307, Visit July 4 to Nurse Cunningham, UNA, UNRRA,
     German Mission, US Zone," vol. 525, PAG 4/3.0.11.3.2:5, UNRRA, UNA;
     "Madeline Taylor, to: Mr J.H. Whiting, Report of Supervisory Nurse Visit,
     Seliqenstad Camp, January 12, 1946," UNRRA, UNA.
131 1944–1945 Diary of Service with UNRRA in Germany, 10, file 2-2, box 2, LC,
     UBC.
132 Ibid., 10.
133 1944–1945 Diary of Service with UNRRA in Germany, 8, file 2-2, box 2, LC,
     UBC. See also "Miscellaneous Nurses Reports to ERO from Camps and Teams,
     Memo: Miss L. Creelman, Chief Nurse, to Dr. Phillips, Chief Medical Officer,
     Nursing Report for the Month of October 1945," 3 Nov. 1945, PAG 4/2.0.6.0:3,
     UNRRA, UNA.
134 Diary of Service with UNRRA in Germany, 9, file 2-2, box 2, LC, UBC.
135 Lyle Creelman to S.J. Haines, deputy chief nurse, 3 Dec. 1945, UNRRA-ERO,
     S-0523-563, UNRRA, UNA.
136 Lyle Creelman to Florence Udell, "Report for November 1945," S-0523-0563,
     UNRRA, UNA.
137 Thorne, "Report for History Project," 6.
138 See L. Creelman to Dr Phillips, "Report for February 1946," PAG 4/3.0.1:
     2.0.2, file 1, box 21, S-0409, UNRRA, UN. The IRO was a specialized agency
     of the UN founded on 20 Aug. 1946 to deal with the massive refugee problem
     after UNRRA was disbanded. A preparatory commission had begun operations
     fourteen months previously. In 1952 its operations ceased, and it was replaced

by the Office of the United Nations High Commissioner for Refugees (UNHCR).

139 In 1946, Creelman requested that Libbie Rutherford, the Canadian who had served as the chief nurse at UNRRA's mobilization centre at Granville, France, be reassigned to a teaching post within the British Zone.

140 Tunis, *In Cap and Gowns*, 82. See also "Canadian Nurses in UNRRA," *Canadian Nurse* 40, no. 10 (1944): 240–2.

141 Thorne, "Report for History Project," 3.

142 Ibid., 7.

143 "Nursing Reports from Germany, Minutes of Conference on Nursing Education for Displaced Persons, British Occupied Zone, Held at the UNRRA Training Centre for Nursing Aides Bergen near Belsen, August 19, 20, 21, 1946," S–0523–0563, UNRRA, UNA.

144 For a full discussion of Cilento's increasing dissatisfaction with UNRRA's official repatriation policy and his attempts to shield the Polish displaced persons from unwanted repatriation, see Fisher, *Raphael Cilento*, 210–15.

145 Creelman, "With UNRRA in Germany," *Canadian Nurse* 43, no. 8 (1947): 610.

146 Creelman, "With UNRRA in Germany," *Canadian Nurse* 43, no. 9 (1947): 711; see also Thorne, "Report for History Project," 8.

147 Thorne, "Report for History Project," 6.

148 Lyle Creelman to Dr W.J.E. Phillips, "Nursing Report for January 1946," Nursing Reports from Germany, PAG 4/2.0.6.0:3, UNRRA, UNA.

149 See, for example, Elizabeth W. Brackett, 22 Mar. 1946, Officers Diaries, 12.1, RF, RFAC. Brackett, who met with Florence Udell after her visit and accompanied Lillian Johnson to the British Zone in the spring of 1946, recorded, "Miss Udell says Miss Creelman is doing a splendid job in [the] British Occupied area Germany." See also Health Division Weekly Staff Meeting, 13 June 1946, ERO 293, S–01518–0700, UNRRA, UNA.

150 Creelman, "Defends UNRRA Camps," *Toronto Daily Star*, 13 June 1946.

151 Creelman, "With UNRRA in Germany," *Canadian Nurse* 43, no. 7 (1947): 607.

152 See Mary Dunn's account of how she reached out to the community to provide more relevant nursing care in an assembly centre of fourteen thousand displaced persons near Hamburg. Mary Dunn, Health Personnel, S–0518–0024, UNRRA, UNA.

153 Lyle Creelman to Dr E. Townsend, "Report for May 1946," PAG 4/2.0.6.0:3, Nursing Reports from Germany, UNRRA, UNA.

154 Field Supervisory Officers, H.Q. Celle; copy attached to L. Creelman to Dr E. Townsend, "Report for May 1946," PAG 4/2.0.6.0:3, Nursing Reports from Germany, UNRRA, UNA.

155 Lyle Creelman to Dr E. Townsend, "Report for May 1946," PAG 4/2.0.6.0:3, Nursing Reports from Germany, UNRRA, UNA.
156 Creelman to Phillips, "Nursing Report for January 1946, " Nursing Reports from Germany, UNRRA, UNA.
157 Mary Elizabeth Tennant, 20 July 1946, 1946, Officers Diaries, 12.1, RF, RFAC.
158 Creelman, "With UNRRA in Germany," *Canadian Nurse* 43, no. 7 (1947): 532.
159 Creelman, "B.C. Nurse Pleads for Refugees," *News Herald*, 21 Nov. 1946; "Refugees Are an Asset," *Sun*, 22 Nov. 1946.

5. Setting a New Course, 1946–1949

1 Lyle Creelman, interview with Audrey Stegen, 3 July 1982, Vancouver, oral history collection, CRNBC.
2 The results of the first phase of the CPHA's inquiry, focusing on the inadequacy of the salary situation, were published in 1946 in the *Report on Salaries and Qualifications of Public Health Personnel in Canada*. It recommended a further study to assess what factors other than salary contributed to the shortage of public health personnel.
3 See Struthers, *No Fault of Their Own* and "Family Allowances." By 1952, federal spending on old-age security and family allowances exceeded its total contribution to unemployment relief during the Great Depression.
4 Struthers, "Family Allowances," 179.
5 Canada, House of Commons, *Debates*, 17 July 1944, 5335, qtd in Struthers, "Family Allowances," 179.
6 The issue had the added constitutional complication that the provinces were responsible for delivering health care but the federal government had the power to tax.
7 Canadian Public Health Association, *Report of the Study Committee on Public Health Practice* (hereafter CPHA, *Report*), 7–8. See also Editorial Section, "Public Health Practice in Canada," *Canadian Journal of Public Health*, February 1953, 75.
8 Lynaugh, Grace, Smith, Sena, Duran de Villalobos, *W.K. Kellogg Foundation*.
9 During her tenure as chair of the CNA Public Health Committee (1942–4), she had to deal with the fallout when the CNA's Public Health Section received a copy of the CPHA's preliminary report, entitled "Recommendations regarding Minimum Requirements for Employment in the Field of Public Health Nursing in the Years 1941–1946," before any arrangements for "the closer collaboration" between the two committees had been worked out. Minutes of the Public Health Section, Canadian Nurses Association, 5 Sept. and 11 Dec. 1940, file: Public Health Section Minute Book, 1921–40, vol. 62, I-248, MG 28, LAC; ibid., minutes of the Public

Health Section, Canadian Nurses Association, 15 Jan. and 5 Feb. 1941, file: Public
Health Section Minute Book, 1941–7, vol. 62.

10 Minutes of the meeting of 27 Sept. 1947, 4, file: Committee on Public Health
Nursing, Minute Book, 1947–52, vol. 62, I-248, MG 28, LAC.

11 The committee was chaired by Dr John Kitching of Hamilton, and Helen McArthur
was chosen to chair the subcommittee studying the practice of public health
nurses.

12 Genevieve K. Bixler was a member of the advisory committee on nursing for the
Kellogg Foundation and a member of the board of directors of the National League
for Nursing Education. Her study "Nursing Resources and Needs in Michigan,"
according to Lynaugh, Grace, Smith, Sena, Duran de Villalobos, became the template for dozens of other state surveys (*W.K. Kellogg Foundation*, 48).

13 Lynaugh, Grace, Smith, Sena, Durán de Villalobos, *W.K. Kellogg Foundation*, 40.

14 For a more detailed discussion of the Kellogg Foundation's decision to invest in the
quality of nursing services, see ibid., 38–40.

15 Newfoundland entered Confederation after the completion of the field studies.

16 No attempt was made to cover all the health agencies serving larger urban areas, on
the grounds that they "did not lend themselves to comparative studies with practices carried out in the smaller urban centres and in the rural districts." For further
details on the committee's pattern of operation in most provinces, see CPHA,
Report, 6.

17 In Quebec, Creelman later learned that, in one case, the chair of the board of a
voluntary agency told the nursing director that she should not have granted permission for Creelman to visit the agency. Diary: Hamilton, Ontario, 17 Jan. 1949
("Related French Agencies"), file 2-4, box 2, LC, UBC.

18 Ibid., 13 Mar. 1948.

19 CPHA, *Report*, 52.

20 The 1934 report, *An Activity Analysis of Nursing*, written for the Committee on the
Grading of Nursing Schools, itemized the characteristics of "good nursing." For
further details, see ibid., 54.

21 Ibid., 18.

22 Ibid., 13.

23 Ibid., 19.

24 Ibid., 20.

25 Diary: Hamilton, Ontario, 18 Mar. 1948, 5, file 2-4, box 2, LC, UBC. For similar
commentary, see ibid., 16 Mar. 1948.

26 Conversely, she noted that, where there was excellent supervision and a well-
planned staff-education program, public health nursing was more positively
viewed as an employment option. See Creelman's discussion with Trenna Hunter,
who had replaced her at the Metropolitan Health Committee: ibid., 28 Sept. 1948.

See also her positive review of Dorothy Percy's leadership under which nurses worked collaboratively on policy development: ibid., 25–8 Feb. 1949.

27 Ibid., 4 Aug. 1948.

28 Ibid., 1 Apr. 1948.

29 See, for example, ibid., 14 Apr. 1948.

30 Ibid., 29 July 1948. Also, ibid., 22 Mar. 1948.

31 CPHA, *Report*, 47.

32 Ibid.

33 Diary: Hamilton, Ontario, 12–19 Aug. 1948, 73, file 2-4, box 2, LC, UBC.

34 Ibid., 1 May 1948.

35 Ibid., 4 June 1948. For other examples, see ibid., 15 Mar. 1948, 16 Mar. 1948, 16 July 1948, 16 July 1948.

36 Green, *Through the Years with Public Health Nursing*, 83.

37 Diary: Hamilton, Ontario, 2 Aug. 1948, 56, file 2-4, box 2, LC, UBC.

38 Ibid.

39 CPHA, *Report*, 43.

40 For other examples, see Diary: Hamilton, Ontario, 15 Mar., 16 Mar., 23 Mar., 31 Mar. 1948, file 2-4, box 2, LC, UBC.

41 Ibid., 24 Mar. 1948.

42 CPHA, *Report*, 28.

43 Creelman again took the opportunity to discuss with the public health nurses the possibility of transferring some of the routine aspects of school service to the teachers in Saskatchewan, and she remained concerned that proposed changes to the teachers' curriculum missed the opportunity to have teachers cover routine screening. Diary: Hamilton, Ontario, 18 Oct. 1948, 98, file 2-4, box 2, LC, UBC.

44 Ibid.

45 Ibid., 29 Sept. 1948.

46 See, for example, Creelman's discussion with the nurses in the Central Island Health Unit, Victoria: ibid., 16 and 17 Sept. 1948.

47 CPHA, *Report*, 30. Creelman suggested that school health services should draw on information provided by the students' own physicians; this would form the basis of the teachers' observations of student's health and development, stressing prevention rather than correction. See also Rands, "Medical Care Programs and Public Health Nursing Practice."

48 CPHA, *Report*, 36.

49 Ibid., 24.

50 Diary: Hamilton, Ontario, 1 Apr. 1948, 13, file 2-4, box 2, LC, UBC; CPHA, *Report*, 34.

51 CPHA, *Report*, 24.

52 Ibid., 34.

53 Diary: Hamilton, Ontario, 1 May 1948, 21b-28, file 2-4, box 2, LC, UBC; CPHA, *Report*, 34.
54 CPHA, *Report*, 40.
55 Ibid., 39–40.
56 See also her diary entry describing her efforts to overcome nursing leaders' reluctance to consider an independent university-based program in Manitoba. Ibid., 29 Nov. 1948.
57 See, for example, the discussion of tuberculosis control in CPHA, *Report*, 43.
58 See CPHA, *Report*, 41.
59 Ibid, 42.
60 Diary: Hamilton, Ontario, 19 Apr. 1948, 19.
61 Ibid., 17 Jan. 1949, 128.
62 See, for example, Toman, "Blood Work."
63 This viewpoint was repeatedly expressed in regard to several visits with industrial nurses; see, for examples, Diary: Hamilton, Ontario, 18 Oct. 1948 (Industrial Nursing, Bell Telephone Company, Montreal), 108–13, file 2-4, box 2, LC, UBC.
64 Ibid., 2 Aug. 1948.
65 CPHA, *Report*, 57.
66 Ibid., 55.
67 Lynaugh, Grace, Smith, Sena, Duran de Villalobos, *W.K. Kellogg Foundation*, 57.
68 CPHA, *Report*, 53.
69 Ibid., 51.
70 Ibid., 23.
71 Diary: Hamilton, Ontario, "Lecture by Dr Bixler: How We Can Solve Our Nursing Problems More Effectively" (notes included after entries for 25–8 Feb. 1949), 140–2, file 2-4, box 2, LC, UBC.
72 For a discussion of the similar transformation of nursing scholarship in the United States, see Fairman, "Context and Contingency."
73 Minutes of Meeting of Sub-Committee on Functions of the Public Health Nurse, National Headquarters, 25 Apr. 1949, file: Committee on Public Health Nursing, Minute Book, vol. 62, I-248, MG 28, LAC.
74 Marsh was hired by the University of British Columbia's School of Social Work in 1947. In 1959, he was named director of research. Cassidy became dean of the School of Social Work at the University of Toronto.
75 "A Beacon Light," *Canadian Nurse* 47, no. 3 (1951): 169.
76 Minutes of the meeting of 22 May 1950, file: Committee on Public Health Nursing, Minute Book, vol. 62, I-248, MG 28, LAC.
77 See ibid., minutes of the meetings of 3 Oct. 1950, 29 Jan. 1951, file: Committee on Public Health Nursing, Minute Book, 1947–52.

78 The Baillie-Creelman Report served as the focus of group discussions at the public health convention held in Alberta in September 1951. See Alberta Association of Registered Nurses (AARN) *Newsletter*, 1951, 18, 19, 29.

79 Green, *Through the Years with Public Health Nursing*, 98, argues that the study directly influenced the provision of public health nursing in British Columbia.

80 Ibid.

81 Journals 1939–52, 29 July 1949, file 2-3, box 2, LC, UBC. Although this diary deals with the years leading up to her UNRRA appointment, a final entry was made in London en route to the WHO in Geneva.

82 Ibid.

6. Joining the WHO, 1949–1951

1 WHO nurses earned unwanted international scrutiny in the political wake of the Soviet Bloc's withdrawal. The WHO's excessive administrative overhead had been cited as a contributing factor to the Soviet Union's dissatisfaction with the WHO's fiscal management. Matters were not helped when the head of the Save the Children Fund wrote to Chisholm in 1953 pointing out that WHO nurses earned more than the Danish prime minister.

2 The cable announcing Russia's resignation caught Chisholm off guard: "I could not believe my eyes," he said when he read it. Since the WHO's constitution made no provisions for withdrawals, he initially refused to accept Russia's decision. "What-Not at WHO," *Time*, 28 Feb. 1949.

3 For a more detailed discussion of the defining events that hardened Cold War attitudes, see Farley, *Brock Chisholm*, chap. 4.

4 A few days after the withdrawal of the Soviet Union, the Ukraine and Byelorussia followed suit; a year later, Albania, Bulgaria, Czechoslovakia, Hungary, and Rumania served notice of their withdrawal.

5 Cueto, *Value of Health*, 92.

6 This viewpoint is developed in Farley, *Brock Chisholm*, chaps 7 and 8.

7 The regional directors and committees developed regional budgets that were then forwarded to the director general for incorporation into the annual budget, "which the Health Assembly rarely questioned." Ibid., 109.

8 Known originally as the Pan American Sanitary Bureau, it had existed since 1902 and had been reorganized, under a new name, in 1947.

9 The U.S. contribution to PASO was to rise from $11,841 in 1948 to a projected $1,226,210 in 1950. The increased funding gave PASO considerably greater leverage in its efforts to resist integration into the WHO. If PASO integrated into the WHO, the separate funding arrangements with PASO would be terminated; the

WHO could not afford the loss of income. See Farley, *Brock Chisholm*, 100–1. See also Cueto, *Value of Health*, 82–91.

10 For a discussion of his controversial ideas about birth control, sterilization practices, negative eugenics, and euthanasia, see Dowbiggin, "Prescription for Survival."

11 Farley, *Brock Chisholm*. A pacifist, Chisholm condemned what he saw as the root causes of war. War, he contended, was a manifestation of collective neurosis: the consequence of poor parenting and social institutions that delivered humanity into a state of perpetual immaturity.

12 Irving, *Brock Chisholm*, 114.

13 Ibid. For a more complete discussion of Chisholm's views of international health work and his advocacy of world federalism, see ibid., 78–90.

14 See Cueto, *Value of Health*, 83.

15 Irving, *Brock Chisholm*, 112.

16 Ibid., 113.

17 Ibid., 114.

18 See, for example, the flattering comments made by John Winslow, cited in Farley, *Brock Chisholm*, 75.

19 Ibid., 111.

20 Ibid.

21 Ibid., 112–13.

22 Ibid., 117.

23 Ibid., 121.

24 For discussion of the challenges and criticism Chisholm faced, see R.R. Struthers Officers' Diary, 16 Jan 1950, 2:1950, series 100, file 3188, box 475, RF, RFA.

25 The term is used in Farley, *Brock Chisholm*, 3.

26 See jot notes for speech undated and untitled, Miscellaneous Notes for Speeches file 2-7, box 2, LC, UBC.

27 Ibid.

28 Ibid.

29 Many of Lyle Creelman's point-form notes for speeches cite Winslow, *Cost of Sickness*. Winslow was a professor of public health at the Yale School of Medicine from 1915 to 1945, where he had been instrumental in the founding of the Yale School of Nursing. He also had worked with the Rockefeller Foundation, the League of Red Cross Societies, and the League of Nations. His teaching at Yale and prolific publications (over six hundred articles and books) emphasized a holistic approach to public health and doubtless influenced Creelman's generation of public health workers in both North America and Europe. For an assessment of his leadership in the public health movement, see Hiscock, "Charles-Edward Amory Winslow."

30 See Audibert, "Fighting Poverty and Disease," 251–2.

31 Van Betten and Moriarty, *Nursing Illuminations*, 49. Lucile Petry Leone was a highly experienced and respected American nursing leader (nursing diploma, Johns Hopkins, 1927; AM, Teachers College, Columbia, 1929; LLD, University of Syracuse, 1945; LHD, Adelphi College, 1945). She taught at the Yale School of Nursing and the University of Minnesota before being appointed founding director of the U.S. Cadet Nurse Corps, which recruited more than 100,000 young women to study nursing in the Second World War. In June 1943 the United States Public Health Service established the Division of Nurse Education within the Office of the Surgeon General to administer the Cadet Nurse Corps program. Petry Leone became its director, the first woman to head a division of the United States Public Health Service. In 1946 the Division of Nurse Education (DNE) was replaced by a broader Division of Nursing, of which, again, Petry Leone was appointed director.

32 Van Betten and Moriarty, *Nursing Illuminations*, 49.

33 Martha M. Eliot was a pioneer in maternal and child health. During her more than twenty-five years with the Children's Bureau, she had established government programs that implemented her ideas about social medicine. In 1934 she drafted most of the Social Security Act's language dealing with maternal and child health. During the Second World War, Eliot was sent to England to study the impact of the evacuation of city children to the countryside. Back home, she ran the Emergency Maternity and Infant Care Program, which served the families of 1.5 million American soldiers, sailors, and airmen. After two years with the WHO, she returned to the bureau as its chief. In 1957 she became chair of the Department of Child and Maternal Health at the Harvard School of Public Health. After retiring in 1960, she acted as a consultant for the WHO and UNICEF. For further information see Wegman, "Martha Eliot and the U.S. Children's Bureau."

34 Farley, *Brock Chisholm*, 70.

35 WHO Diary entries, 31 July 1949, file 2-5, box 2, LC, UBC.

36 Lyle Creelman, interview with Kay Dier, 27 May 1985. Vancouver, KD.

37 Ibid.; WHO Diary entries, 26 Oct. 1949, file 2-5, box 2, LC, UBC.

38 WHO Diary entries, 26 Oct. 1949, file 2-5, box 2, LC, UBC.

39 Verna Huffman Splane, interview with the author, 15 Apr. 2008.

40 Creelman had her own contacts with American and Canadian nursing leaders through Teachers College, the Rockefeller Foundation, the Canadian Nurses Association, UNRRA, and the Kellogg Foundation.

41 The work of the UNRRA nursing brigade in Greece under Olive Baggallay's direction is covered more extensively in Armstrong-Reid and Murray, *Armies of Peace*, 242–3.

42 Verna Huffman Splane, interview with Susan Armstrong-Reid, 15 Apr. 2008, Vancouver. See also Lapeyre and Nelson, "'The Old Internationals.'"

43 During the first year alone, Baggallay and Creelman had to recruit and monitor the nurses and midwives required to assist in over fifty free-standing maternal and child health-care projects spread over twenty-eight countries. WHO, *First Ten Years of the World Health Organization*, 399.

44 See, for example, Creelman's discussion of the pressure she faced to appoint more East European personnel to WHO's nursing staff. Interviews: 27–30 Oct. 1962, 235, file 2, box 1, VA, UBHGARC.

45 See Lyle Creelman to Dame Elizabeth Cockayne, 31 Aug. 1962; Lyle Creelman to R.L. van Voorthuijsen, Netherland Institute for Preventative Medicine, 8 June 1964, Membership of WHO Expert Panel on Nursing, JKT2, N2-136-3, WHOHQ, World Health Organization/Organisation mondiale del la Santé (WHO/OMS).

46 See Report of Sub Committee by the Fifth Assembly of the Regional Committee for the Eastern Mediterranean, 26 Oct. 1955, 14, RC5/EM/19, WHO. It recommended that the nursing program follow the guidelines set down by the expert committees on nursing.

47 WHO, Expert Committee on Nursing, *Report of the First Session*, World Health Technical Report Series, no. 24 (Geneva: WHO, 1950), 3.

48 There is a rich literature on the matrix of technological, political, and socio-economic factors that shaped nursing's place within the post-war health-care landscape. In the American context, see D'Antonio, *American Nursing*; Fairman and Lynaugh, *Critical Care Nursing*; Keeling, "Blurring the Boundaries between Medicine and Nursing." In the Canadian-British context, see Kathryn McPherson, *Bedside Matters*; Flynn, *Moving beyond Borders*; and Toman, "Blood Work."

49 Creelman discussed how all these factors inhibited the development of nursing education and services in Egypt. See "Lyle Creelman Writes," *Canadian Nurse*, 46 no. 9 (1950): 139–40.

50 WHO, Expert Committee on Nursing, *Report of the First Session*, World Health Technical Report Series, no. 24 (Geneva: WHO, 1950), 5.

51 Ibid., 4.

52 See McGann, "Collaboration and Conflict in International Nursing, 1920–1939."

53 Lyle Creelman to Margaret Kerr, 2 May 1950, file 3-3, box 3, LC, UBC.

54 WHO, Expert Committee on Nursing, *Report of the First Session*, World Health Technical Report Series, no. 24 (Geneva: WHO, 1950), 7.

55 See Splane, *Halfway to Poona*, 107–8.

56 WHO, Expert Committee on Nursing, *Report of the First Session*, 14.

57 Ibid.

58 Ibid., 5.

59 See, for example, Lynaugh, Grace, Smith, Sena, Duran de Villalobos, *W.K. Kellogg Foundation*, 55–81, for a discussion of the Kellogg Foundation's role in the direction of nursing education in the post-war era.

60 WHO, Expert Committee on Nursing, *Report of the First Session*, 28.

61 "Draft Item for the Canadian Nurse," 2, file 4-2, box 4, LC, UBC. The contents, undated, describe work with first expert committee on nursing (1950) and the expert committee on health care (1951).

62 WHO, Expert Committee on Nursing, *Report of the First Session*, 28.

63 Lyle Creelman to Margaret Kerr, 2 May 1950, file 3-3, box 3, LC, UBC.

64 See WHO, Expert Committee on Nursing, *Report of the First Session*, 10.

65 Ibid, 20.

66 Lyle Creelman to Margaret Kerr, 2 May 1950, file 3-3, box 3, LC, UBC.

67 Ibid.

68 Ibid.

69 Draft "Item for the Canadian Nurse," 16 Nov. 1951, 3, file 4-2, box 4, LC, UBC. The article appeared as "Lyle Creelman Writes," *Canadian Nurse* 48, no. 1 (1952).

70 WHO diary, 13 Dec. 1951, file 2-5, box 2, LC, UBC.

71 May 1950, EB5.R38, WHO/OMS; The Third World Assembly, May 1950, WHA.6.

72 WHO, Expert Committee on Nursing, *Report of the First Session*, 7.

73 Ibid., 21.

74 "Convention Report," *Canadian Nurse* 48, no. 5 (1952): 337–42.

75 Olive Baggallay to Lyle Creelman, 30 Sept. [no year], file 3-3, box 3, LC, UBC.

76 Draft of an article for the December 1951 issue of *Canadian Nurse*, file 4-2, box 4, LC, UBC.

77 WHO, Expert Committee on Nursing, *Report of the First Session*.

78 Ibid.

79 Lyle Creelman to Margaret Kerr, 2 May 1950, file 3-3, box 3, LC, UBC.

80 Ibid.

81 Elizabeth Barton, in interview with the author, 26 Aug. 2007, Maiden Newton, England. Barton confirmed that Creelman was active in negotiating better salaries for nurses. When Creelman discovered that the salaries of nurses who, like Barton, had trained as midwives had not been increased, she took steps to correct the situation. See also draft of an article for the December 1951 issue of *Canadian Nurse*, file 4-2, box 4, LC, UBC.

82 Draft of an article for the December 1951 issue of *Canadian Nurse*, file 4-2, box 4, LC, UBC; Creelman, "Lyle Creelman Writes," *Canadian Nurse* 48, no. 2 (1952).

83 Quinn, "Social and Economic Welfare," 35.

84 Margaret Kruse to Lyle Creelman, 24 July 1968, file 3-6, box 3, LC, UBC.

85 From 2 to 6 July 1950, she attended the Quadrennial Congress of the Northern Nurses Association in Göteborg, situated on the southwest coast of Sweden. There, 1,250 nurses from Denmark, Finland, Iceland, Norway, and Sweden gathered to discuss the integration of public health into both undergraduate and postgraduate curriculum and to consider the relationship of the national association with trade unions.

86 Elizabeth Brackett Officers Diaries, 13 Sept. 1949, 12.1, file 1948–1949, box 20, RF, RFA.
87 Elizabeth Brackett to M.E. Tennant, 2 Feb 1950, 2; 1950, series 100, file 3179, box 473, RF RFA.
88 Mary Elizabeth Tennant, 5 Mar. 1950, 12.1, RF, RFAC.
89 See, for example, Mary Elizabeth Tennant, Officers Diaries, 28 May 1951, 12.1, RF, RFAC.
90 Journal, 14 Jan. 1951, 1951–2, file 2-3, box 2, LC, UBC.
91 "Draft Item for the *Canadian Nurse*" (Apr. 1951 issue), file 4-2, box 4, LC, UBC; Creelman, "Lyle Creelman Writes," *Canadian Nurse* 47, no. 4 (1951).
92 See CPHA, *Report*, 74.
93 Ibid., 74.
94 Diary, 28 Nov. 1949, file 2-3, box 2, LC, UBC.
95 Lyle Creelman, interview with Kay Dier, 27 May 1985, Vancouver.
96 WHO/OMS, *The World Needs Nurses / le Monde a besoin d'Infirmière* (Geneva, n.d.). Recruiting bulletin found in the Margaret McLean Private Papers.
97 Creelman, "Lyle Creelman Writes," *Canadian Nurse* 46, no. 8 (1950): 659.
98 Lyle Creelman, "Observations on Nursing in Egypt, December 1949–January 1950," 14, file 4-2, box 2, LC, UBC.
99 Ibid., 21–2.
100 "Draft Item for *the Canadian Nurse*" (Sept. 1950 issue), file 4-2, box 4, LC, UBC; Creelman, "Lyle Creelman Writes," *Canadian Nurse* 46, no. 9 (1950): 739.
101 Lyle Creelman, "Recommendations in Relation to Nursing [Nursing, Egypt]," 7 Mar. 1951 (MH/182.50) (MH/AS/172.52) WHO/IMO.

7. Establishing the Nursing Section, 1951–1952

1 Charles, "Origins, History and Achievements of the World Health Organization," 295.
2 WHO, Expert Committee on Nursing, *Report of the Second Session*, 3.
3 This aspect reflected Baggallay's experience as a member of a badly divided UNRRA team posted to Athens that abandoned the organization's policy of strict neutrality during the Greek civil war. See Armstrong-Reid and Murray, *Soldiers of Peace*, chap. 8.
4 Mary Elizabeth Tennant, 14–23 Oct. 1951, Officers Diaries, 12.1, RF, RFAC.
5 T.K. Adranvala (India), Daisy Bridges (ICN), L.A. de Illueca (Panama), Maria Rosa Pinhairo (Brazil), Gladys Peake (Chile), A. Tuer (Turkey), and Lyle Creelman (WHO). In addition, Katherine Leahy, a special consultant WHO for the second expert committee, was a former fellow. Mary Elizabeth Tennant, October 14 through October 23 1951, Officers Diaries, 12.1, RF, RFAC.

6 For a discussion of the nurse's responsibility to her community, see WHO, Expert Committee on Nursing, *Report of the Second Session*, 8.

7 See ibid., 20.

8 "Expert Committee on Nursing by [the] World Health Organization," *American Journal of Nursing* 52, no. 9 (1952): 114.

9 WHO, Expert Committee on Nursing, *Report of the Second Session*, 8. In particular, as the prestige of science, medical technology, and hospital medicine increased, the public health nurse as independent social reformer and community advocate could not withstand "medical dominance and the pull of professional ideology." Melosh, *Physician's Hand*, 143.

10 WHO, Expert Committee on Nursing, *Report of the Second Session*, 8.

11 Mary Elizabeth Tennant, October 14 through October 23 1951, Officers Diaries, 12.1, RF, RFAC.

12 WHO, Expert Committee on Nursing, *Report of the Second Session*, 17.

13 Ibid.

14 Ibid., 14.

15 Ibid., 15.

16 Mary Elizabeth Tennant, Officers Diaries, 12.1, RF, RFAC.

17 Elizabeth Brackett to Olive Baggallay, 5 July 2 1951, series 100, file 3433, box 513, 1955, RF, RFAC.

18 The conference grew out of the recommendation of the first expert committee that basic programs of nursing education needed to be reviewed to ensure that they prepared nurses for "the continuous evolution of modern health work and that the WHO should sponsor international seminars on particular nursing issues." WHO, *Working Conference on Nursing Education*, 3.

19 A graduate of Stanford University School of Nursing (1921), Leahy had obtained an AB from the University of Oregon with preparation in public health and social work and later received an MSc from the University of Washington, majoring in nutrition.

20 WHO, *Working Conference on Nursing Education*, 18.

21 "Nursing," *Chronicle of the World Health Organization* 7, no. 3 (1953): 74.

22 Boschma, "Ambivalence about Nursing's Expertise," 169–70.

23 Journals 1939–52, 5 Apr. 1952, file 3-2, box 2, LC, UBC.

24 Ellen Broe, "Florence Nightingale International Foundation," AARN (Alberta Association of Registered Nurses), *Newsletter*, 1952, 9.

25 Lyle Creelman to Prescott [Creelman], 29 June 1952, file 3-3, box 3, LC, UBC.

26 Journals 1939–52, 21 Aug. 1952, file 2-3, box 2, LC, UBC.

27 Lyle Creelman, "Common Elements in In-Service Training in Public Health and Social Welfare," 1, file 4-3, box 4, LC, UBC.

28 Ibid., 6.

29　Ibid., 8.

30　Ibid., 16.

31　Ibid.

32　WHO Diary entries, 1949–1952, 4 Jan. 1951, file 2-5, box 2, LC, UBC.

33　"Draft Item for the *Canadian Nurse*," n.d., file 42, box 4, LC, UBC.

34　Diary, 4 Jan. 1951, file 2-3, box 2, LC, UBC.

35　See Lyle Creelman, "Lyle Creelman Writes," *Canadian Nurse* 47, no. 3 (1951).

36　"Draft Item for the Canadian Nurse," 14 Mar. 1951, file 4-2, box 4, LC, UBC. See also Lyle Creelman, "Lyle Creelman Writes," *Canadian Nurse*, 47, no. 7 (1951).

37　EWB Dairy, 5–11 Dec. 1950, 12.1, file 1950–1951, box 20, RF, RFAC.

38　Creelman, "Lyle Creelman Writes," *Canadian Nurse* 47, no. 3 (1951): 575.

39　Ibid., 573.

40　For a more detailed description of the Canadian government's cautious attitudes towards Washington's Latin American policy, see Farley, *Brock Chisholm*, 101–9.

41　"Draft Item for the *Canadian Nurse*," 1 (n.d., but describes events from August to November 1951), file 4-2, box 4, LC, UBC. See also Lyle Creelman, "Lyle Creelman Writes," *Canadian Nurse* 47, no. 10 (1951): 723.

42　See Healey, '"Seeds That May Have Been Planted May Take Root."'

43　Fernanda Alves Diniz graduated from the Escola Teenica de Enfermeiras in Lisbon and studied nursing education at the University of Toronto before returning to Lisbon to assume the post of director of nursing for sick children and subsequently the directorship of the School of Nursing.

44　Creelman drew this to her fellow Canadian nurses' attention in the *Canadian Nurse*. "Draft Item for the *Canadian Nurse*," 1, n.d., file 4-2, box 4, LC, UBC. See also Lyle Creelman, "Lyle Creelman Writes," *Canadian Nurse* 47, no. 10 (1951): 724.

45　Bacillus Calmette-Guérin (BCG) was first used against tuberculosis in 1921 and was soon fairly widely used in Canada. It was used to protect student nurses and other health professionals in Canada against the disease, and Creelman would have been familiar with it in her public-health work in Canada. Its introduction internationally, first by the Health Committee of the League of Nations, however, remained controversial in the 1950s, despite its efficacy following the Second World War.

46　Farley, *Brock Chisholm*, 139.

47　"Draft Item for the *Canadian Nurse*," 1, n.d., file 4-2, box 4, LC, UBC. See also Creelman, "Lyle Creelman Writes," *Canadian Nurse* 47, no. 10 (1951): 725.

48　WHO diary entries, 31 Oct. 1949, file 2-5, box 2, LC, UBC.

49　Ibid.

50　See Craddock, *Retired Except on Demand*.

51 "Draft Item for the *Canadian Nurse*," 1 (n.d., but describes a 1952 or 1953 SEARO field trip), file 4-2, box 4, box 4, LC, UBC; Lyle Creelman, "Lyle Creelman Writes," *Canadian Nurse* 48, no. 6 (1952): 470.

52 "Draft Item for the *Canadian Nurse*," 2, file 4-2, box 4, LC, UBC. See also Lyle Creelman, "Lyle Creelman Writes," *Canadian Nurse* 48, no. 4 (1952): 288.

53 Lyle Creelman to Olive Baggallay, 31 Jan. 1952 (letter with diary of field trip to Southeast Asia), file 2-5, box 5, LC, UBC.

54 WHO Diary entries, "Field Trip – South East Asia 1952," 1, file 2-5, box 2, LC, UBC.

55 Ibid., 4.

56 Ibid., 2.

57 Ibid., 11.

58 Ibid., 7.

59 Ibid., 10.

60 Ibid., 7.

61 Ibid., 10.

62 Ibid., 2.

63 Ibid.

64 Ibid., 8.

65 Ibid., 6.

66 Ibid., 5.

67 Ibid., 13.

68 Ibid., 14.

69 Ibid., 8.

70 Ibid.

71 Born in 1891 in China to American medical missionary parents, Ruth Ingram graduated from the Pennsylvania Hospital in 1918 and then served on an American Red Cross expedition to Siberia in 1919. She received a master's degree from Teachers College, Columbia, in 1924, and then joined the staff of the Nursing School of the Peking Medical College and served as dean of the school. Afterwards, she joined the staff of Barnes Hospital in St Louis, She served as director, Washington [DC] University School of Nursing, from 1931 to 1938 before serving with UNRRA and later the WHO in China from 1945 to 1950. See Bernard Becker Medical Library, http://beckerexhibits.wustl.edu/mowihsp/bios/wusndirectors.htm#ingram.

72 Diary of field trip to Southeast Asia, 22 Jan. 1952, 3, 27 Feb. 1952, 34, 0000, file 2-5, box 2, LC, UBC.

73 Taylor, "Nursing at Vellore, South India," 816.

74 See Amrith, "Aspects of the Social History of Medicine," 117.

75 *International Organizations and India Health Programs*, 1.
76 The Colombo Plan to aid India, Pakistan, Ceylon, Sarawak, and Borneo was presented at meetings of the British Commonwealth; it envisaged an £8-billion economic program over six years, starting on 1 July 1951. The Point Four Program – the fourth of I.S. President Harry Truman's foreign-policy objectives – was announced in his inaugural address on 20 January 1949 and aimed at providing technical assistance to encourage flow of private capital to these regions.
77 Diary of field trip to Southeast Asia, 22 Jan. 1952, 1 Feb. 1952, 15, file 2-5, box 2, LC, UBC.
78 Ibid., 15.
79 Ibid., 16.
80 Ibid., 22.
81 Ibid., 28.
82 Ibid., 20.
83 Ibid., 45.
84 Ibid., 37.
85 Approximately seven million Hindus and Sikhs from Bangladesh and Pakistan moved to India after the partition of Pakistan and India in 1947.
86 "Item for the Canadian Nurse" (n.d., but describes a 1952 or 1953 SEARO field trip), file 4-2, box 4, LC, UBC. See Creelman, "Lyle Creelman Writes," *Canadian Nurse* 48, no. 6 (1952): 470.
87 WHO, *Care of the Umbilical Cord Reproductive Health*.
88 Lyle Creelman, "Lyle Creelman Writes," *Canadian Nurse* 47, no. 5 (1951): 338.
89 Ibid., 339.
90 "Lyle Creelman Writes." *Canadian Nurse* 48, no. 2 (1952): 32.
91 Lyle Creelman to Eleanor Graham, 17 Jan. 1955, file 3-3, box 3, LC, UBC
92 Diary of field trip to Southeast Asia, 24 Feb. 1952, 33, file 2-5, box 2, LC, UBC.
93 Ibid., 29.
94 Ibid., 30.
95 Ibid., 40.
96 Ibid., 41.
97 Ibid., 26 Feb. 1952. They also met the following year. See EWB Diary, 17 Nov. 1953, 2.1, file 594, box 64, RF, RFAC.
98 Diary of field trip to Southeast Asia, 44, 23 Feb. 1952, file 2-5, box 2, LC, UBC.
99 She was educated at Bates College in Maine and at Yale and Harvard.
100 WHO Diary Entries, file 2-5, box 2, LC, UBC.
101 "Dr A. Helen Martikainen Receives 1978 APHA International Award for Excellence."

102 Lyle Creelman to Prescott and Frieda [Creelman], 3 Jan. 1952, file 3-3, box 3, LC, UBC.
103 Lyle Creelman's handwritten journal (1961–1969), 7 Sept. 1962, 1961–1969, file 5-3, box 5, LC, UBC.
104 Journals, 1939–52, 17 Sept. 1952, file 2-3, box 2, LC, UBC.

8. From Deputy to Chief, 1953–1960

1 Candau was born across the bay from Rio de Janeiro. After graduating in medicine in 1933 and then completing further studies in public health work at Johns Hopkins, he served for seventeen years with the Brazilian Public Health Service. During this time he worked with Fred Soper on a Rockefeller Foundation–funded project to eradicate the mosquito. Soper was a strong supporter of Candau's candidacy. See Lee, *Global Institutions*.
2 While both of Chisholm's biographers argue that the decision not to seek a second term as director general was taken by Chisholm without duress, Farley deals with the issue at greater length. He rejects the idea that the deadlock over birth control at the World Health Assembly in 1952 probably cost Chisholm a second term as director general. In fact, Farley views Chisholm – who conveniently set aside his own principle that the WHO's staff should be apolitical to campaign vigorously for Candau – as the kingmaker who brokered the political deadlock. See Farley, *Brock Chisholm*, 190–5.
3 Journals 1939–1952, 14 Mar. 1954, file 2-3, box 2, LC, UBC.
4 Farley, *Brock Chisholm*, 194; Cueto, *Value of Health*, 96.
5 Packard, "Malaria Dreams," 17.
6 Cueto, "Origins of Primary Health Care and Selective Primary Health Care," 6.
7 Ibid. The same view is expressed in Packard and Brown, "Rethinking Health Development and Malaria."
8 "In Memory of Dr M.G. Candau," WHO *Chronicle* 37 (1983): 145, Collection of Papers, Marcolino Gomes Candau, WHO/OMS.
9 Miscellaneous Notes for Speeches, Vancouver, chapter 11, May 1953, file 7, box 2, LC, UBC.
10 "Léon Bernard Foundation Award," WHO *Chronicle* 28 (1974): 354, Collection of Papers, Marcolino Gomes Candau, WHO/OMS.
11 "In Memory of Dr M.G. Candau," 146, Collection of Papers, Marcolino Gomes Candau, WHO/OMS.
12 Candau, quoted in ibid., 146.
13 Ibid. See also Brockington, *World Health*.
14 Creelman, "Lyle Creelman Writes," *Canadian Nurse* 47, no. 5 (1951): 339.

15 See Meier, "Highest Attainable Standard."

16 Robert Berkov praised the move to further decentralization, while others, including John Farley, have been more guarded in their assessment of its outcome for
the WHO's ability to viewed as the single directing voice for global health. He and
Ascher concurred that the regional approach allowed the WHO programs to be
tailored to specific health problems within the region. See Berkov, *World Health
Organization*; Ascher, "Current Problems in the World Health Organization's
Program."

17 Lyle Creelman to Prescott and Frieda [Creelman], 27 June 1954, file 3-3, box 3, LC,
UBC.

18 WHO, *First Ten Years of the World Health Organization*, 401. See also "ICN: An
Account of Its Relationship with the World Health Organization," 6 Dec. 1968,
WHOHQ N2-348-2, WHO-OMS. The four studies were "An International List of
Advanced Programs in Nursing Education," "How to Survey a Nursing School,"
"Principles and Practices of Nursing Education," and "Principles of Nursing
Education and Principles of Administration as Applied to Advanced Programs in
Nursing Education."

19 Creelman, "The Relationship between the World Health Organization and
Professional Nursing," 38.

20 Ibid., 39.

21 Journals 1939–1952, 18 Dec. 1954, file 2-3, box 2, LC, UBC.

22 "Draft Article for *Canadian Nurse*" (submitted Nov. 1953), file 4-2, box 4, LC,
UBC.

23 Ibid.

24 Creelman, "Trends in Nursing," 603–4.

25 Ibid.

26 WHO, *First Ten Years*, 400.

27 Elizabeth Cockayne to Lyle Creelman, 22 May 1956, file 3-4, box 3, LC, UBC.

28 In July 1945, when the first nurses were commissioned in the USPHS, Pearl McIver
and Lucile Petry Leone were among those included. Van Betten and Moriarty,
Nursing Illuminations, 365.

29 Ann to "Dear Helen" [Martikainen] and Lyle [Creelman], 13 June 1956, file 3-4,
box 3, LC, UBC.

30 WHO, "Nurses: Their Education and Their Role," *Chronicle of the World Health
Organization* 10, no. 7 (1956): 214. The experiment of including nurses in national
delegations was not destined to be repeated during Creelman's time, as she herself
predicted.

31 Journals 1939–1952, 21 Apr. 1956, file 2-3, box 2, LC, UBC.

32 Prior to her appointment to the Department of National Health and Welfare, Percy
had served as the second assistant superintendent of the Victorian Order of Nurses

at the national office in Ottawa and held a teaching appointment at the School of Nursing, University of Toronto. She became the first chief nursing consultant for that Department – a position that she held until her retirement in 1966.

33 Percy, "Signpost at Geneva," 798.

34 WHO, "Nurses: Their Education and Their Role," 218.

35 Alice Wright and Creelman worked together when Creelman was on the Registered Nurses Association of British Columbia executive before joining UNRRA; Wright was the registrar and executive director of the RNABC from 1943 to 1960 and is regarded as one of Canada's pioneers in labour relations for nurses.

36 Elizabeth Hill graduated from the University of California School of Nursing, Berkeley, and later obtained an MA from Teachers College, Columbia University; she became the first executive director of the Visiting Nurses Association of Los Angeles and served in the U.S. Army Nurse Corps in Washington during the Second World War.

37 "Diary of a Trip, 14 April to 13 May 1956," Alice Wright Fonds, UBC. I am indebted to Dr Glennis Zilm for bringing this diary to my attention.

38 Arnstein had already directed similar field studies in hospitals, urban ghettos, and rural Appalachia designed to improve patient care.

39 Journals 1939–1952, 6 Oct. 1956, file 2-3, box 2, LC, UBC.

40 Margaret Arnstein to Lyle Creelman, 30 Nov. 1956, file 3-4, box 3, LC, UBC.

41 "Report on an Analysis of Replies from 34 Conference Participants to a Follow-up Questionnaire on the Conference, Circulated on 26th November 1957," file 94, box 12, Margaret Arnstein Papers, Boston University, Howard Gotlieb Archival Centre (BUHGARC). International Conference on Planning of Nursing Studies, held at Centre International, Études Pedagogiques, Sèvres, France, 12–24 Nov. 1956. Twenty-one of the thirty-five respondents indicated that the conference changed the way they approached nursing research.

42 Lyle Creelman to Elizabeth Hill, 10 May 1955, file 3-3, box 3, LC, UBC.

43 "News," Toronto Star, 14 June 1958.

44 Candau, "World Health Catalysts," 676.

45 Meier, "Highest Attainable Standard," 77.

46 WHO, Expert Committee on Nursing, Report of the Fourth Session, 4.

47 "Public Health Nursing," WHO Chronicle 15, no. 3 (1961): 79.

48 WHO, Expert Committee on Nursing, Report of the Fourth Session, 14–20.

49 For a list of recommendations that followed those of the earlier expert committees, see ibid., 27–35.

50 Ibid., 30–1.

51 Dorothy M. Percy to Dr Layton, "Expert Committee on Nursing – W.H.O. – 'Public Health Nursing,'" 30 Dec. 1958, file 485-5-9, vol. 762, RG 29, LAC.

52 Percy, "From Where I Sit."
53 "Daft Item for the *Canadian Nurse*," n.d., file 4-2, box 4, LC, UBC; Lyle Creelman, "Lyle Creelman Writes," *Canadian Nurse* 50, no. 8 (1954): 638.
54 Educated at the Royal Victoria Hospital, Montreal, Justine Delmotte joined the South African Nursing Sisters at the start of the Second World War. After the war, she served with UNRRA and the IRO before studying public health at McGill University's School for Graduate Nurses in 1948.
55 Yaws was one of the first diseases to claim the WHO's attention. For a more detailed account of the UNICEF/WHO yaws-control program, see WHO, *Four Decades of Achievement*, 1–2.
56 Hill served in UNRRA's China mission. *American Journal of Nursing* 46, no. 3 (1946): 300; *American Journal of Nursing* 55 no. 4 (1955): 406.
57 "Item for the Canadian Nurse," n.d., file 4-2, box 4, LC, UBC; Creelman, "Lyle Creelman Writes," *Canadian Nurse* 50, no. 8 (1954): 639.
58 Journals 1939–1952, 8–19 Jan. 1954, file 2-3, box 2, LC, UBC. (Note: Journals include entries after 1952.)
59 Journals 1939–1952, 22–9 Jan. 1954, file 2-3, box 2, LC, UBC.
60 Ibid., 29 Jan.–4 Feb. 1954.
61 Ibid., 4 Feb. 1954.
62 Script of Tape Recording, WHO, 17 Mar. 1954, 5, file 4-3, box 4, LC, UBC.
63 Ibid., 6.
64 Helena Friesen Reimer received her R.N. (Registered Nurse) from Winnipeg General Hospital in 1937 where she held various positions ranging from nurse to instructor and supervisor before joining UNRRA. Helena then returned to Winnipeg for a few years where she was the Assistant Superintendent of Nursing at Winnipeg General Hospital. During this time, she completed her Bachelor of Nursing from McGill before resuming her work overseas with the WHO in 1951.
65 Wilhelmina Visscher was a well-educated and experienced international nurse. Originally trained in Holland, she took a midwifery course in Johannesburg, South Africa, and completed a public health course at McGill in 1948 and a course in administration and supervision at the University of Toronto from 1959 to 1960. She had served as a military nurse with the South African Military Nursing Services during the Second World War before her UNRRA appointment as the chief nurse for the American and French zones of Austria. Vischer, Wilhelmina, file 54, vol. 160, I-248, MG 28, LAC. Alice Talbot was originally from Montreal but had worked in the United States for years.
66 Script of Tape Recording, WHO, 17 Mar. 1954, 3, file 4-3, box 4, LC, UBC. Creelman article in the *Canadian Nurse* also empathized the "experimental" nature of the program there. Lyle Creelman, "Lyle Creelman Writes," *Canadian Nurse* 48, no. 10 (1952): 808.
67 WHO, *First Ten Years*, 394–5.

68 Reimer, "My Job in Cambodia," *WHO Newsletter* 10 (1952), HR.
69 "Item for the *Canadian Nurse*," 3, 1952, file 4-2, box 4, LC, UBC; Creelman, "Lyle Creelman Writes," *Canadian Nurse* 48, no. 10 (1952): 808.
70 Copy of *Nursing News*, July 1952, appendix 1, Helena Reimer Private Papers (HR).
71 Ibid., 2. Other WHO workers in Cambodia carried on that approach until "the sad subsequent history" of a country engulfed in war eroded the organization's work. See, for example, Barton, "Notes from the Field," where she argues that the nurses attempted to devise programs and techniques that could be carried out by rural health workers.
72 Helena Reimer to Lyle Creelman, 1 Aug. 1952, file 3-3, box 3, LC, UBC.
73 Ibid.
74 Alice Talbot, Reimer's colleague, was also forced to return home on sick leave.
75 Helena Reimer to family, 2 Jan. 1952, HR.
76 Journals 1939–1952, 10 Mar. 1955, file 2-3, box 2, LC, UBC.
77 Lyle Creelman and Inge Götsche, "Report on Tour to Iran, Syria, Lebanon and Jordon," 6–26 Feb. 1956, 2, N2/418/2 EMA, WHO.
78 Lyle Creelman and Inge Götsche, "Report on Tour to Cyprus, Lebanon, Syria, Jordan, Iraq and Egypt," 9 Mar.–9 Apr. 1955, 5.
79 Ibid., 6.
80 Queenie Donaldson, with a certificate in public health nursing from UBC (1954), worked for the Division of Venereal Disease Control in Vancouver before joining the WHO.
81 Creelman and Götsche, "Report on Tour to Cyprus, Lebanon, Syria, Jordan, Iraq and Egypt," 11.
82 For a discussion of the role of nurses in controlling TB in British Columbia between 1895 and 1945, see Zilm and Warbinek, "Early Tuberculosis Nursing in British Columbia."
83 Queenie Donaldson to Lyle Creelman, 24 May 1955, file 3-3, box 3, LC, UBC.
84 Ibid., 2.
85 "Quarterly Field Report: Fourth Quarter 1954," 10 Jan. 1955, HR.
86 See also "A Philosophy of Life, Education and Nursing," in Helena Reimer, "A Basic Professional Nursing Curriculum for an Arab Country of the Eastern Mediterranean Region," *Report: Higher Institute of Nursing WMRO* 5 (1956): 18, HR. Her Canadian colleagues were expected to follow the same process during their initial orientation. See, for example, Lara Thordarson to Lyle Creelman, 17 Oct. 1954, file 3-3, box 3, LC, UBC.
87 Reimer, "Basic Professional Nursing Curriculum," 40, HR.
88 "Quarterly Report: First Quarter Report," 30 Mar. 1955, 6, HR.
89 "College of Nursing: Narrative Monthly Report No. 2," 30 Nov. 1950, 5, HR. Reimer acknowledged the efforts of national nurses to improve nursing standards. See "Helena Friesen Reimer Biographical Notes 1978," 17, HR.

90 Letter from Margaret Murray Campbell Jackson to her mother and father, 28 Apr. 1956, file 11-22, Margaret Murray Campbell Jackson Fonds (MMJC), BCHNGA, where she reported receiving a letter from Lara Thordarson explaining what had led to the three team members' resignations.

91 It should be noted that Creelman received requests for assistance from nurses within more advanced Commonwealth countries experiencing the same problems. In both Australia and New Zealand, for example, there was considerable opposition to the introduction of university-based nursing programs. Once again, she sent well-respected Canadian nursing leaders – Helen Gemeroy to New Zealand and Rae Chittick to Australia – as consultants to help launch the new initiatives. See the extensive correspondence between Lyle Creelman and Bea Salmon dealing with issue: file 3–5, box 3, LC, UBC.

92 "Helena Friesen Reimer Biographical Notes 1978," 20, HR.

93 See, for example, Lyle Creelman to Joan A. Monnik, 15 Oct. 1954, file 3-3, box 3, LC, UBC.

94 Joan A. Monnick to Mrs Mallik, 4 Nov. 1954, file 3-3, box 3, LC, UBC.

95 Joan Monnick, Mary Saunders, and Ingrid Stavnem to Lyle Creelman, 19 Nov. 1955, file 3-3, box 3, LC, UBC.

96 Ibid.

97 Inge Götsche to Lyle Creelman, 11 Oct. 1954, file 3-3, box 3, LC, UBC.

98 Joan A. Monnick to Mrs Mallik, 4 Nov. 1954, file 3-3, box 3, LC, UBC.

99 Lyle Creelman to M. Bertrand, 14 Oct. 1954, file 3-3, box 3, LC, UBC.

100 Lyle Creelman to her mother [Mrs S.P. Creelman], 11 Feb. 1958, file 3-4, box 3, LC, UBC.

101 Lyle Creelman to her mother, 7 July 1956, file 3-4, box 3, LC, UBC.

102 Lyle Creelman to her mother, 5 July 1956, file 3-4, box 3, LC, UBC.

103 Lyle Creelman, "Report on Visit to Gambia, 19–25 January 1958," 6, AFR/Nurs/11 (D68.AF 227), WHO/OMS.

104 Ibid., 7–8.

105 Lyle Creelman to her mother, 21 Jan. 1958, file 3-4, box 3, LC, UBC.

106 Lyle Creelman, "Report on Visit to La Reunion," 7–11 July 1956, AFR/NURS/5 1956 (D68.AF223), WHO/OMS.

107 Lyle Creelman to her mother, 17 July 1956, file 3-4, box 3, LC, UBC.

108 Lyle Creelman, "Report of Visit to Mauritius," 11–18 July 1956, AFN/NURS/6 1956 (D68.AF224), WHO/OMS.

109 Lyle Creelman to her mother, 1 July 1956, file 3-4, box 3, LC, UBC.

110 Lyle Creelman, "Report on Visit to Zanzibar," 27 June–3 July 1956, AFR/NURS/4 1956 (D68.AF222), WHO/OMS.

111 Lyle Creelman to her mother, 1 July 1956, file 3-4, box 3, LC, UBC.

112 Lyle Creelman, "Report on Visit to Uganda," 17–23 June 1956, 3, AFR/NURS/5 1956 (D68. F221), WHO/OMS.

113 Creelman, "Report on Visit to Uganda." See "Nursing Education," draft of 14 July 1967, Uganda 37, WHO/OMS.
114 Lyle Creelman to her mother, 23 June 1956, file 3-4, box 3, LC, UBC.
115 Lyle Creelman to her mother, 19 Jan. 1958, file 3-4, box 3, LC, UBC.
116 Lyle Creelman to her mother, 21 Jan. 1958, file 3-4, box 3, LC, UBC.
117 Ibid.
118 Lyle Creelman, "Report on Visit to Gambia," 19–25 Jan. 1958, 5, AFR/ NURS/11 (D68.AF227), WHO/OMS.
119 Ibid., 4–5.
120 Lyle Creelman to her mother, 28 Jan. 1958, file 3-4, box 3, LC, UBC.
121 Lyle Creelman, "Report on Visit to Sierra Lione," 25 Jan.–1 Feb. 1958, 1, AFR/ NURS/10/1958 (D68.AF228), WHO/OMS.
122 Lyle Creelman to her mother, 2 Feb. 1958, file 3-4, box 3, LC, UBC.
123 Lyle Creelman, "Report on Visit to Sierra Leone," 25 Jan.–1 Feb. 1958, 4, AFP/ NURS/10 (D68.AF228), WHO/OMS.
124 Ibid., 4–6.
125 It remained a British protectorate in the north part of the Horn of Africa until 1960.
126 Lyle Creelman, "Report on a Visit to Somaliland Protectorate," 8–16 June 1965, AFR/NURS/7 (D68.AF220), WHO/OMS. The average age of girls expressing an interest in nursing in the first school for girls, opened in 1953, was twelve. A special language course for more mature students had been established to raise the literacy rate.
127 Lyle Creelman to her mother, 10 June 1956, file 3-4, box 3, LC, UBC.
128 Lyle Creelman, "Report on Visit to Ghana," 2–9 Feb. 1958, AFR/NURS11 1958 (D68.AF229), WHO/OMS.
129 Lyle Creelman to her mother, 9 Feb. 1958, file 3-4, box 3, LC, UBC.
130 See Opare and Mill, "The Evolution of Nursing Education," 938–9.
131 Lyle Creelman, "Report on Visit to Ghana," 2–9 Feb. 1958, 4, AFR/NURS11 1958 (D68.AF229), WHO/OMS.
132 Ibid., 9.
133 Lyle Creelman to her mother, 2 Mar. 1958, file 3-4, box 3, LC, UBC.
134 Lyle Creelman to her mother, 23 June 1956, file 3-4, box 3, LC, UBC.
135 The Mau Mau uprising, an insurgency by Kenyan rebels against the British colonial administration, lasted from 1952 to 1960. The core of the resistance was formed by members of the Kikuyu ethnic group, along with smaller numbers of Embu and Meru. The uprising failed militarily, though it may have set the stage for Kenyan independence in 1963.
136 Lyle Creelman to Mrs Samuel Creelman, 27 Jan. 1956, file 3-4, box 3, LC, UBC.
137 Journals 1939–1952, 20 July 1956, file 2-3, box 2, LC, UBC.
138 Lyle Creelman to her mother, 10 July 1956, file 3-4, box 3, LC, UBC.

139 Lyle Creelman to her mother, 1 July 1956, file 3-4, box 3, LC, UBC.
140 Lyle Creelman to her mother, 20 July 1956, file 3-4, box 3, LC, UBC.
141 Lyle Creelman to her mother, 12 Mar. 1958, file 3-4, box 3, LC, UBC.
142 Ibid.
143 Ibid.
144 Lyle Creelman to her mother, 11 Feb. 1958, file 3-4, box 3, LC, UBC.
145 WHO, *Former WHO Nurses Remember*, 114.

9. Lyle's Secret Service, 1954–1968

1 Virginia Arnold to Lyle Creelman, 13 Nov. 1958, file 3-4, box 3, LC, UBC.
2 "In Memory of Dr M.G. Candau," *WHO Chronicle* 37 (1983): 144–7, Collection of Papers, Marcolinio Gomes Candau, WHO/OMS.
3 Elizabeth Barton, interview with Susan Armstrong-Reid, 26 Aug. 2007, Maiden Newton, England.
4 Lyle Creelman to Elizabeth Hill, 9 Feb. 1955, file 3-3, box 3, LC, UBC.
5 Lillian Turnbull did her initial nursing training at the Regina General Hospital before obtaining a BScN from McGill in teaching and supervision; she subsequently studied advanced nursing education at the University of Toronto.
6 Elizabeth Hill to Lyle Creelman, 21 Jan.1955, file 3-6, box 3, LC, UBC.
7 See, for example, Lyle Creelman to Inge Götsche, 13 Sept. 1955, file 3-6, box 3, LC, UBC.
8 It was not uncommon for WHO nurses recruited for one project to be reassigned for political reasons. Cammaert, for example, was deemed "acceptable to Mexico" after being rejected by another country and after a protracted time when she was still being considered by India. Margaret Cammaert, interview with Susan Armstrong-Reid, 18 Apr. 2008, Victoria.
9 Lillian Turnbull to Lyle Creelman, 5 May 1966, file 3-3, box 3, LC, UBC.
10 Journals 1939–1952, 2 Jan. 1952, file 2-3, box 2, LC, UBC.
11 Ibid., 22 Nov. 1949.
12 Ibid.
13 Lyle Creelman to Elizabeth Hill, 10 May 1955, file 3-3, box, LC, UBC.
14 Elizabeth Hill to Lyle Creelman, 28 May 1957, file 3-6, box 3, LC, UBC.
15 While on home leave in the spring of 1954, she recruited and interviewed prospective candidates and, for the same purpose, visited the WHO's Regional Office in New York. Lyle Creelman to Inge Götzsche, 22 Nov. 1954, file 3-3, box 3, LC, UBC.
16 Lyle Creelman to Inge [Götzsche], 15 Oct. 1954, file 3-3, box 3, LC, UBC.
17 Journals 1939–1952, 28 Oct. 1949, file 2-3, box 2, box 3, LC, UBC.
18 Lyle Creelman, interview with Kay Dier, Vancouver, 27 May 1985, KD.

19 Ibid.
20 Lyle Creelman to Eleanor Graham, 17 Jan. 1955, file 3-3, box 3, LC, UBC.
21 The *Canadian Nurse* reported that the CNA had appointed an advisory committee on placements for the WHO. "C.N.A. Convention Reports," *Canadian Nurse* 48, no. 5 (1952): 337–42. See, for example, Creelman's correspondence with Trenna Hunter on the suitability of a prospective WHO candidate. Trenna Hunter to Lyle Creelman, 11 July [no year], file 3-10, box 3, LC, UBC.
22 Lyle Creelman, interview, KD.
23 Ruth Pinkus, "Quality of Dedication Top Requisite for Job," clipping, *Vancouver Sun*, 21 May 1958, file 1-7, box 1, LC, UBC.
24 Lyle Creelman to Dick [Pullen], 6 July 1958, file 3-4, box 3, LC, UBC.
25 Memo: Nursing Section to Director, OPHS, 22 Oct. 1957, Meeting of the Canadian Nurses Association, N2-86-10, WHOHQ, WHO/OMS.
26 "Distinguished Nurses at CNA Meeting," *Globe and Mail*, 24 June 1958, file 1-7, box 1, LC, UBC. She made the same point before the Prince George Rotary Club: Lyle Creelman, Prince George Rotary, 24 April, "Citizens of the World," file 2-7, box 2, LC, UBC.
27 Lyle Creelman's notes for speech, undated and untitled, file 2-7, box 2, LC, UBC.
28 See, for example, Final Report, Midwifery, Nurses' Training – Calcutta India, Nursing India, 19 Feb. 1955. The report indicated that WHO nurses designed a program only after taking the time to "understand the different methods of nursing being taught and practiced" but still faced initial resistance from the physicians in the hospital.
29 See Eleanor Graham private letter to Lyle Creelman. She wrote that a WHO nurse going through Geneva "would be able to tell you some things about the project that we were not able to write about" and complained that the report they had written had been edited. 24 May 1964, file 3-5, box 5, LC, UBC.
30 WHO, *Former WHO Nurses Remember*, 9.
31 Kay Dier, interview with Susan Armstrong-Reid, 7 Apr. 2008, Edmonton.
32 Mary Abbott, interview with Susan Armstrong-Reid, 25 and 27 June 2007, St Andrews, Fife, Scotland.
33 Ibid.
34 Splane received a diploma in public health nursing from the University of Toronto (1939) and then completed a BSc at Columbia (1957) and a master's at the University of Michigan School of Public Health (1964) before undertaking her first WHO nursing assignment in the Caribbean, as a nursing consultant to the ministries of health of British Guiana, Barbados, and Trinidad (1959–62).
35 Splane, *Halfway to Poona*, 69.
36 Ibid., 108.
37 Lyle Creelman to Prescott [Creelman], 24 Oct. 1953, file 3-3, box 3, LC, UBC.

38 Eva Moody Williamson to "Dear Edythe," 20 Aug. 1954, Eva Moody Williamson Private Papers (EMW). In the same vein, another British Columbia recruit wrote home recounting her social outings with Creelman: Margaret Murray Campbell Jackson to her mother and father, 19 Nov. 1954, file 11-18, MMCJ, BCHNGA.

39 Kay Dier, interview with Susan Armstrong-Reid; and Margaret Cammaert, interview with Susan Armstrong-Reid. The same point was made in earlier interviews; see Audrey Stegen, 26 Oct. 1987, Eleanor Kunderman Tape 1, 2, no. 1, Oral Histories, CRNBC.

40 For example, Creelman informed one of her regional nursing advisers that, when a Mrs Johnstone came through Geneva, she would take "her home with me for lunch … and will add a bit at the end of this as to how I feel about her potential as a team leader." Lyle Creelman to Inge Götzsche, 11 May 1955, file 3-3, box 3, LC, UBC.

41 WHO, *Former WHO Nurses Remember*, 7.

42 Elizabeth Barton, interview with Susan Armstrong-Reid.

43 Dorothy Hall, interview with Susan Armstrong-Reid, 11 June 2007, at her farm near Mount Forrest, Ontario.

44 See D.M. Ross to Lyle Creelman, n.d.; Elizabeth Hilborn to Lyle Creelman, 20 Mar. [no year], file 3-5, box 3, LC, UBC; Louise Bell to Lyle Creelman, 1 Feb. 1960, file 3-10, box 3, LC, UBC.

45 Unknown [WHO nurse in Gambia] to Lyle Creelman, 20 Feb. 1963, file 3-5, box 3, LC, UBC.

46 Lyle Creelman to Joan Monnik, 15 Oct. 1954, file 3-3, box 3, LC, UBC.

47 Fernanda [Alves-Diniz] to Lyle Creelman, 13 Feb. 1957, file 3-4, box 3, LC, UBC.

48 Rita Hill to Lyle Creelman, 15 Aug. 1963, file 3-5, box 3, LC, UBC.

49 Ibid., unknown author to Lyle Creelman, 27 Oct. 1963, file 3-5, box 3, LC, UBC.

50 See also Eleanor Kunderman to Lyle Creelman, 2 Nov. 1960, file 3-5, box 3, LC, UBC.

51 Eleanor Graham to Lyle Creelman, 29 July 29 [no year], file 3-3, box 2, LC, UBC; Eleanor Graham to Lyle Creelman, 27 Apr. [no year], file 3-10, box 3, LC, UBC.

52 Eleanor Graham to Lyle Creelman, 3 Jan. 1955, file 3-10, box 3, LC, UBC.

53 Ibid., Lyle Creelman to Eleanor Graham 17 Jan. 1955.

54 Ibid., Lyle Creelman to Elizabeth Hill, 27 Jan. 1955.

55 Olive Baggallay to Lyle Creelman, 20 Nov. [no year], file 3-10, box 3, LC, UBC. Olive Baggallay shared Creelman's reservations about Pedersen and wrote Creelman that she would have a poor opinion of Dr Mani if he did not terminate her contract in March.

56 Doris Pedersen to Lyle Creelman, 2 Feb. 1956, file 3-10, box 3, LC, UBC.

57 From 1954 to 1958, the Krishak Sramik and the Awami League waged a ceaseless battle for control of East Pakistan's provincial government.

58 Dorothy Potts, interview with Kay Dier, KD.
59 Sister tutors and nurse-teachers received specialized post-registration training courses. Interview with Lyle Creelman; interview with Kay Dier, KD.
60 Dorothy Potts to Lyle Creelman, 1 Feb. 1956, file 3-4, box 3, LC, UBC.
61 Dorothy Potts, interview with Kay Dier, KD.
62 Elizabeth Barton to Lyle Creelman, 20 Oct. 1954, file 3-3, box 3, LC, UBC.
63 Fanny Annette (Nan) Kennedy (VGH 1933) received her public health nursing diploma in 1945 and her BScN in 1954 from UBC. Prior to joining the WHO, she was a supervisor of nursing from 1949 to 1952 with the Upper Fraser Valley Health Unit. F.A. [Nan] Kennedy, interview with S. Coates, Jan. 1987, Oral History no. 10, CRNBC.
64 See Steltzer, "In Iran"; Khomeira and Deans, "Nursing Education in Iran."
65 Green, *Through the Years with Public Health Nursing*, 78.
66 Maryam Hazarti, G. Mirzabeigy, and Ahmad Nejatian. "The History of Nursing in the Islamic Republic of Iran." *Nursing History Review* 19 (2011): 171–4.
67 On 19 August 1953, the democratically elected government, headed by Prime Minister Mohammad Mosaddegh, was overthrown. The coup was orchestrated by the United States and Great Britain to re-secure the oil reserves that had been nationalized.
68 See Campbell Jackson's letters home describing the hurdles she faced in trying to implement change along Western lines in file 11-18, MMCJ, BCHNGA.
69 Margaret Murray Campbell Jackson to her mother and father, 24 July 1955, file 11-20, MMCJ, BCHNGA.
70 Margaret Murray Campbell Jackson to her mother and father, 19 Oct. 1955, file 11-19, MMCJ, BCHNGA.
71 Margaret Murray Campbell Jackson to "Mary, Bill and Ruth," 6 Jan. 1955, file 11-19, MMCJ, BCHNGA.
72 Margaret Murray Campbell Jackson to her mother and father, 21 Jan. 1955, file 11-19, MMCJ, BCHNGA.
73 Margaret Murray Campbell Jackson to her mother and father, 29 Jan. 1955, file 11-19, MMCJ, BCHNGA. See also Margaret Murray Campbell Jackson to her mother and father, 21 Feb. 1955, where she again writes, "I don't think Miss Creelman has a clue what conditions are like here."
74 Margaret Murray Campbell Jackson to "Mary, Bill and Ruth," 25 Mar. 1955, file 11-20, MMCJ, BCHNGA.
75 Margaret Murray Campbell Jackson to "Mary, Bill and Ruth," 12 July 1955, file 11-20, MMCJ, BCHNGA.
76 Margaret Murray Campbell Jackson to her mother and father, 24 July 1955, file 11-20, MMCJ, BCHNGA.

77 For a more detailed description of Campbell's political manoeuvring in determin-
    ing budget lines, to obtain students, or the ultimatum to threating to request the
    team's withdrawal to overcoming the bureaucratic inertia in setting up a new
    clinic, see, for examples, Margaret Murray Campbell Jackson to her mother
    and father, 24 Aug. 1955, file 11-20, MMCJ, BCHNGA; Margaret Murray
    Campbell Jackson to her mother and father, 10 Jan. 1956; file 11-22, MMJC,
    BCHNGA.
78 Lillian [Turnbull] to Lyle Creelman, 17 Feb. [no year], file 3-10, box 3, LC, UBC.
79 Ibid. In 1967 Creelman would urge Turnbull's appointment as regional nursing
    adviser for EMRO over Evelyn Matheson, who had been holding down the job
    until a permanent appointment was made. Turnbull wrote privately to Creelman
    that she preferred to apply for study leave and, moreover, believed that Matheson
    should be appointed because she knew the region far better. In all likelihood,
    Creelman wanted Turnbull to acquire wider experience so as to improve her
    chances of succeeding her as CNO, but in the end she respected her wishes, per-
    haps remembering that she herself had taken a study leave before replacing Olive
    Baggallay.
80 Lillian Turnbull to Lyle Creelman, 11 Sept. [no year], file 3-10, box 3, LC, UBC.
81 Lillian Turnbull to Lyle Creelman, 27 Feb. 1957, file 3-4, box 3, LC, UBC.
82 Lillian [Turnbull] to Lyle Creelman, 15 Aug. [no year but contents indicate 1968],
    file 3-10, LC, UBC.
83 "Ethopia" (excerpt from E.M.'s [Evelyn Matheson] report): "It is very important
    that the building up of professional nurses who are going to tackle these problems
    must have a training which will prepare them to handle the specific problems of
    Ethiopia and not just training imported from England, the United States or other
    countries," file 2-7, box 2, LC, UBC.
84 "Cambodia" (excerpt from E.H.'s [Elizabeth Hill] early reports), file 2-7, box 2, LC,
    UBC.
85 Lillian [Turnbull] to Lyle Creelman, 15 Aug. [no year, but contents indicate 1968],
    file 3-10, box 3, LC UBC.
86 Barbara Darbyshire Bubb (British WHO nurse, who worked closely with Hall
    in SEARO), interview with Susan Armstrong-Reid, 21–2 Aug. 2007, Old School
    House, East Marden, Chichester, England. Dorothy Hall graduated from Victoria
    Hospital in London, Ontario, and obtained her BScN at the University of Western
    Ontario. She worked as an outpost nurse in rural Ontario before joining the WHO
    in 1950.
87 Dorothy Potts to Lyle Creelman, 10 Aug. 1954, file 3-3, box 3, LC, UBC; Elizabeth
    Hill to Lyle Creelman, 26 May 1957, file 3-4, box 3, LC, UBC.
88 Elizabeth Hill to Lyle Creelman, 26 May 1957, file 3-4, box 3, LC, UBC.

89 Several former WHO nurses commented on Creelman's ability to size up her nurses' current and future contribution to the WHO and take decisive action, even when that involved a friend. Verna Huffman Splane, interview with Susan Armstrong-Reid, 15 Apr. 2008, Vancouver; and Barbara Darbyshire Bubb, interview with Susan Armstrong-Reid.

90 Inge Götzsche to Lyle Creelman, 22 Sept. 1955, file 3-3, box 3, LC, UBC.

91 A graduate of St Paul's Hospital, Vancouver, Kunderman later received a diploma in public health nursing (1945) and a certificate in teaching and supervision (1947) from UBC before obtaining a BScN in 1956.

92 Margaret Cammaert received a BScN from the University of Alberta (1944), a master's in public health from Johns Hopkins (1951), and an honorary doctorate from the University of Alberta (1996).

93 Margaret Cammaert, interview with Susan Armstrong-Reid.

94 WHO, *Former WHO Nurses Remember*, 5.

95 Eleanor Kunderman received her initial training at St Paul's Hospital, Vancouver, in 1944. Later she obtained a diploma in public health nursing from the UBC School of Nursing (1945) and then completed a UBC certificate program in teaching and supervision in 1947 before receiving her BScN in 1956. She also obtained a master's degree from Teachers College, Columbia, during her first study leave from the WHO. From 1947 to 1951, she was head nurse at St Paul's. In 1952 she was appointed as travelling instructor in British Columbia to teach on radiation nursing under a grant from the federal government. She then became a nursing instructor at Vancouver's Willow Chest Centre. In 1956 she was made supervisor of nursing education in the Division of TB Control in Vancouver.

96 Eleanor Kunderman to Lyle Creelman, 26 Apr. 1959, file 3-4, box 3, LC, UBC.

97 Ibid.

98 Ibid.

99 Eleanor [Kunderman] to Lyle Creelman, 8 June 1959, file 3-4, box 3, LC, UBC.

100 Eleanor Kunderman, interview with Audrey Stegen, 26 Oct. 1987, tapes 1, 2, Oral Histories no. 1, CRNBC.

101 Eleanor Kunderman to Lyle Creelman, 20 May 1966, file 3-5, box 3, LC, UBC. See also the letter from Beatrice Salmon, Nursing Department, University of Ghana, to Lyle Creelman, 23 Oct. 1964, file 3-5, box 3, LC, UBC, where she described a similar reaction to her time at Lyle's chalet: "My visit to Switzerland was quite the most enjoyable part of my seven weeks' vacation and particularly my few days at Sam Suphy. I often sit in my tropical surroundings and think of that beautiful spot and wish I might wake up one morning to the sound of cowbells rather than the insistent rhythm of African drums." See also Monique Arseneau [WHO nurse, Côte d'Ivoire] to Lyle Creelman, 10 Mar. 1963, file 3-5, box 3, LC, UBC;

D.M. Ross to Lyle Creelman, 20 Oct. 1960, file 3-5, box 3, LC, UBC; and Elizabeth Hilborn to Lyle Creelman, 20 Mar. [no year], file 3-10, box 3, LC, UBC.

102 Eleanor Kunderman, "For Lyle," "One Year Later," May 1966, file 3-5, box 3, LC, UBC.

103 Katherine Lyman to Lyle Creelman, 8 Jan. 1961, file 3-5, box 3, LC, UBC. See also Katherine Lyman to "Miss Creelman," 20 Jan. 1955, file 3-3, box 3, LC, UBC, where she again thanks Creelman for the advice and "friendly touches" during her initial briefing in Geneva.

104 Lyle Creelman, interview with Kay Dier, 27 May 1985, Vancouver, KD.

105 Olive Manning to Lyle Creelman, 5 Dec. 1962, file 3-5, box 3, LC, UBC.

106 Ibid.

107 Lyle Creelman to Eleanor [Graham], 16 Sept. 1957, file 3-4, box 3, LC, UBC.

108 Typically, this letter was done "hastily so that Elizabeth Gillespie [a fellow Canadian] can take it with her." Lyle Creelman to Eleanor [Graham], 16 Sept. 1957, file 3-4, box 3, LC, UBC.

109 Eve Moody (Billie) Williamson, interview with Susan Armstrong-Reid, 5 Nov. 2007, Vancouver.

110 Barbara Darbyshire Bubb, interview with Susan Armstrong-Reid.

111 Elizabeth Barton, interview with Susan Armstrong-Reid.

112 Lyle Creelman often relied upon Canadian nurses to launch new programs; she sent Marion Pennington, a UNRRA veteran and UBC graduate, to pilot the postgraduate programs in Turkey, the first European country to receive WHO assistance. Joan Webster from Vancouver headed nursing in the first health-demonstration area in El Salvador, training auxiliary personnel as the first step to establishing public health nursing in the country. It should be noted, too, that Creelman frequently chose British-trained midwives for the MCH placements, often in remote or troubled locations.

113 Office of the Chief Nursing Consultant, file 485-5-9ptz, vol. 762, RG 29, LAC. This was a harbinger of the contemporary international network of WHO Collaborative Centres that carry out activities in support of WHO's mandate for international health work and its current program priorities.

114 Bothwell, *Alliance and Illusions*, 8.

115 See Officers Dairy, Elizabeth W. Brackett, 17 Nov. 1953, 12.1, file 1952-4, box 21, RF, RFAC.

116 WHO, *Former WHO Nurses Remember*, 2.

117 Ibid.

118 Ibid., 9.

119 Journal, 10 May 1953, file 2-3, box 2, LC, UBC.

120 Journal, 14 Mar. 1954, file 2-3, box 2, LC, UBC.

121 Lyle Creelman to Dick [Pullen], 6 July 1958, file 3-4, box 3, LC, UB.

10. The Voice of International Nursing, 1960–1968

1 Creelman, "Quality Care," 169–70.
2 WHO, *The Second Ten Years*, 401.
3 Creelman, "Nursing in the World Health Organization," 18.
4 WHO, *The Second Ten Years*, 94–5.
5 Lyle Creelman to Dame Elizabeth Cockayne, 31 Aug. 1962, Membership of the Expert Panel on Nursing, N2-136-3, WHOHQ, WHO/OMS; see also Olive Baggallay to Dr Candau, April 1962, Membership of the Expert Panel on Nursing, WHOHQ N2-136-3, WHO/OMS.
6 Quinn joined the ICN staff in 1961 as the director of the social and economic welfare division of the ICN and was appointed executive director in 1967. Throughout her long and distinguished career, Quinn was a vital figure in both the ICN and British nursing. She served as president of the Royal College of Nursing from 1982 to 1986 and regional nursing officer, Wessex Regional Health Authority 1978–83, and as UK member of the Permanent Committee of Nurses in Liaison with the EEC (PCN) formed in 1971, subsequently referred to as the Standing Committee (SCN), of which she also served as president 1983–91. In May 1979 Dame Sheila was elected the first president of the EEC Advisory Committee on Training in Nursing.
7 Dame Sheila Quinn, interview with Susan Armstrong-Reid, 27 Aug. 2007, Chandler's Ford, UK.
8 "From the Executive Desk, Lyle Creelman – an Appreciation," *ICN Calling* 9 (Oct. 1968): 1, file 1-7, box 1, LC, UBC.
9 Quinn, *A Dame Abroad*, 75.
10 Dame Sheila Quinn, interview with Susan Armstrong-Reid.
11 "Nursing – Co-ordination with the International Council of Nurses – ICN – General, Lyle Creelman to Katharine Lyman," 30 Jan. 1962, 1, WHOHQ N2-372-4, WHO/OMS.
12 Creelman to Lyman, 30 Jan. 1962, 2–3, WHOHQ N2-372-4, WHO/OMS.
13 Lyle Creelman to Ellen Broe, 30 Jan. 1962, 2–3, WHOHQ N2-372-4, WHO/OMS.
14 Dame Sheila Quinn interview with Susan Armstrong-Reid.
15 See Meier's discussion of the WHO's abrogation of leadership on human rights, children's rights, discrimination against women, and racial discrimination: Meier, "Highest Attainable Standard," 80–100.
16 "WHO/ILO Collaboration – International Instrument on the Status of Nursing Personnel with Special Reference to Nurses. Memorandum: International Instrument on Nurses," 27 Sept. 1967, WHOHQ N2-372-5, WHO/OMS.
17 Lillian Turnbull, interview with Kay Dier, 15 June 1989, KD.
18 Lyle Creelman, interview with Kay Dier, Vancouver, 27 May 1985, KD.

19 Dame Sheila Quinn, interview with Susan Armstrong-Reid.

20 Lyle Creelman to F.S. Beck [director of Nursing Services, ICN], 15 Aug. 1963, N2-109-Z, WHOHQ, WHO/OMS.

21 Lyle Creelman to F.S. Beck, 10 Mar. 1959, WHOHQ N2-372-5, WHO/OMS.

22 Diary, 18 Jan. 1965, box 3, VA, N 86, BUHGARC. See also Diary, 24 Jan. 1958, box 1, VA, N 86, BUHGARC.

23 Virginia Arnold, Meeting of Nurse Representatives from Agencies with International Health Programs, 30, 31 Jan. 1964, 12.2 Officers' Diaries, VA, file 1964, box 5, RFA.

24 Lyle Creelman to Lucile Petry Leone, 19 Jan. 1966, box 2, Lucile Petry Leone Papers, BUHGARC.

25 See Diary, 8 and 9 Oct. 1961, Geneva, box 2, VA.

26 At times Arnold provided Creelman with an unsolicited opinion of a WHO nurse. On one such occasion, Arnold complained that the WHO regional nursing adviser in Copenhagen, Fernanda Alves Diniz of Portugal, was interfering in Rockefeller business. Creelman already knew that the autocratic Alves Diniz could be "somewhat of a loose cannon." Diary, 1 May 1958, box 1, VA, N 86, BUHGARC. Conversely, Arnold apologized in 1958 for advancing Maria P. Tito de Moraes, another Portuguese WHO nurse, for Rockefeller fellowships outside the regular WHO application channels. Diary, 27 Apr. 1958, box 1, VA, N 86, BUHGARC. This kind of candid exchange averted potential conflicts that might compromise Creelman's ability to secure Arnold's official backing for a contentious WHO appointment or Rockefeller financial support for a future joint nursing project.

27 As a member of UNRRA, Arnold served in Yugoslavian refugee camps in Egypt and Greece. She was a member of the WHO expert advisory panel from 1962 to 1974.

28 Shortly after her appointment, Arnold learned that there had been a significant power struggle over continuing support for nursing. Virginia Arnold, interview with Mary Ann Garrigan, 28 Jan. 1971, folder 1, box 3, VA, N 86, BUHGARC.

29 Virginia Arnold to Lyle Creelman 11 Nov. [no year], file 3-10, box 3, LC, UBC.

30 Virginia Arnold to Lyle Creelman, 23 Jan. [no year], file 3-10, box 3, LC, UBC.

31 Virginia Arnold to Lyle Creelman, 7 Aug. 1968, file 3-6, box 3, LC, UBC.

32 See, for example, their discussions on nursing in Chile: Diary, Santiago, Chile, 13–18 1959, box 1, folder 1, box 3, VA, N 86, BUHGARC.

33 Virginia Arnold to Lyle Creelman [n.d., but report is dated 1959], file 3-4, box 3, LC, UBC.

34 Garrigan, interview with Virginia Arnold, folder 1, box 3, VA, N 86, BUHGARC.

35 Diary, 8 and 9 Oct. 1961, file 2, box 1, VA, N 86, BUHGARC.

36 Virginia Arnold to Lyle Creelman, 14 Feb. 1963, file 3-5, box 3, LC, UBC.

37 Diary, 16–28 Apr. 1961, 112, file 2, box 1, VA, N 86, BUHGARC.
38 Diary, 15–18 Sept. 1960, 182, file 1, box 1, VA, N 86, BUHGARC.
39 Diary, 16–28 Apr. 1961, 112, file 2, box 1, VA, N 86, BUHGARC.
40 Interview, 27–30 Oct. 1962, 235, file 2, box 1, VA, N 86, BUHGARC.
41 Ibid., 65. There are many other examples of Creelman approaching the RF for
    funding through Virginia Arnold. See, for example, Diary, 1 May 1958, file 1,
    box 1, VA, N 86, BUHGARC.
42 Diary, 27–30 Oct. 1962, 2, file 2, box 1, VA, N 86, BUHGARC.
43 The United States had agreed to assume the additional costs involved, up to
    $400,000. Beigbeder, Nashat, Orsini, and Tiercy, *The World Health Organization*,
    42.
44 Virginia Arnold to Lyle Creelman, 13 Nov. 1958, file 3-4, box 3, LC, UBC.
45 Lyle Creelman to Virginia Arnold, 19 Nov. 1958, file 3-4, box 3, LC, UBC.
46 Ibid.
47 Ibid.
48 WHO Diary, 3 July 1965, 1961–9 [not currently catalogued], LC, UBC.
49 Girard had been the first bilingual president of the CNA (1958–60) and the only
    woman to be named to the 1961 Royal Commission on Health Services.
50 Lyle Creelman to Ruth Freeman, 20 Jan. 1965, file 2-6, box 2, LC, UBC.
51 Lyle Creelman to Ruth Freeman, 10 Jan. 1962, file 2-6, box 2, LC, UBC.
52 Lyle Creelman to Ruth Freeman, 2 Dec. 1962, file 2-6, box 2, LC, UBC.
53 Lyle Creelman to Ruth Freeman, 5 Dec. 1962, file 2-6, box 2, LC, UBC.
54 Lyle Creelman to all WHO nurses, "Study of Nursing in WHO," 28 Jan. 1963, file 6,
    box 2, LC, UBC.
55 Lyle Creelman, "Nursing in the World Health Organization," 8, file 4-8, box 4, LC,
    UBC.
56 Lyle Creelman to Ruth Freeman, 28 Nov. 1962, LC, UBC.
57 Lyle Creelman to Ruth Freeman, 3 July 1963, LC, UBC.
58 Lyle Creelman to Ruth Freeman, 12 July 1963, LC, UBC.
59 Lyle Creelman to Ruth Freeman, 12 Sept. 1963, LC, UBC.
60 Margaret Arnstein Papers, BUHGARC; a copy of the summary of the responses
    is found in file 161, box 1. Of the 531 questionnaires sent out, responses were
    received from 346 nurses (66 per cent).
61 Creelman, "Nursing in the World Health Organization," 16.
62 Ibid., 11.
63 Ibid., 19.
64 Ibid., 27.
65 Murphy, "Group Teaching in Public Health."
66 Alvim, "The Visitadora Sanitá," 163.

67 Hence, the article explored public health education in Nigeria, the role of the *assistant sociale* in France, the work and training of *feldshers* and nurses in the USSR, and the Brazilian approach to the use of auxiliary public health workers.

68 Margaret C. Cammaert to Dr M. Candau, "Report on the Meeting of the Zone Nurse Advisors and the Opinion of the Group on Miss Freeman's Report," 22 Mar. 1966, WHO/OMS.

69 Meeting of Zone Nurse Advisors, Final Report, Washington, DC, 28 Feb.–11 Mar. 1966, WHO/OMS.

70 Marion Murphy, Background Paper, Fifth Expert Committee on Nursing, Geneva, 26 Apr.–2 May 1966, 23–4, file D, box 1, Marion Murphy Papers, BUHGARC.

71 Ibid., 26.

72 Ibid.

73 Ibid., 33.

74 WHO, Expert Committee on Nursing, *Report of the Fifth Session*, 6.

75 On this point, see Boschma, "Ambivalence about Nursing's Expertise," 169–70.

76 Ibid., 5. See also Lyle Creelman, "There Is No Change without Challenge." The speech foreshadowed many of the themes that underscored the work of the fifth expert committee on nursing.

77 WHO, Expert Committee on Nursing, *Report of the Fifth Session*, 6–7.

78 Ibid.

79 Ibid., 8.

80 Ibid., 9.

81 Ibid., 31.

82 Schlotfeldt, *"Teachers as Exemplars."*

83 WHO, Expert Committee on Nursing, *Report of the Fifth Session*, 22.

84 Ibid., 14.

85 Guidelines for the Development of Post-Basic Education for Nurses, 5, WHO/Nurs/tech.Guide/69.4, WHO/OMS.

86 Ibid., 8. See also ibid., 13, where the document reiterates the expert committee's warning against importing nursing-education programs from other countries.

87 Ibid., 14.

88 Ibid., 5.

89 VA Officers Diaries, 1966, no. 84, box 3, VA, N 86, BUHGARC.

90 Margaret Mclean, a graduate of the University of Western Ontario (BScN) and of Teachers College, Columbia, had served as the WHO consultant to the ten-day nursing seminar in Tehran in 1967. For more detailed biographical information, see file 18, vol. 158, I-248, MG 28, LAC.

91 "Nurses and the Practice of Nursing: Reaction to the W.H.O. Expert Committee on Nursing, Fifth Report, Paper Presented at the International Congress of Nurses, Montreal 25 June 1969," Margaret D. Mclean Private Papers.

92 Barbara Darbyshire Bubb, interview with Susan Armstrong-Reid, 21 Aug. 2007, East Marden, U.K.

93 Louise Bell to Lyle Creelman, 1 Feb. 1960, file 3-5, box 3, LC, UBC.

94 Letter of complaint about Louise Bell's lack of decorum during duty travel: E. Losonczi to Dr J. Camournac, 23 Nov. 1959, file 3-5, box 3, LC, UBC.

95 Louise Bell to Lyle Creelman, 1 Feb. 1960, file 3-5, box 3, LC, UBC.

96 Interviews: VA, 14 Mar. 1962, 65, file 2, box 1, VA, N 86, BUHGARC.

97 See Virginia Arnold, 23, 24, 29 May 1963, Officers Diaries, 12.2, file 1963, box 5, RF, RFAC.

98 Ibid.

99 Ibid.

100 Memo: Virginia Arnold to Mildred Gottdank, 18 Sept. 1963, subseries c-nursing, series 497, file 90, box 8 1.2, RF, RFAC.

101 Pratt, the president of the Professional Association of Trained Nurses of Nigeria, had led the first two Nigerian delegations to the INC meetings in 1957 and in 1961 would be appointed a member of the WHO's expert panel on nursing in 1970.

102 Akinsanya, *African Florence Nightingale*, 196.

103 Ibid., 110.

104 Ibid., 113.

105 Louise Bell to Lyle Creelman, 13 Dec. 1961, file 3-5, box 3, LC, UBC.

106 Louise Bell to Lyle Creelman, 22 Jan. 1962, file 3-5, box 3, LC, UBC.

107 Virginia Arnold to Lyle Creelman, 26 Apr. 1962, file 3-5, box 3, LC, UBC; see also memo Virginia Arnold, 5–11 Apr. 1962 [Ibdan], 1.2 series 497-c nursing, file 89, box 8, LC, UBC.

108 See Virginia Arnold, 23, 24 May 1963, Officers Diaries, 12.2, RF, RFAC.

109 Lyle Creelman's handwritten diary (1960s WHO diary), 23 Mar. 1963, 1961–9, file 5-3, box 5, LC, UBC.

110 Ibid.

111 Ferguson, "Visit to the Middle East," 768.

112 Lyle Creelman's handwritten diary, 23 Mar. 1963, 27 Nov. 1964, 1961–9, file 5-3, box 5, LC, UBC.

113 Creelman, "Quality Care in the Right Quantity."

114 Lyle Creelman, "Some Notes on Nursing and Midwifery in the USSR," n.d., file 25-19, vol. 25, R-8293, LAC.

115 Lyle Creelman's handwritten diary, 3 Dec. 1964, file 5-3, box 5, LC, UBC.

116 There is only a passing reference to this trip in Creelman's WHO diary of the period. See Lyle Creelman, "Report of Visit to the USSR, Moscow," 11–15 Mar. 1966. Copy found in file 25-21, vol. 25, R-8293, LAC.

117 Dame Sheila Quinn, interview with Susan Armstrong-Reid.

118 Ibid.

119　Lyle Creelman's handwritten diary, 17 Oct. 1966, 1961–9, file 5-3, box 5, LC, UBC.

120　Dame Sheila Quinn, interview with Susan Armstrong-Reid.

121　Helen Mussallem to "Dear Mother and family," 10 Oct. 1966, Helen Mussallem Fonds (HM). (I am indebted to Helen Mussallem for sharing her private letters.)

122　Helen Mussallem to "Mother and family," 20 Oct. 1966, HM.

123　Lyle Creelman, "How Can Nursing Meet the Challenges of Expanding Health Services, Traveling Seminar on Nursing, USSR," 6–8 Oct. 1966, 1–4 (PA/66.181), WHO/OMS Library.

124　Ibid., 7.

125　For a more detailed elaboration of these ideas, see ibid., 7–10.

126　*Report of the Traveling Seminar on Nursing in the USSR* (Geneva, 1967), 6–8 Oct. 1966, 18, WHO/NURS/67.77, WHO/OMS Library.

127　Ibid., 21.

128　Lyle Creelman to Helen Mussallem, 7 Dec. 1966, file 25-22, vol. 25, R-8293, LAC.

129　See, for example, a range of correspondence dealing with gifts received and hospitality extended by Creelman or advice sought on potential WHO candidates: Helen Mussallem to Lyle Creelman 5 Dec. 1963; Helen Mussallem to Lyle Creelman, 1 Mar. 1965; and Helen Mussallem to Lyle Creelman, 3 Aug. 1968, file 7-13, R 8293-0-4-E HM, LAC. See also "CNA Executive Director in West Indies," 767.

130　Helen Mussallem to "Dear Mother and family," 14 Oct. 1966, file 13, box 7, HM, LAC.

131　Helen Mussallem to Lyle Creelman, 22 Nov. 1966, file 13, box 7, R 8293-0-4-E, HM, LAC.

132　Lyle Creelman to Helen Mussallem, 24 Jan. 1967, file 13, box 7, R 8293, HM, LAC. See also Creelman to Mussallem, 7 Dec. 1966, file 13, box 7, R 8293-0-4-E, HM, LAC. Years later, Dame Sheila Quinn remained unconvinced that the seminar had been a success. Dame Sheila Quinn, interview with Susan Armstrong-Reid.

133　Lyle Creelman to Prescott and Frieda Creelman, 3 Jan. 1952, file 3-3, box 3, LC, UBC.

134　Lyle Creelman to Dr Anderson, 15 May 1952, file 3-3, box 3, LC, UBC.

135　Journals 1939–1952, 14 Mar. 1954, file 2-3, box 2, LC, UBC.

136　Journals 1939–1952, 11–12 Jan. 1956, file 2-3, box 2, LC, UBC.

137　Ibid.

138　Ibid., 9 Feb. 1959.

139　Lyle Creelman's handwritten diary, Dec.–Jan. 1961, file 5-3, box 5, LC, UBC.

140　Nursing – Co-ordination with the International Council of Nurses, N2-372-4, WHOHQ, WHO/OMS.

141　Lyle Creelman's handwritten diary, 19 May 1962, file 5-3, box 5, LC, UBC.

142　Ibid.

143 Ibid., 26–9 July 1962.

144 Ibid., 5 Sept. 1961.

145 Lyle Creelman, interview with Kay Dier.

146 Lyle Creelman to Ruth Freeman, 3 July 1963, file 6, box 2, Ruth Freeman Papers, BUHGARC.

11. A Chance for Retrospection, 1968

1 See the discussion of the debates over family planning that nearly proved fatal to the organization and perhaps Chisholm's career in Farley, *Brock Chisholm*, 173–84.

2 "Report of Visit to African Region," 8, file 4-3, box 4, LC, UBC.

3 Lyle Creelman's handwritten diary, 7 June 1964, 1961–9, file 5-3, box 5, LC, UBC.

4 Trained at the Royal Jubilee School of Nursing and a graduate of UBC (1936), Hodgson had served as the assistant superintendent of nurses and then director at the Tranquille Sanatorium and later still as the assistant supervisor of the Vancouver Unit, TB Division, before joining the WHO.

5 For a more extensive discussion of the politics of African development in the 1960s, see Grubbs, *Secular Missionaries*.

6 Notes for a speech, n.d., file 2-7, box 2, LC, UBC.

7 "Visit to Kenya: 26 February–2 March 1968," 13, file 4-3, box 4, LC, UBC.

8 Ibid.

9 Grubbs, *Secular Missionaries*, 74.

10 "Report of Visit to Congo-Kinshasa," 6, file 4-3, box 4, LC, UBC.

11 "Visit to Regional Office," 4, file 4-3, box 4, LC, UBC.

12 In the latter country, Dr Kwame Nkrumah had been ousted by a military coup in February 1966 and Creelman was now scheduled to meet the new head of state, Lieutenant-General Joseph Arthur Ankrah, who had been the first commander of the Ghanaian army.

13 "Visit to Ghana," 3–4, file 4-3, box 4, LC, UBC.

14 Chittick helped launch the first two-year basic nursing program in Canada. As director of the McGill School of Graduate Nurses from 1953 to 1963, she set up a master's program as well as a basic nursing course leading to a BSc in nursing. For additional information on her achievements, see "Nursing Profiles," *Canadian Nurse* 59, no. 8 (1963): 743.

15 Opare and Mill, "Evolution of Nursing Education."

16 Barbara Darbyshire Bubb, interview with Susan Armstrong-Reid, 21 Aug. 2007, East Marden, U.K.

17 "Visit to Ghana," 3, file 4-3, box 4, LC, UBC.

18 Ibid., 3–4.

19 "Report of Visit to African Region," 4, file 4-3, box 4, LC, UBC. See also "Visit to Ghana: 15–19 March 1968," 1, file 4-3, box 4, LC, UBC. See also Lyle Creelman's handwritten diary, file 5-3, box 5, LC, UBC.
20 Lyle Creelman's handwritten diary, file 5-3, box 5, LC, UBC.
21 The nursing consultant chosen by Lyle Creelman, Rae Chittick, shared her view in this respect. Opare and Mill, "Evolution of Nursing Education"; Chittick, "Post-Basic Nursing in Ghana."
22 Kay Dier, interview with Susan Armstrong-Reid.
23 See Agbese, "Maintaining Power"; Akinsanya, *An African "Florence Nightingale."*
24 This project was also financially supported by the Rockefeller Foundation, which funded the construction of a modern, spacious, and architecturally beautiful building, and UNICEF, which provided equipment, supplies, salary supplements, and stipends.
25 Lyle Creelman's handwritten diary, 15 Mar. 1968, file 5-3, box 5, LC, UBC. See also Field Diaries, 1967 and 1968, Mary Abbott Private Papers (MA), for a more detailed account of the stand-off over the appointment of counterparts.
26 See Diary, 19 Mar. 1968, 1968, MA: "Not a specially pleasant faculty meeting. I wish I were more able to foster some kind of unity among the WHO team." In Abbott's view, certain members of the team saw themselves as faculty members, not WHO representatives. See Diary, 25 July 1968.
27 Lyle Creelman's handwritten journal, 15 Mar. 1968, file 5-3, box 5, LC, UBC.
28 Ibid., 14.
29 "Report of Visit to African Region," 12, file 4-3, box 4, LC, UBC. See also "Visit to Kenya," 9, file 4-3, box 4, LC, UBC.
30 Lyle Creelman's handwritten diary, 3 Mar. 1968, 1961–9, file 5-3, box 5, LC, UBC.
31 Ibid., 3 Mar. 1968.
32 "Report of Visit to African Region," 12, file 4-3, box 4, LC, UBC. For a somewhat more cautious opinion of the work done, see "Visit to Ghana," 6, file 4-3, box 4, LC, UBC.
33 "Visit to Ghana," 6, file 4-3, box 4, LC, UBC.
34 "Visit to Niger: 21–25 March 1968," file 4-3, box 4, LC, UBC.
35 Ibid.
36 Ibid.
37 "Visit to Dakar," 3, file 4-3, box 4, LC, UBC.
38 Ibid., 5.
39 Ibid., 6.
40 Ibid., 7.
41 Ibid., 6.
42 Lyle Creelman's handwritten diary, 15 Apr. 1968, 1961–9, file 5-3, box 5, LC, UBC.
43 Ibid.
44 Ibid., 6 Jan. 1964.

45 Ibid., end of 1967.
46 Lyle Creelman to Helen Mussallem, 31 Oct. 1968, file 7-13, HM, LAC.
47 "From the Executive Desk, Lyle Creelman – An Appreciation," *ICN Calling* 9 (Oct. 1968): 1, file 1-7, box 1, LC, UBC.
48 Lyle Creelman to Helen Mussallem, 7 Nov. 1968, file 7-13, HM, LAC.
49 Lyle Creelman to Helen Mussallem, 4 Nov. 1968, file 7-13, HM, LAC.
50 Lyle Creelman's handwritten diary, 6 Oct. 1968, 1961–9, file 5-3, box 5, LC, UBC.
51 When the first World Health Assembly met in Geneva in June 1948 and formally created the World Health Organization, the Office Internationale d'Hygiène Publique, the League of Nations Health Organization, and UNRRA merged into the new agency.
52 Irving, *Brock Chisholm*, 91.
53 For an overview of the position of chief nursing officer in the immediate post-war period, see Splane and Huffman Splane, *Chief Nursing Officer Positions*, 96–106.
54 Madelaine Healey's recent work has offered a more critical view of the WHO's efforts in developing nursing programs in India, efforts that "attempted to institutionalise the values and infrastructure of the nurse professionalism that had evolved in the early twentieth century North America." She argues that focusing on professionalism diverted attention from the underlying social-economic systemic factors that hindered the sustainable indigenous development of nursing within the Indian health-care system. See "'I'm the Gal That Can Do It If They Let Me.'"
55 Tennant's, Brackett's, and Arnold's assistance was frequently sought to recruit and screen prospective WHO staff. See, for examples, Elizabeth Brackett, 29 June 1950, Officers Diaries, 12.1, file 1950–1951, box 20, RF, RFAC; Interviews: VA, 21–2 Mar. 1962, file 2, box 1, VA, BUHGARC.
56 My thinking has been influenced by Peter Haas's work analysing their shared values, causal beliefs, and notions of validating knowledge as well as their contribution to the emergence and character of cooperation at the international level. See Hass, "Epistemic Communities and International Policy Coordination."
57 For a more detailed analysis see Keck and Sikkink, "Transnational Advocacy Networks in International Politics."
58 "Public Health Nursing," 81, file 4-9, box 4, LC, UBC.
59 M. Lourdes [Verderese] to Lyle Creelman, 3 Dec. 1962, file 3-5, box 3, LC, UBC.
60 Elizabeth Hill [regional nursing adviser] to Lyle Creelman, 2 May 1955, file 3-3, box 3, LC, UBC. Well-used copies of all five of the expert committee on nursing reports are contained in the private papers of Evelyn Matheson and of the regional nursing adviser. Mary Abbott, both in interviews and in her private memoir, cited the expert committee reports as a source for the principles of curriculum development. Mary Abbott, interview with Susan Armstrong-Reid, 25 and 27 June 2007, St Andrews, Fife, Scotland.
61 Elizabeth Hill to Lyle Creelman, 2 May 1955, file 3-3, box 3, LC, UBC.

62 Lyle Creelman, interview with Kay Dier, Vancouver, 27 May 1985, KD.
63 WP/RC7/5, Part I, WPRO, WHO Archives.
64 Miscellaneous Notes, "Nursing around the World," 4, LC, UBC. See also Katherine
    Lyman to Lyle Creelman, 22 Oct. 1958, file 3-4, box 3, LC, UBC. Many WHO
    nurses made similar comments on teaching students or working with their
    counterparts.
65 VA Officer's diary, interviews 7–8 Dec. 1960, 12.2, file 1960, box 3, RF, RFA.
66 Creelman, "Nursing around the World"; Creelman, "Draft Item for the Canadian
    Nurse" (Mar. issue), file 4-2, box 4, LC, UBC.
67 Creelman, "Nursing around the World."
68 "Draft Item for the Canadian Nurse" (Mar. issue), file 4-2, box 4, LC, UBC.
69 My thinking about an alternative feminine perspective on power has been influ-
    enced by Peterson and Runyan, *Global Gender Issues in the New Millennium*
    (quotation is on p. 50).
70 Ingrid Nyman, "Assignment Report, Nursing Education, Chittagong (East
    Pakistan), August 1963–June 1965," Aug. 1965, Pakistan 4401, Project file, WHO/
    OMS.
71 Assistance to Institute of Nursing-Medical College, Calcutta, Final Report
    Midwifery, 1955, India 19, Project file, WHO/OMS.
72 See, for example, "Nursing around the World," 816, LC, UBC.
73 Dorothy Cox Final Report on Assistance in Nursing Given to the Christian
    Medical College, Ludhiana, Punjab, India, 30 April 1958, Final Report, Nursing
    Training Project, Ludhiana, India 381953-1958, Project files, WHO/OMS.
74 Creelman, "Nursing in the World."
75 Creelman, "Lyle Creelman Writes," *Canadian Nurse* 47, no. 3 (1951): 181.
76 Creelman, "UN Needs Nurses."
77 Ibid.
78 Quoted in Creelman, "The Seventh Nursing Mirror Lecture," 4, file 4-1, box 4, LC,
    UBC.
79 Creelman, Chagnas, and Arnold, "WHO and Professional Nursing," 448.
80 Ibid., 449.
81 Miscellaneous Notes for a Speech, "What Is Nursing?," LC, UBC.
82 Working Conference on Nursing Education, WHO, Technical Report Series,
    no. 60, 18.
83 WHO, "Postbasic Nursing Education Programmes for Foreign Students: Report
    on A Conference, Geneva, 5–14 Oct. 1958," World Health Organization Technical
    Reports Series 199 (Geneva: WHO, 1960).
84 See Healey, "Seeds That May Have Been Planted May Take Root." Healey's assess-
    ment of the WHO position, based on secondary sources, excludes Creelman's
    views.

85 Quoted in Creelman, "The Seventh Nursing Mirror Lecture," 5, file 4-1, box 4, LC, UBC.
86 Creelman, "Nursing in the World," 819.
87 Miscellaneous Notes for a Speech, "World Health," Richmond PTA, 12 Mar. 1953, LC, UBC.
88 "In relation to health, a rights-based approach means integrating human rights norms and principles in the design, implementation, monitoring, and evaluation of health-related policies and programmes. These include human dignity, attention to the needs and rights of vulnerable groups, and an emphasis on ensuring that health systems are made accessible to all. The principle of equality and freedom from discrimination is central, including discrimination on the basis of sex and gender roles. Integrating human rights into development also means empowering poor people, ensuring their participation in decision-making processes which concern them and incorporating accountability mechanisms which they can access." WHO, "Human Rights-Based Approach to Health."
89 WHO, *Third Ten Years of the World Health Organization*, 1.
90 "Report of the International Conference on Primary Health Care, Alma Ata, USSR, 6–12 September 1978" (Geneva: WHO, 1978).
91 WHO, *Third Ten Years of the World Health Organization*, 2.
92 Several scholars have used the notion of "hybridity" within the "contact zone" (a social space where cultures meet, clash and accommodate each other, often in the context of asymmetrical relations of power), to situate women's agency experience within the broader landscape of colonial and imperial history. Pickles and Rutherdale, *Contact Zones*; Aschcroft, Griffiths, and Tiffin, *Key Concepts in Postcolonial Studies*.
93 Scholars have noted that American and other international health-care agencies' aspirations to cultural hegemony ushered in a new era of imperialism. John Farley contends that the U.S. drive to contain communism within the former colonies distorted the WHO's policy priorities, favouring the bio-medical model. Madeline Healy raises doubts as to whether the system of elite nursing education introduced in India was suited to needs of a country emerging from colonialism. Both offer important perspectives, but not a complete picture. See Farley, *Brock Chisholm*; and Healey, "'I'm the Gal That Can Do It If They Let Me.'"

Epilogue, 1968–2007

1 Lyle Creelman to Helen K. Mussallem, 4 Nov. 1968, R-8293, file 7-13, vol. 25 HM, LAC.
2 Hopper, "Miss Lyle Creelman."
3 M.G. Candau to Lyle Creelman, 22 Aug. 1968, file 3-6, box 3, LC, UBC.

4 Dorothy Hall to Lyle Creelman, 26 Aug. 1968, file 3-6, box 3, LC, UBC.
5 Genevieve Richardson to Lyle Creelman, 8 July 1968, file 3-6, box 3, LC, UBC.
6 Mary Abbott to Lyle Creelman, 15 Aug. 1968, file 3-6, box 3, LC, UBC.
7 Virginia Arnold to Lyle Creelman, 7 Aug. 1968, file 3-6, box 3, LC, UBC. See also
   I.M. Lovedee to Lyle Creelman, 21 Aug. 1968.
8 M.G. Candau to Lyle Creelman, 22 Aug. 1968, file 3-6, box 3, LC, UBC.
9 Lyle Creelman to Helen Mussallem, Apr. 1968, R-8293, file 7-13, vol. 25, HN, LAC.
10 Lyle Creelman to Helen Mussallem, 4 Nov., R-8293, file 7-13, vol. 25, HN, LAC.
11 Helen K. Mussallem to Lyle Creelman, 23 Aug. 1968, file 3-6, box 3, LC, UBC; Lyle
   Creelman to Helen K. Mussallem, 14 Aug. 1968.
12 Lyle Creelman's handwritten journal (1961–9), 23 Jan. 1969, file 5-3, box 5, LC,
   UBC.
13 Ibid., 31 Oct. 1968.
14 Lyle Creelman to Helen K. Mussallem, 10 Jan. 1969, R-8293, file 7-13, box 25, HM,
   LAC.
15 Ibid.
16 Lyle Creelman's handwritten journal (1961–9), 23 Jan. 1969, file 5-3, box 5,
   LC, UBC.
17 Journals 1969–1983, 24 Apr. 1969, file 2-6, box 2, LC, UBC.
18 Ibid., 3 May 1969.
19 An epidemiologist, Hugh Russell had worked for the World Health Organization
   in its early days, initially in the eastern Mediterranean and then in Southeast Asia.
   "Obituaries," *British Medical Journal*.
20 Organizational Chart, 1 Aug. 1969, Annexes, SEA/RC22/2, SEARO, WHO.
21 Journals 1969–1983, 25 May 1969, 1969, file 2-6, box 2, LC, UBC.
22 Ibid., 14 May 1969.
23 Ibid., 1 June 1969.
24 Ibid., 25 June 1969.
25 Ibid., 23 July 1969.
26 Ibid., 3 May 1969.
27 Ibid.
28 Ibid., 1 June 1969.
29 Ibid., 25 June 1969.
30 Ibid., 15 July 1969.
31 See Cueto, *Value of Health*.
32 Diary of 1973 ICN trip, "Miscellaneous Notes by Lyle Creelman," file 2-7, box 2,
   LC, UBC.
33 Lillian Turnbull, interview with Kay Dier, 15 June 1989, KD.
34 Ibid.

35 Bea (Salmon) to Lyle Creelman, 21 June 1970, file 3-7, box 3, LC, UBC.
36 Lyle Creelman, Christmas greeting to friends, Christmas 1970, file 3-7, box 3, LC, UBC.
37 Verna Huffman Splane's contributions to the nursing profession were recognized through the RNABC Award of Merit (1987), the Order of Canada (1996), the Queen's Silver Jubilee Medal and Gold Jubilee Medal (1977, 2002), the Jeanne Mance Award (1982), the Canadian Red Cross Distinguished Service Award (1975), the Lillian Carter Center for International Nursing Award (shared with her husband Richard) (2001), and the Emily Gleason Sargent Award (date unknown).
38 Journals 1969–1983, 16 May 1982, 21 Sept. 1983, 30 Apr. 1983, 1979–83, file 2-6, box 2, LC, UBC.
39 Ibid., 7 May 1981.
40 Journals 1969–1983, 5 Apr. 1974, file 2-6, box 2, LC, UBC.
41 Verna Huffman Splane, interview with Susan Armstrong-Reid, 15 Apr. 2008, Vancouver.
42 UBC, http://www.library.ubc.ca/archives/hdcites/hdcites10.html.
43 Lyle Creelman, "Season's Greetings," 1971, file 2-6, box 2, LC, UBC.
44 Verna Huffman Splane, interview with Susan Armstrong-Reid.
45 Lyle Creelman, interview with Kay Dier, Vancouver, 27 May 1985, KD.
46 Melchior, "Feminist Approaches to Nursing History," 346.
47 Journals 1969–1983, 23 Aug. 1971, file 2-6, box 2, LC, UBC.
48 Lyle Creelman, Christmas greeting to friends, Christmas 1970, file 3-7, box 3, LC, UBC.
49 Eleanor Hill and Louise Brooks, interview Susan Armstrong-Reid, May 2007, Hollyburn House, Vancouver. Both had been part of Lyle's bridge group in Vancouver and on Bowen Island.
50 Journals 1969–1983, 3 Apr. 1975, 1974–9, file 2-6, box 2, LC, UBC; 12 Feb. 1979, 1979–83, file 2-6, box 2, LC, UBC.
51 Journals 1969–1983, 3 Oct. 1977, 1974–9, file 2-6, box 2, LC, UBC.
52 Ibid., 29 Nov. 1977.
53 Journals 1969–1983, 4 Mar. 1979, 1979–83, file 2-6, box 2, LC, UBC. See also 25 May 1980.
54 Creelman, "Season's Greetings," 1971, file 3-7, box 3,.LC, UBC.
55 Journals 1969–1983, 18 Mar. 1975, 1974–9, file 2-6, box 2, LC, UBC.
56 Ibid., 11 Feb. 1974, 24 Oct. 1974.
57 Ibid., 4 Sept. 1975.
58 Ibid., 26 Sept. 1975.
59 Her journal noted that the decision to buy the property was taken in early December 1976. Ibid., 9 Dec. 1976, 14 Jan. 1977. A subsequent journal entry on

20 Jan. 1977 noted, "Meeting of Historians. Good turn out: First report of purchase of property." Creelman's record dates this purchase three years after other informal accounts compiled by the Bowen Island Historians.

60　Minutes of the directors meeting, 8 Sept. 1975, Bowen Island Historians, Bowen Island Museum and Archives.

61　Minutes of directors meeting, 28 Nov. 1978, Bowen Island Historians, Bowen Island Museum and Archives.

62　Journals 1969–1983, 21 Feb. 1979, 1979–83, file 2-6, box 2, LC, UBC.

63　Ibid., 7 June 1980.

64　Lyle Creelman, "Dear Katherine," 30 Nov. 1973, file 3-7, box 3, LC, UBC.

65　Ibid.

66　Lyle Creelman, Christmas letter, Dec. 1978, file 3-7, box 3, LC, UBC.

67　Louise Brooks, interview with Susan Armstrong-Reid.

68　Journals 1969–1983, 21 July 1980, file 2-6, box 2, LC, UBC.

69　Ibid., 2 Mar. 1981.

70　Ibid., 4 June 1981.

71　Ibid., 20 Apr. 1982.

72　Ibid., 3 Feb. 1983.

73　Ibid., 7 Feb. 1983.

74　Ibid.

75　Ibid.

76　Lyle Creelman, Christmas letter, 1983, file 3-8, box 3, LC, UBC.

77　Ibid.

78　Ibid.

79　Correspondence by e-mail with Glennis Zilm providing an account of Lyle Creelman's memorial tea, 15 Mar. 2007.

80　I am indebted to one of the external readers of this manuscript for bringing this point to my attention.

81　Fairman, "History for the Future (of Nursing)"; CNA, *Toward 2020: Visions for Nursing.*

82　An important work, from a feminist, international-relations perspective, on this subject is Peterson and Runyan, *Global Gender Issues in the New Millennium.* The authors argue that, without deconstructing the "power of gender," the contemporary crises of "reproduction, resources and security" will not be resolved. The third edition of this book stimulated my thinking on the historical antecedents of the contemporary struggle for social justice, including gender equality.

83　WHO, *Global Strategy for Health for All by the Year 2000.*

84　Kirton and Mannell argue that the G-8 might be better positioned than the WHO of old to take the lead in the field of global-health governance: "The G8 and Global Health Governance," 115–46. See also Osterholm, "Preparing for the Next

Pandemic." The challenges faced in international transcultural nursing and the wider debate being waged within the contemporary nursing world bear striking parallels to bygone days. See Gennaro, "The Past 25 Years and Beyond."

85 For a fuller discussion, see Iriye, *Global Community*.
86 Kickbusch and de Leeuw, "Global Public Health," 287.
87 Chan makes this case in "Cross-cultural Civility," 232–52. See also Kickbusch and de Leeuw, "Global Public Health," which argues that allowing non-government actors into new networks was an important step in developing the frameworks required to reconcile national health sovereignty with globalization.
88 The Nightingale Initiative for Global Health is a grassroots, nurse-inspired movement to raise global public awareness about the priority of health and to empower nurses and concerned citizens to stand for a healthy world everywhere.
89 This organization strengthens people's health movements around the globe by organizing and supporting a variety of learning, sharing, and planning opportunities for activists.

Bibliography

Archival Sources

Boston University, Howard Gotlieb Archival Research Center, Boston

Virginia Arnold Fonds
Margaret Arnstein Fonds
Ruth Freeman Fonds
Marion Murphy Fonds

Bowen Island Museum and Archives, BC

Bowen Island Historians Fonds

BC History of Nursing Society, UBC, Vancouver

Margaret Murray Campbell Jackson Fonds
Ester Paulson Fonds
Alice Wright Fonds

City of Richmond Archives, Richmond, BC

City of Richmond Directories, 1924–8

City of Vancouver Archives

Medical Health Officers Annual Report of the Greater Vancouver
    Metropolitan Health Committee

College of Registered Nurses of British Columbia, Vancouver

BIOGRAPHICAL FILES
Elizabeth Breeze
Margaret Campbell
Lyle Creelman
Beverly Witter DuGas
Grace M. Fairley
Helen May Gemeroy
Eleanor Scott Graham
Mabel Gray
Mary E. Henderson
Lorna May Horwood
Treena Hunter
Nan Kennedy
Margaret E. Kerr
Heather Kilpatrick
Eleanor Kunderman
Geraldine Langton (Homfray)
Ruth Morrison
Frances McQuarrie
Helen Kathleen Mussallem
Eva Moody (Billie) Williamson

MEMORIAL BOOK
Treena Hunter
Heather Kilpatrick
Frances McQuarrie

ORAL HISTORY INTERVIEWS
Lyle Creelman, 3 July 1987, by Audrey Stegen
Beverly DuGas, 1987
Mary Henderson, 27 April 1988, by Audrey Stegen
Treena Hunter, March 1987, by Sheila Zerr, transcribed 26 March 1993 by
    Ethel Warbinek
Geraldine Langton (Homfray), August 1988 (tape no. 120 and transcript)
F.A. (Nan) Kennedy, January 1987, by S. Coates
Eleanor Kunderman, 26 October 1987, by Audrey Stegen

REGISTERED NURSES OF BRITISH COLUMBIA FONDS
Minute books

Harvard University, Schlesinger Library, Boston

Peplau Hildegard Papers

Library and Archives Canada, Ottawa

GOVERNMENT RECORDS
Department of External Affairs
Health Services and Promotions Branch
Office of the Chief Nursing Consultant, Department of Health and Welfare

PRIVATE PAPERS
Canadian Nurses Association
Frank and Libbie Park
Victorian Order of Nurses for Canada

National Archives, Washington

GOVERNMENT RECORDS
United States Public Health Service

PRIVATE PAPERS
Mary Abbott
Elizabeth Barton
Joan Bentley
Mardi Brown
Kay Dier
Beverly DuGas
Evelyn Matheson
Margaret McLean
Helen Mussallem
Edna Osborne Private Family Papers
Helena Reimer
Eva Moody Williamson

Queen's University Archives, Kingston, Ontario

John Alexander Edmison Fonds

Revelstoke Museum and Archives, BC

Revelstoke Review

Rockefeller Foundation Archives, Sleepy Hollow, New York

MINUTES AND ANNUAL REPORTS

ROCKEFELLER FOUNDATION FONDS
Elizabeth Brackett Fonds
Fellowship Recorder Cards
R.R. Struthers Fonds
Mary Elizabeth Tennant Fonds

Royal College of Nursing, Edinburgh

ORAL HISTORY INTERVIEW
Mary Abbott

United Nations Archive, New York

UNRRA

University of British Columbia, Rare Books and Special Collections, Vancouver

Totem

UBC Undergraduate Calendar

Ubyssey

University of British Columbia Undergraduate Calendars

University of British Columbia Archives, Vancouver

PRIVATE PAPERS
Lyle Creelman Fonds
Mabel F. Gray Fonds

SCHOOL OF NURSING FONDS
Minutes of the Science Girls Clubs

*University of New Brunswick, Harriet Irving
Library, Archives and Special Collections*

Faculty of Nursing
Presidents Papers

University of Toronto Archives

Margaret M. Allemang Centre for the History of Nursing Fonds
University of Toronto, School of Nursing

Vancouver General Hospital Archives

Vancouver General Hospital Annual Report

World Health Organization

Development Programme (Geneva, June 1998)
Former WHO Nurses Remember: Stories from the Field (Geneva: World
   Health Systems)

NURSING NEWS
UNRRA Fonds

WHO CHRONICLE
WHO Fonds

WHO NEWSLETTER

Correspondence and Interviews

Mary Abbott
Elizabeth Barton
Louise Brooks
Margaret Cammaert
Lois Myers Carter
Kay Creelman
Lyle Creelman
Barbara Bubb Darbyshire
Graham Dawson
Kay Dier
Joan Dorrie
Beverly DuGas
Dorothy Hall
Eleanor Hill
Helen Mussallem
Leith Nance
Lorna Creelman Nauss

Rudi and Patricia North
Dame Sheila Quinn
Sonja Sanguinetti
Verna Huffman Splane
Shirley Stinson
Eva Moody Williamson

Secondary Sources

"A Tribute to Our Editor and Executive Director on Her Retirement: Margaret E. Kerr." *Canadian Nurse* 61, no. 9 (1963): 705–7.

Abrams, Sarah Elise. "Seeking Jurisdiction: A Sociological Perspective on Rockefeller Foundation Activities in Nursing in the 1920's." In *Nursing History and the Politics of Welfare*, edited by Anne Marie Rafferty, Jane Robinson, and Ruth Elkan, 207-225 New York: Routledge, 2007.

Agbese, Aje-Ori. "Maintaining Power in the Face of Political, Economic and Social Discrimination: The Tale of Nigerian Women." *Women and Language*, 22 Mar. 2003. http://www.highbeam.com

Akinsanya, Justus A. *An African "Florence Nightingale": A Biography of Chief (Dr) Mrs Kofoworola Abeni Pratt*. Ibadan: Vintage Publishers, 1987.

Alves Diniz, Fernanda. "WHO's European Program in Nursing." *International Nursing Review* (Apr. 1958): 17–18.

Alvim, Ermengarda M. J de F. "The Visitadora Sanitá: A Brazilian Approach to the Use of Auxiliary Public Health Workers; Aspects of Public Health Nursing." World Health Organization Public Health Papers, no. 4 (Geneva: WHO, 1961).

Amrith, Sunil. "Aspects of the Social History of Medicine: Political Culture of Health in India; A Historical Perspective." *Economic and Political Weekly*, Jan. 2007, 13.

Araki, Iyro. "Nursing in Japan: Its Origins and Development." *American Journal of Nursing* 28, no. 10 (1928): 1003–6.

Armstrong-Reid, Susan. "'Go Anywhere Do Anything': Nursing with the Friends Ambulance Unit, China Convoy." Paper presented to Canadian Association for the History of Nursing, 2011.

Armstrong-Reid, Susan, and David Murray. *Armies of Peace: Canada and the UNRRA Years*. Toronto: University of Toronto Press, 2008.

Ascher, Charles S. "Current Problems in the World Health Organization's Program." *International Organization* 6, no. 1 (Feb. 1952): 27. http://dx.doi.org/10.1017/S0020818300016179.

Ashcroft, Bill Gareth Griffiths, and Helen Tiffin. *Key Concepts in Post-colonial Studies*. London: Routledge, 2000.

"Association News: Dr A. Helen Martikainen Receives 1978 APHA International Award for Excellence." *American Journal of Public Health* 69, no. 1 (1979): 92.

Audibert, M. "Fighting Poverty and Disease in an Integrated Approach." *Bulletin of the World Health Organization* 84, no. 2 (2006).

Baggallay, Olive. "Our Nurses Serve the World." *Canadian Nurse* 50, no. 4 (Apr. 1954): 281–3. Medline:13150300.

"Nursing in the World Health Organization." *International Nursing Bulletin* 6, no. 1 (1950): 9–10.

Bandy, J., and J. Smith. "Factors Affecting Conflict and Cooperation in Transnational Social Movement Networks." In *Coalitions across Borders: Transnational Protest and the Neoliberal Order*, edited by J. Bandy and J. Smith, 129–31 Lanham, MD: Rowman and Littlefield, 2005.

Barton, Elizabeth. "Notes from the Field: Maternal and Child Health in the 1950's and 1960's." *World Health Forum* 19 (1998): 19.

"BC Nurse Pleads for Refugees." *News-Herald* (Vancouver), 21 Nov. 1946.

Beigbeder, Yves, Mahyar Nashat, Marie-Antoinette Orsini, and J.F. Tiercy. *The World Health Organization*. Geneva: Societa italiana per l'organizzazione internazionale / Graduate Institute of International Studies, 1998.

Berkov, R. *The World Health Organization: A Study in Decentralized International Administration*. Geneva: Librairie E. Droz, 1957.

Betten, Patricia Van, and Melisa Moriarty. *Nursing Illuminations: A Book of Days*. St Louis, MO: Mosby, 2004.

Birth, Edith. "Report of the Labour Relations Committee." *Canadian Nurse* 40, no. 9 (1944): 693–5.

Boschma, Geertje. "Ambivalence about Nursing's Expertise: The Role of Gendered Holistic Ideology, 1890–1990." In *Nursing History and the Politics of Welfare*, edited by Anne Marie Rafferty, June Robinson, and Ruth Elkan, 164–76. New York: Routledge, 2007.

– "A Family Point of View: Negotiating Asylum Care in Alberta, 1905–1930." *CBMH/BCHM* 25, no. 2 (2008): 367–89.

– "Writing International Nursing History: What Does It Mean?" *Nursing History Review* 16, no. 1 (2008): 9–12. http://dx.doi.org/10.1891/1062-8061.16.9. Medline:18595338.

Bothwell, Robert. *Alliance and Illusions: Canada and the World, 1945–1984*. Vancouver: UBC Press, 2007.

Brockington, Colin Fraser. *World Health*. London: Penguin Books, 1958.

Broe, Ellen. "Florence Nightingale International Foundation." *AARN* (Alberta Association of Registered Nurses), 1952.

Bolduan, Charles. "Haven Emerson: the Public Health Statesman." *American Journal of Public Health Nations Health* 40, no. 1 (1950): 1–4.

Brush, Barbara L., Joan E. Lynaugh, and Geertje Boschma, eds. *Nurses of All Nations: A History of the International Council of Nurses, 1899–1999*. New York: Lippincott, 1999.

Buhler-Wilkerson, Karen. "Bringing Care to the People: Lillian Wald's Legacy to Public Health Nursing." *American Journal of Public Health* 83, no. 12 (Dec. 1993): 1778–86. http://dx.doi.org/10.2105/AJPH.83.12.1778. Medline:7695663.

Burns, Anne. "The Eleventh World Health Assembly: A Report by the Nurse Adviser to the United States Delegation." *American Journal of Nursing* 58, no. 9 (Sept. 1958): 1278–9. Medline:13559311.

Calhoun, Eva D. "Public Health Activities in the Province of British Columbia." *Public Health Nurse* 14 (June 1922): 334–41.

Canadian Nurses Association. *Toward 2020: Visions for Nursing*. Ottawa: CNA, 2006.

"Canadian Nurses in UNRRA." *Canadian Nurse* 40, no. 10 (1944): 240–2.

Canadian Public Health Association. *Report of the Study Committee on Public Health Practice in Canada*. Toronto: CPHA, 1950.

Candau, M.G. "World Health Catalysts." *American Journal of Public Health and the Nation's Health* 47, no. 6 (June 1957): 675–81. http://dx.doi.org/10.2105/AJPH.47.6.675. Medline:13424811.

Cassidy, Harry. *Social Security and Reconstruction in Canada*. Toronto: Ryerson, 1943.

Caughley, Jill. *Sixty Years of Collaboration: International Council of Nurses and the World Health Organization*. Geneva: ICN, 2009.

Chan, Stephanie. "Cross-Cultural Civility in Global Civil Society: Transnational Cooperation in Chinese NGOs." *Global Net World* 8, no. 2 (2008): 232–52. http://dx.doi.org/10.1111/j.1471-0374.2008.00193.x.

Charles, J. "Origins, History and Achievements of the World Health Organization." *British Medical Journal* 2 (4 May 1968): 293–6.

Christy, Teresa E. *Cornerstone for Nursing Education: A History of Nursing Education at Teachers College, Columbia University 1899–1947*. New York: Teachers College Press, 1969.

Chittick, Rae "Post-Basic Nursing in Ghana." *International Journal of Nursing Studies* 2 no. 1 (Aug. 1965): 39–42.

Choy, Catherine Ceniza. *Empire of Care: Nursing and Migration I Filipino American History*. Durham, NC: Duke University Press, 2003.

"City Nurse Appointed Chief." *Province*, 8 Apr. 1954.

Clarke, Emma de V. "Mental Hygiene in Public Health Nursing." *Canadian Nurse* 27, no. 9 (1931): 451–7.

Clarke, Harvey. "Mental Hygiene for Nurses." *Canadian Nurse* 27, no. 2 (1931): 70–1.

Clarke, Nic. "Sacred Daemons: Exploring British Columbian Society's Perceptions of Mentally Deficient Children, 1870–1930." *BC Studies* 144 (Winter 2004/5): 61–89.

Comacchio, Cynthia. *"Nations Are Built for Care Saving": Ontario's Mothers and Children 1900–1940*. Montreal and Kingston: McGill-Queen's University Press, 1993.

Connolly, Cynthia A. "Nurses: The Early Twentieth-Century Tuberculosis Preventorium's 'Connecting Link.'" In *Nurses' Work: Issues across Time and Place*, edited by Patricia D'Antonio Ellen Baer, Sylvia Rinker, and Joan E. Lynaugh, 173–203. New York: Springer Publishing, 2007.

Copp, Terry. *Cinderella Army: The Canadians in Northwest Europe, 1944–1945*. Toronto: University of Toronto Press, 2006.

Craddock, Sally. *Retired Except on Demand: The Life of Dr Cicely Williams*. Oxford: Green College, 1983.

Creelman, Dave. *Stewiacke Valley Sketchbook to Commemorate the Stewiacke Valley Bicentennial, 1780–1980*. Printed by author, 1980.

Creelman, Lyle. "First Monthly Infant Weighing Station Held." *Revelstoke Review*, 19 Mar. 1937.

– "Guardian of World Health." *International Nursing Review* 15, no. 2 (1968): 101–10. Medline:5185773.

– Letter to the editor. *Canadian Nurse* 41, no. 6 (1945): 476–80.

– "Lyle Creelman Writes." *Canadian Nurse* 46, no. 6 (1950): 477–8.

– "Lyle Creelman Writes." *Canadian Nurse* 46, no. 7 (1950): 565–6.

– "Lyle Creelman Writes." *Canadian Nurse* 46, no. 8 (1950): 658–9.

– "Lyle Creelman Writes." *Canadian Nurse* 46, no. 9 (1950): 739–40.

– "Lyle Creelman Writes." *Canadian Nurse* 46, no. 10 (1950): 799–802.

– "Lyle Creelman Writes." *Canadian Nurse* 46, no. 11 (1950): 888–90.

– "Lyle Creelman Writes." *Canadian Nurse* 46, no. 12 (1950): 976–7.

– "Lyle Creelman Writes," *Canadian Nurse* 47, no. 1 (1951): 33–4.

– "Lyle Creelman Writes," *Canadian Nurse* 47, no. 3 (1951): 180–2.

– "Lyle Creelman Writes," *Canadian Nurse* 47, no. 4 (1951): 269–70.

– "Lyle Creelman Writes," *Canadian Nurse* 47, no. 5 (1951): 338–40.

– "Lyle Creelman Writes." *Canadian Nurse* 47, no. 7 (1951): 495–6.

– "Lyle Creelman Writes," *Canadian Nurse* 47, no. 8 (1951): 577–9.

– "Lyle Creelman Writes," *Canadian Nurse* 47, no. 10 (1951): 723–4.

– "Lyle Creelman Writes." *Canadian Nurse* 48, no. 1 (1952): 495–6.

– "Lyle Creelman Writes." *Canadian Nurse* 48, no. 2 (1952): 116–18.

– "Lyle Creelman Writes." *Canadian Nurse* 48, no. 4 (1952): 286–88. Medline:14916404.

– "Lyle Creelman Writes." *Canadian Nurse* 48, no. 6 (1952): 469–71.

– "Lyle Creelman Writes." *Canadian Nurse* 48, no. 10 (1952): 807–09.
– "Lyle Creelman Writes." *Canadian Nurse* 49, no. 1 (1953): 28–9.
– "Lyle Creelman Writes." *Canadian Nurse* 50, no. 8 (1954): 638–41.
– "Mental Hygiene in the Public Health Program." *Canadian Nurse* 36, no. 10 (1940): 679–84.
– "Nursing in the World Health Organization." *Canadian Nurse* 54, no. 9 (Sept. 1958): 814–9.
– "Protect Your Child from Diptheria." *Relevstoke Review*, 11 Sept. 1936.
– "Public School Health Report." *Revelstoke Review*, 19 Feb. 1937.
– "Quality Care in the Right Quantity." *International Nursing Review* 15, no. 2 (Apr. 1968): 102–12.
– "The Relationship between the World Health Organization and Professional Nursing." *International Nursing Review* 1, no. 1 (1954).
– "Report of the Public Health Section." *Canadian Nurse* 40, no. 9 (1944): 682–85.
– "Revelstoke Reflections." *Public Health Nurse's Bulletin* 2, no. 4 (1937): 11–14.
– "There Is No Change without Challenge." *Nursing Mirror,* repr. 7 and 14 May 1965.
– "Trends in Nursing and Public Health Having Implications for Health Visitors." *Journal of the Royal Society for the Promotion of Health* 75, no. 8 (1955): 602.
– "UN Needs Nurses to Aid Those in Other Countries." *Toronto Star*, Mar. 1954.
– "What Is Public Health Nursing?" *Canadian Nurse* 37, no. 2 (1941): 111–13.
– "What of the Future?" *Canadian Nurse* 39, no. 1 (1943): 35–8.
– "With UNRRA in Germany." *Canadian Nurse* 43, no. 7 (1947): 552–6.
– "With UNRRA in Germany." *Canadian Nurse* 43, no. 8 (1947): 605–10.
– "With UNRRA in Germany: Repatriation of DP's." *Canadian Nurse* 43, no. 9 (1947): 710–12.
Creelman, Lyle, Agnes W. Chagnas, and Virginia Arnold. "WHO and Professional Nursing." *American Journal of Nursing* 54, no. 4 (1954): 448–9.
Cueto, Marcos. "The Origins of Primary Health Care and Selective Primary Health Care." *American Journal of Public Health* 94, no. 11 (Nov. 2004): 1864–74. http://dx.doi.org/10.2105/AJPH.94.11.1864. Medline:15514221.
– *The Value of Health: History of the Pan American Health Organization*. Rochester, NY: University of Rochester Press, 2007.
D'Antonio, Patricia. *American Nursing: A History of Knowledge, Authority and the Meaning of Work*. Baltimore: Johns Hopkins University Press, 2010.
– "Preface." In *Nurses' Work: Issues across Time and Place*, edited by Patricia D'Antonio, Ellen Baer, Sylvia Rinker, and Joan E. Lynaugh, xv–xvii. New York: Springer Publishing, 2007.
– "Rethinking and Rewriting of Nursing History." *Bulletin of the History of Medicine* 73, no. 2 (1999): 268–90.

– "Thinking about Place: Researching and Reading the Global History of Nursing." *Texto & Conteto Enfermagem* 18, no. 4 (2009): 767–72.

D'Antonio, Patricia, Ellen Baer, Sylvia Rinker, and Joan E. Lynaugh. *Nurses' Work: Issues across Time and Place.* New York: Springer Publishing, 2007.

Davidson, Geo. A. "Mental Hygiene and Nursing." *Canadian Nurse* 25 (May 1929): 243–4.

Davies, Megan J. "Competent Professionals and Modern Methods: State Medicine in British Columbia during the 1930s." *Bulletin of the History of Medicine* 76, no. 1 (Spring 2002): 56–83. http://dx.doi.org/10.1353/bhm.2002.0016. Medline:11875244.

"Defends UNRRA Camps." *Daily Star* (Toronto), 13 June 1946.

Dehli, Kari. "Health Scouts for the State?" *Historical Studies in Education / Revue d'histoire de l'éducation* 2, no. 2 (1990): 247–64.

Dodd, Diane. "Nurses' Residence: Using the Built Environment as Evidence." *Nursing History Review* 9 (2001): 187.

Doherty, Muriel Knox. *Letters from Belsen 1945: An Australian Nurse's Experiences with the Survivors of War.* St Leonards, Australia: Allen and Unwin, 2000.

Donahue, M.P. "Isabel Maitland Stewart's Philosophy of Education." *Nursing Research* 32, no. 3 (May–June 1983): 140–6. http://dx.doi.org/10.1097/00006199-198305000-00003. Medline:6341966.

Dowbiggin, I. "Prescription for Survival: Brock Chisholm, Sterilization and Mental Health in the Cold War Era." In *Mental Health in Canadian Society: Historical Perspectives*, edited by J. Moran and D. Wright, 176–92. Montreal and Kingston: McGill-Queen's University Press, 2005.

"Dr Creelman Works to Quit." *Vancouver Sun*, 3 Jan. 1968.

Duranti, Marco. "Utopia, Nostalgia and the World War at the 1939–40 New York World's Fair." *Journal of Contemporary History* 41, no. 4 (2006): 663–83. http://dx.doi.org/10.1177/0022009406067749.

– "Editorials." *Canadian Nurse* 25, no. 11 (1929): 660–1.

Elliott, Jane, Meryn Stuart, and Cynthia Toman. *Place and Practice in Canadian Nursing History.* Vancouver: UBC Press, 2008.

Ellis, Kathleen. "Grace M. Fairley." *Canadian Nurse* 38, no. 6 (1942): 383–4.

– "Review of the *Modern Trend of Nursing Education*." *Canadian Nurse* 23, no. 2 (1927): 59–62.

Eschle, Catherine. *Global Democracy, Social Movements and Feminism.* New York: Basic Books, 2000.

Ewan, Mark, and John Blatherwick, eds. *History of Public Health in B.C.* Vancouver: FJB Air, 1980.

"Expert Committee on Nursing by [the] World Health Organization." *American Journal of Nursing* 52, no. 9 (1952): 1144.

Fairman, Julie. "Context and Contingency in the History of Post World War II Nursing Scholarship in the United States." *Journal of Nursing Scholarship* 40, no. 1 (2008): 4–11. http://dx.doi.org/10.1111/j.1547-5069.2007.00199.x. Medline:18302585.

– "History for the Future (of Nursing)." *Nursing History Review* 20, no. 1 (2012): 10–3. http://dx.doi.org/10.1891/1062-8061.20.10. Medline:22359996.

Falk-Rafael, Adeline. "Globalization and Global Health: Toward Nursing Praxis in the Global Community." *ANS: Advances in Nursing Science* 29, no. 1 (Jan.–Mar. 2006): 2–14. Medline:16495684.

Fairley, Grace M. "Report of Conference on University Courses in Nursing." *Canadian Nurse* 25, no. 3 (1928): 141–3.

Farley, John. *Brock Chisholm: The World Health Organization and the Cold War.* Vancouver: UBC Press, 2008.

Faville, Katharine. "The Second World Health Assembly." *American Journal of Nursing* 49, no. 12 (1949): 766–7.

Fennimore, Martha, and Kathryn Sikkink. "International Norm Dynamics and Political Change." In *Exploration and Contestation in the Study of World Politics,* edited by Peter J. Katzenstein, Robert O. Keohane, and Stephen D. Krasner, 247–79. Cambridge, MA: MIT Press, 1999.

Ferguson, June. "A Visit to the Middle East." *Canadian Nurse* 60, no. 8 (Aug. 1964): 768–9. Medline:14178675.

Fisher, Fedora Gould. *Raphael Cilento: A Biography.* St Lucia, Australia: University of Queensland Press, 1994.

Flynn, Karen. "I'm Glad That Someone Is Telling the Nursing Story: Writing Black Canadian Women's History." *Journal of Black Studies* 38, no. 3 (2008): 443–60.

– *Moving beyond Borders: A History of Black Canadian and Caribbean Women in the Diaspora.* Toronto: University of Toronto Press, 2011.

"From the Executive Director's Desk." *News Letter of the International Council of Nurses* 9 (Oct. 1968).

Goostry, Stella. "Isabel Maitland Stewart: The Story of a National and International Nursing Leader in Education." *American Journal of Nursing* 54, no. 3 (1954): 302–305.

Gray, Mabel F. "Nurses' Undergraduate Study." *Totem,* 1935, 54.

– "Nurses' Undergraduate Study." *Totem,* 1936, 52.

Green, Monica. *Through the Years with Public Health Nursing: A History of Public Health Nursing in the Provincial Government Jurisdiction British Columbia.* Ottawa: Canadian Public Health Association, 1984.

Grubbs, Larry. *Secular Missionaries: Americans and African Development in the 1960's.* Amherst: University of Massachusetts Press, 2010.

Grypma, Sonya. "Critical Issues in the Use of Biographic Methods in Nursing History." In *Capturing Nursing History: A Guide to Historical Methods in Research*, edited by Sandra B. Lewenson and Eleanor Krohn Herrmann, 63–78. New York: Springer, 2008.

– *Healing Henan: Canadian Nurses in the North China Mission, 1888–1947.* Vancouver: UBC Press, 2008.

Gunn, S.W.A. "The Canadian Contribution to the World Health Organization." *Canadian Medical Association Journal* 99 (7 Dec. 1968): 1080–8.

Haas, Peter M. "Epistemic Communities and International Policy Coordination." *International Organization* 46, no. 1 (1992): 1–35. http://dx.doi.org/10.1017/S0020818300001442.

Hall, Jacquelyn David. "Second Thoughts on Writing a Feminist Biography." *Feminist Studies* 13, no. 1 (1987): 19. http://dx.doi.org/10.2307/3177833.

Hazarti, Maryam, G. Mirzabeigy, and Ahmad Nejatian. "The History of Nursing in the Islamic Republic of Iran." *Nursing History Review* 19 (2011): 171–4.

Healey, Madelaine. "'I'm the Gal That Can Do It If They Let Me': International Nurse Advisers and Notions of Professionalisms in Indian Nursing, 1947–1965." http://coombs.anu.edu.au/SpecialProj/ASAA/biennial-conference/2006/Healey-Madelaine-ASAA2006.pdf.

– "'Seeds That May Have Been Planted May Take Root': International Aid Nurses and Projects of Professionalism in Post Independence India." *Nursing History Review* 16 (2008): 8–90.

Henderson, Virginia A. "The Development of a Personal Concept." In *Nurses' Work: Issues across Time and Place*, edited by Patricia D'Antonio , Ellen Baer, Sylvia Rinker, and Joan E. Lynaugh, 307–26. New York: Springer Publishing, 2007.

Hey, Richard N. "Ernest G. Osbourne, Family Life Educator." *Journal of Marriage and the Family* 27, no. 2 (1965): 134. http://dx.doi.org/10.2307/350062.

Hiscock, I.. "Charles-Edward Amory Winslow: February 4, 1877–January 8, 1957." *Journal of Bacteriology* 73, no. 3 (Mar. 1957): 295–6. Medline:13416187.

Hopper, Doris. "Miss Lyle Creelman: Devoted to Ministering to Ills of the World." *Province* (Vancouver), 12 Apr. 1969.

Hulme, Kathryn. *The Wild Place.* Boston: Little Brown, 1953.

International Council of Nurses. "Who Is Missing at the WHO? The Nursing Voice Excluded from Policy at World Health Organization." News release, 7 May 2011. http://www.icn.ch/images/stories/documents/news/press_releases/2011_PR_07_Emergency_WHO_resolution.pdf.

– "Going, Going Gone: The Nursing Presence in the World Health Organization." *International Nursing Review* 59, no. 2 (June 2012): 155–8.

India. Central Health Education Bureau. *International Organizations and India Health Programs.* New Delhi: Government of India CHEB, 1961.

"Interesting People: Lillian J. Johnston." *Canadian Nurse* 41, no. 9 (1945): 723.

International Council of Nurses. *The Basic Education of the Professional Nurse.* London: ICN, 1949.

International Organizations and India Health Programs. New Delhi: Government of India Central Health Education Bureau, 1961.

Iriye, Akira. *Global Community: The Role of International Organizations in the Making of the Contemporary World.* Berkeley, Los Angeles: University of California Press, 2002.

Irving, Allan. *Brock Chisholm: Doctor to the World.* Markham, ON: Associated Medical Services / Fitzhenry and Whiteside, 1998.

Irwin, Julia F. "Nurses without Borders: The History of Nursing as U.S. International History." *Nursing History Review* 19, no. 1 (2011): 78–102. http://dx.doi.org/ 10.1891/1062-8061.19.78. Medline:21329146.

Jennissen, Thérèse, and Colleen Lundy. "'Keeping Sight of Social Justice': 80 Years of Building CSWA." n.d. http://www.casw-acts.ca/sites/default/files/attachements/ CASW%20History.pdf.

Johns, Ethel. "Canada Looks at the Neighbours." *Canadian Nurse* 26, no. 1 (1930): 11–13.

Jones, M. "Heroines of Lonely Outposts or Tools of Empire? British Nurses in Britain's Model Colony, 1878–1948." *Nursing Inquiry* 11, no. 3 (2004): 148–60.

Keck, Margret, and Kathryn Sikkink. *Activists beyond Borders: Advocacy Networks in International Politics.* Ithaca, NY: Cornell University Press, 1998.

Keohane, Robert O. "Introduction: From Interdependence and Institutions to Globalization and Governance." In *Power and Governance in a Partially Globalized World*, edited by Robert O. Keohane, 1–24. London: Routledge 2002.

Kerr, Margaret. "The Importance of Post-Graduate Public Health Training." *Canadian Nurse* 26, no. 3 (1930): 135–7.

– "Kla-How-Ya, Tillicum." *Canadian Nurse* 38, no. 1 (1942): 42–3.

Kerr, Margaret, and Lyle Creelman. "Public Health Nurses in Canada." *Canadian Nurse* 38, no. 1 (1942): 42–3.

Khomeira, R., and C. Deans. "Nursing Education in Iran." *Nurse Education Today* 27 no. 7 (2007): 708–14.

Kickbusch, Ilone, and Evelyne de Leeuw. "Global Public Health: Revisiting Healthy Public Policy at the Global Level." *Health Promotion International* 14, no. 4 (1999): 285–8. http://dx.doi.org/10.1093/heapro/14.4.285.

Kinnear, Julia L. "The Professionalization of Canadian Nursing, 1924-32: views in the CN and the CMAJ." *Canadian Bulletin of Medical Health* 11 (1966): 153–74.

Kirkwood, Rondalyn. "Blending Vigorous Leadership and Womanly Virtues: Edith Kathleen Russell at the University of Toronto, 1920–52." *CBMH/BCHM* 11 (1994): 175–205.

– "Florence Emory." *Registered Nurse* (Oct./Nov. 1994): 32–5.

Kirton, John, and Jenilee Guebert. "The Field of Global Governance: Past, Present and Future." Paper presented at annual convention of the International Studies Association, New York, 15–18 Feb. 2009.

Kirton, John, and Jenevieve Mannell. "The G8 and Global Health Governance." In *Governing Global Health: Challenge, Response, Innovation*, edited by Andrew F. Cooper, John J. Kirton, and Ted Schrecker, 115–47. Aldershot, UK: Ashgate, 2007.

Klassen, Donni. "Camp Alexandra: A Brief History." 2012. http://www.surreyhistory.ca/campalexandra.html.

Lagerway, Mary Deane. "Third Reich, Nursing and the AJN." *American Journal of Nursing* 109, no. 8 (2009): 44–9.

Langton, Geraldine, and Isabelle Chodat. "Planning Field Experience for Postgraduate Course in Public Health Nursing." *Canadian Nurse* 39, no. 11 (1943): 739–44.

Lapeyre, Jaime, and Sioban Nelson. "'The Old Internationals': Canadian Nurses in an International Nursing Community." *Canadian Journal of Nursing Leadership* 23, no. 4 (2010): 33–44.

Lawrence, Ida L. "Mental Hygiene from the Standpoint of a Social Nurse." *Canadian Nurse* 19, no. 4 (1923): 220–6.

Lawson, Mabel G. "German Nursing Services 1945–1946." *Canadian Nurse* 43, no. 4 (1947): 285–8.

Laycock, S.R. "Mental Hygiene and Public Health." *Canadian Nurse* 26, no. 1 (1930): 29–33.

Lee, Kelly. *Global Institutions: The World Health Organization*. London: Routledge, 2009.

Lerner, Gerda. "Placing Women in History." In *Major Problems in American Women's History*, edited by Mary Beth Norton, 1–7. Toronto: D.C. Heath, 1989.

– "The Necessity of History and the Professional Historian." *Journal of American History* 69, no. 1 (June 1982): 7–20.

Lewis, Norah. "'Creating the Little Machine'": Child Rearing in British Columbia, 1919–1939." *BC Studies* 56 (Winter 1982–3): 44–60.

Lynaugh, Joan E., Helen K. Grace, Gloria R. Smith, Roseni R. Sena, and Maria Mercedes Duran de Villalobos. *The W.K. Kellogg Foundation and the Nursing Profession: Shared Values, Shared Legacy*. Indianapolis: Sigma Theta Tau International, Honor Society of Nursing, 2007.

Mackie, Janet W., and Olive Baggallay. "Nursing Education in Africa." *American Journal of Nursing* 54, no. 8 (Aug. 1954): 984–5. http://dx.doi.org/10.2307/3460742. Medline:13180551.

Marsh, Leonard. *Report on Social Security for Canada*. Toronto: University of Toronto Press, 1943.

Mathers, A.T. "Mental Hygiene and Nursing." *Canadian Nurse* 24 (1928): 425–31.

Maxwell, Jennifer. "Children and State Intervention: Developing a Coherent Historical Perspective." In *Nursing History and the Politics of Welfare*, edited by Anne Marie Rafferty, Jane Robinson, and Ruth Elkan, 226–41. New York: Routledge, 2007.

McCreary, John F. *The Empire Club of Canada Speeches 1946–1947.* Toronto: Empire Club Foundation, 1947.

McGann, Susan. "Collaboration and Conflict in International Nursing, 1920–1939." *Nursing History Review* 16 (2008): 29–57.

McLaren, Angus. *Our Own Master Race: Eugenics in Canada, 1885–1945.* Toronto: McClelland and Stewart, 1990.

McPherson, Kathryn. *Bedside Matters: The Transformation of Canadian Nursing, 1900–1990.* Toronto: Oxford University Press, 1996.

Meier, Benjamin Mason. "The Highest Attainable Standard: The World Health Organization, Global Health Governance, and the Contentious Politics of Human Rights." PhD diss., Columbia University, 2009.

Melchior, F. "Feminist Approaches to Nursing History." *Western Journal of Nursing Research* 26, no. 3 (Apr. 2004): 340–55. http://dx.doi.org/10.1177/0193945903261030. Medline:15068556.

Melosh, Barbara. *The Physician's Hand: Work Culture and Conflict in American Nursing.* Philadelphia: Temple University Press, 1982.

"The Mental Hygiene Movement in Canada." *Canadian Nurse* 30, no. 2 (1929): 59–62.

"Miss Gray Retires." *Canadian Nurse* 37, no. 11 (1941): 755–6.

"Miss Lyle Creelman." *Province* (Vancouver), 12 Apr. 1969.

Mitchell, W.T.B. "The Importance of Mental Hygiene in the Curriculum of Schools of Nursing." *Canadian Nurse* 26, no. 3 (1930): 123–7.

Mitchinson, Wendy. *Giving Birth in Canada, 1900–1950.* Toronto: University of Toronto Press, 2002.

Mitrany, David. *A Working Peace System.* Chicago: Quadrangle Books, 1944.

Montgomery, S.R. "The Mental Health Clinic." *Canadian Nurse* 28, no. 3 (1932): 146–8.

Mott, G.A. "Mental Hygiene in a Public Health Department." *Public Health* 74, no. 8 (May 1960): 283–93. http://dx.doi.org/10.1016/S0033-3506(60)80087-X.

Murphy, Marion. "Group Teaching in Public Health: Aspects of Public Health Nursing." World Health Organization Public Health Papers, no. 4 (Geneva: WHO, 1961).

"Names." *Canadian Nurse* 29, no. 10 (1966): 18.

"Names: Eva M. Williamson; Trenna G. Hunter." *Canadian Nurse* 62, no. 10 (1966): 18.

"Names: Grace M. Fairley." *Canadian Nurse* 65, no. 5 (1969): 18.

"Names: Ruth Ingram; Alice Girard." *Canadian Nurse* 64, no. 9 (1968): 24–5.

"N.F. 'Dick' Pullen." *Observer* (Cariboo), 3 Jan. 1963.

"Nurse School on Government Basis Urged." *Vancouver Sun*, May 1958.

"Nursing Profiles." *Canadian Nurse* 55, no. 9 (1956): 1032.

"Nursing Profiles." *Canadian Nurse* 54, no. 10 (1958): 931.

"Nursing Profiles." *Canadian Nurse* 54, no. 3 (1958): 230.

"Nursing Profiles: Isabel Maitland Stewart." *Canadian Nurse* 59, no 8. (1963): 638.

"Obituaries." *British Medical Journal*, (2 December 2006): 333.

"One Nurse to 18,000 People." *Daily Colonialist*, 30 May 1953.

Opare, Mary, and Judy E. Mill. "The Evolution of Nursing Education in a Post Independence Context." *Western Journal of Nursing Research* 22 (2000): 936–44.

Ormsby, Margaret. *British Columbia: A History*. Vancouver: Evergreen, 1958.

Osborne, Ernest G., and Mary Rideout Osborne. "Parent Education and the Nurse." *American Journal of Nursing* 41, no. 11 (1941): 1257–60.

Osterholm, Michael. "Preparing for the Next Pandemic." *Foreign Affairs* 84, no. 4 (July/August 2005): 24–37. http://dx.doi.org/10.2307/20034418.

Packard, Randall M. "Malaria Dreams: Postwar Visions of Health and Development in the Third World." *Medical Anthropology* 17, no. 3 (May 1997): 279–96. http://dx.doi.org/10.1080/01459740.1997.9966141.

Packard, Randall M., and Peter J. Brown. "Rethinking Health, Development, and Malaria: Historicizing a Cultural Model in International Health." *Medical Anthropology* 17, no. 3 (May 1997): 181–94. http://dx.doi.org/10.1080/01459740.19 97.9966136.

Palmer, Helen. "There Are Good Jobs for Nurses Who Have a Yen to Travel." *Daily Star* (Toronto), 13 Jan. 1961, Women's Section.

Percy, Dorothy. "From Where I Sit." *Canadian Nurse* 61, no. 9 (1965): 608.

– "Signpost at Geneva." *Canadian Nurse* 52, no. 10 (1956): 790–8.

Peterson, V. Spike, and Anne Sisson Ryan. *Global Gender Issues in the New Millennium*. Boulder, CO: Westview, 2010.

Pickles, Kate, and Myra Rutherdale, eds. *Contact Zones: Aboriginal and Settler Women in Canada's Colonial Past*. Vancouver: University of British Columbia Press, 2005.

"Professor Margaret Scott Wright: Nursing Leader Whose Intellectual and Organisational Prowess Led to Her Appointment as the UK's First Professor of Nursing." *Times*, 20 May 2008. http://www.thetimes.co.uk/tto/opinion/obituaries/article2081555.ece.

Prowd, Pat. "City Nurse Appointed Chief." *Province*, 8 Apr. 1964.

Quinn, Sheila. *A Dame Abroad*. Stanhope, UK: Memoir Club, 2004.

– "Social and Economic Welfare: An International Approach." *Canadian Nurse* 64, no. 8 (Aug. 1968): 34–7.

Rafferty, Anne Marie, and D. Solano. "The Rise and Demise of the Colonial Nursing Service: British Nurses in the Colonies, 1896–1966." *Nursing History Review* 15, no. 1 (2006): 147–54. http://dx.doi.org/10.1891/1062-8061.15.147.

Rands, Stanley. "Medical Care Programs and Public Health Nursing Practice." *Canadian Nurse* 47, no. 12 (Dec. 1951): 875–80.

"Refugees Are Assets." *Sun* (Vancouver), 22 Nov. 1946.

Riddell, Susan. "Curing Society's Ills: Public Health Nurses and Public Health Nursing in Rural British Columbia, 1919–1946." MA thesis, Simon Fraser University, 1991.

Robinson, P. "Maternal and Child Health Services in S.E. Asia." *Journal of Tropical Paediatrics* 5 no.4(Sept. 1956): 130–1.

Rosen, George. "Public Health, Then and Now: The First Neighborhood Health Center Movement – Its Rise and Fall." *American Journal of Public Health* 61, no. 8 (Aug. 1971): 1620–37. http://dx.doi.org/10.2105/AJPH.61.8.1620. Medline:4935169.

Rosenfield, Allan. "The View from the Dean's Office." *American Journal of Epidemiology* 147, no. 3 (1998): 201–2.

Ross-Kerr, Janet C. "Innovation in Public Health Nursing in Canada: The Rockefeller Foundation and the University of Toronto." n.d. http://www.rockarch.org/publications/conferences/rosskerr.pdf.

Roy, Patricia E. " 'Due to Their Keenness regarding Education They Will Get the Utmost out of the Whole Plan': The Education of Japanese Children in the British Columbia Interior Housing Settlements during World War Two." *Historical Studies in Education / Revue d'histoire de l'éducation* 4, no. 2 (1992): 211–31

Russell, Kathleen Edith. "The Canadian University and the Canadian School of Nursing." *Canadian Nurse* 34, no. 12 (1928): 627–30.

Saunier, Pierre-Yves. "World of Nursing: The Rockefeller Moment." Rockefeller Archive Center. 2008. http://www.rockarch.org/publications/resrep/pdf/saunier.pdf.

Schlotfeldt, R.M. *"Teachers as Exemplars of Nursing Practice." Teacher-Practitioner: Collaborators for Improving Nursing Care.* New York: National League on Nursing Education, 1965.

Schouten, Hank. "Ted Metcalfe: The Adventurous Nurse." *Dominion Post* (Wellington), 14 Aug. 2009.

Setzler, Lorraine. "Nursing and Nursing Education in Germany." *American Journal of Nursing* 45, no. 12 (Dec. 1945): 993–5.

– "In Iran: The Development of a Nursing School in Shiraz." *American Journal of Nursing* 41, no. 5 (1941): 58–63.

Sherlock, Leona. *UBC Chronicle* 6, no. 4 (1952).

Shiers, Kelly. "A World-Class Health Professional." *Chronicle Herald*, 7 Mar. 2007.

Sleeper, Ruth. "The Sixth World Health Assembly." *American Journal of Nursing* 53, no. 12 (Dec. 1953): 1463–4. Medline:13104485.

Solano, D., and A.M. Rafferty. "Can Lessons Be Learned from History? The Origins of the British Imperial Nurse Labour Market: A Discussion Paper." *International Journal of Nursing Studies* 44, no. 6 (Aug. 2007): 1055–63. http://dx.doi.org/10.1016/j.ijnurstu.2006.07.004.

Splane, Richard B., and Verna Huffman Splane. *Chief Nursing Officer Positions in National Ministries of Health: Focal Points for Nursing Leadership*. San Francisco: University of California Regents, 1994.

Splane, Verna Huffman. *Halfway to Poona: A Public Health Nurse's Journey; A Work in Progress*. Vancouver: Rhino Print Solutions, 2007.

Steppe, Hilde. "Nursing in the Third Reich." *History of Nursing Journal* 3, no. 4 (1991): 23, 24, 25–6.

Stewart, Isabel Maitland. "Isabel Maitland Stewart Recalls the Early Years." *American Journal of Nursing* 60, no. 10 (1960): 1426–30. http://dx.doi.org/10.1097/00000446-196060100-00015.

– "The Philosophy of the Collegiate School of Nursing." *American Journal of Nursing* 40, no. 9 (1940): 1033–5.

Strong-Boag, Veronica. "A Beacon of Light." *Canadian Nurse* 47, no. 3 (1951): 169–70.

– "Making a Difference: The History of Canada's Nurses." *Canadian Bulletin of Medical History / Bulletin canadien d'histoire de la médecin* 8, no. 2 (1991): 231–48. Medline:11612614.

Struthers, James. "Family Allowances, Old Age Security and the Construction of Entitlement in Canadian Welfare, 1943–1951." In *The Veterans Charter and Post–World War II Canada*, edited by Peter Neary and J.L. Granatstein, 179–205 Montreal and Kingston: McGill-Queen's University Press, 1998.

– *No Fault of Their Own: Unemployment and the Canadian Welfare State, 1914–1941*. Toronto: University of Toronto Press, 1983.

Sweet, Helen. "'Wanted: 16 Nurses of the Better Educated Type': Provision of Nurses to South Africa in the Late Nineteenth and Early Twentieth Centuries." *Nursing Inquiry* 11, no. 3 (Sept. 2004): 176–84. http://dx.doi.org/10.1111/j.1440-1800.2004.00228.x. Medline:15327657.

Taylor, Effie J. "Isabel Maitland Stewart: Educator." *American Journal of Nursing* 36, no. 1 (1936): 38–44.

Taylor, Florence. "Nursing at Vellore, South India." *Canadian Nurse* 47, no. 11 (Nov. 1951): 816–18. Medline:14879349.

Taylor, Ruth. "[Fifth World Health Assembly]." *American Journal of Nursing* 52, no. 12 (Dec. 1952): 1463–4.

Thom, Agnes. "Nurse Thom's Report." *Revelstoke Review*, 26 June 1936.

Thomson, Gerald E. "'Not an Attempt to Coddle Children': Dr Charles Hegler Gundy and the Mental Hygiene Division of the Vancouver School Board, 1939–1969." *Historical Studies in Education / Revue histoire d'éducation* 4, no. 6 (2002): 247–78.

Toman, Cynthia. "Blood Work: Canadian Nursing and Blood Transfusion, 1942–1990." *Nursing History Review* 9 (2001): 51–78.

– *An Officer and a Lady: Canadian Military Nursing and the Second World War.* Vancouver: UBC Press, 2007.

– "The Trained Nurse as a Storm Centre of Discussion." *Canadian Medical Association Journal (CMAJ)* 16 (Dec. 1926): 359.

Tunis, Barbara Logan. *In Cap and Gowns: The Story of the School for Graduate Nurses, McGill University, 1920–1964.* Montreal and Kingston: McGill-Queen's University Press, 1966.

"UN: What-Not at WHO." *Time* 28 Feb. 1949.

Van Betten, Patricia, and Melisa Moriarty. *Nursing Illuminations: A Book of Days.* St Louis, MO: Mosby, 2004.

Wegman, M.E. "Martha Eliot and the U.S. Children's Bureau." *Pediatrics* 19, no. 4 Part 1 (Apr. 1957): 651–6. Medline:13419437.

Williams, Eileen. "Public Health Nursing in a Japanese Community in British Columbia." *Canadian Nurse* 37, no. 5 (1941): 339.

Williams, Jeffery. *The Long Left Flank: The Hard Fought Way to the Reich, 1944–194.* Toronto: Stoddart Publishing, 1988.

Wilson, Jean S. "Notes from the National Office." *Canadian Nurse* 38, no. 4 (1942): 171–7.

Winslow, C.E.A. *The Cost of Sickness.* Geneva: World Health Organization, 1951.

Wodlinger, David. "A UNRRA Field Supervisor Looks Back." *CW, Canadian Welfare* (Apr. 1948): 24.

Woodbridge, George. *UNRRA: The History of the United Nations Relief and Rehabilitation Administration.* 3 vols. New York: Columbia University Press, 1950.

– "Words of Peace, Words of War," Ibiblio. http://www.ibiblio.org/pha/policy/index.html.

World Health Organization. *Care of the Umbilical Cord Reproductive Health.* Geneva: WHO Reproductive Health (Technical Support) Maternal and Newborn Health / Safe Motherhood, 1999. https://apps.who.int/rht/documents/MSM98-4/MSM-98-4.htm.

– *The First Ten Years of the World Health Organization.* Geneva: WHO, 1950.

– *Four Decades of Achievement: The Highlights of the Work of WHO*. Geneva: WHO, 1988.
– "Human Rights–Based Approach to Health." 2013. http://www.who.int/trade/glossary/story054/en/.
– "Nurses, Their Education and Their Role in Health Programmes: Report of the Technical Discussions at the Ninth World Health Assembly." *Chronicle of the World Health Organization* 10, no. 7 (1956): 339–42.
– *Report of the International Conference on Primary Health Care, Alma Ata, USSR, 6–12 September 1978*. Geneva: WHO, 1978).
– *The Second Ten Years, 1958–1968*. Geneva: WHO, 1968.
– *The Third Ten Years of the World Health Organization*, 1968-1977. Geneva: WHO, 2008.
– *Strategic Directions for Strengthening Nursing and Midwifery Services: 2011–2015*. Geneva: WHO, 2011.
– *Working Conference on Nursing Education*. World Health Technical Report Series, no. 60. Geneva: WHO, 1953.
World Health Organization, Expert Committee on Nursing. *Report of the Fifth Session*. World Health Technical Report Series, no. 347. Geneva: WHO, 1966.
– *Report of the First Session*. World Health Technical Report Series, no. 24. Geneva: WHO, 1958.
– *Report of the Fourth Session*. World Health Technical Report Series, no. 167. Geneva: WHO, 1959.
– *Report of the Second Session*. World Health Technical Report Series, no. 49. Geneva: WHO, 1952.
– *Report of the Third Session*. World Health Technical Report Series no. 91. Geneva: WHO, 1954.
"The World of Nursing: CNA Executive Director in West Indies." *Canadian Nurse* 60, no. 8 (1964): 766.
Zilm, Glennis. "Lyle Morrison Creelman, 1908." In *American Nursing: A Biographical Dictionary*. Vol. 3, edited by Sharon Richardson, L. Sentz, and W.L. Bullough 91–3. New York: Springer Publishing, 2000.
Zilm, Glennis, and Ethel Warbinek. "Early Tuberculosis Nursing in British Columbia." *Canadian Journal of Nursing Research* 27, no. 3 (Fall 1995): 65–81.
– *Legacy: History of Nursing Education at the University of British Columbia, 1919–1994*. Vancouver: University of British Columbia, School of Nursing, 1994.

Index

Abbott, Mary, 198, 208, 248
Adranvala, Tehmina, 144, 159–60, 171–2
Africa: French-speaking nurses in, 214;
  LC in, 183–92; nationalism in, 192;
  post-basic nursing education in, 243,
  250; regime changes in, 245; WHO
  nurses in, 245–6
African nurses, 190
Akwei, Eustace, 189
Alexandra Fresh Air Camp, 20–1, 23–4
Allied Control Commission (ACC), 83,
  84–5, 93, 104
Alma Ata Declaration, viii, 263–4
Alves Diniz, Fernanda, 152, 214, 223,
  267, 342n26
American Association of Nurses, 77
Amyot, Grégoire, 8, 9, 20, 21, 25, 55, 56
Anderson, Susan Sontag, 222
Ankrah, Joseph Arthur, 347n12
Armstrong-Reid, Susan, *Armies of Peace,*
  xii–xiii
army cadet nurses, 77
Arnold, Virginia, 221–4, 233, 266
Arnstein, Margaret, 75, 81, 82, 150–1, 172
Asmara nursing school, 235
"Aspects of Public Health Nursing"
  (WHO), 228

assembly centres, 83, 84, 94, 95, 99
assistantes sociales, 139
Atlantic Charter, 123
autonomy: in international nursing, 213;
  for nurses, 10, 23, 35, 132; for public
  health nurses, 31, 108, 180; regional,
  194, 213
auxiliary nursing personnel: in developing countries, 257; education of, 231,
  248, 260–1; in Egypt, 142; expert
  committees and, 174, 256, 257; in
  Gambia, 187; in health teams, 260–1;
  international nursing and, 135, 136,
  228; in Kenya, 248; nursing shortage
  and, 132, 142; in Pakistan, 204; role of,
  228; in SEARO, 267–9; supervision of
  work by, 174; in TB projects, 180

Bacillus Calmette-Guérin (BCG),
  152, 155
Baggallay, Olive: about, 130–1; and
  alliances among nursing leaders,
  138–9; and chief nursing officer, 143;
  climbing with LC, 162; and expert
  committees on nursing, 131; and
  Florence Nightingale International
  Foundation, 83, 131; leaves WHO, 170;